Nutrition in the
Life Span

Nutrition in the
Life Span

Virginia A. Beal
University of Massachusetts

JOHN WILEY AND SONS
New York · Chichester · Brisbane · Toronto

Library of Congress Cataloging in Publication Data

Beal, Virginia A.
    Nutrition in the Life Span.

    Includes bibliographies and index.
    1. Nutrition. I. Title.

QP141.B28   613.2   79-24610
ISBN 0-471-03664-1

Printed in the United States of America

10 9 8 7 6 5 4 3 2 1

Preface

The stimulus to write this book arose from the problems of teaching a course in nutrition in the life span without the convenience of a single inclusive text. Instructors of similar courses in other institutions have also been forced to use abbreviated chapters in the final section of basic nutrition texts, books devoted to specific age periods, or journal articles. As a result, teaching has been more difficult and the student has been required either to buy several textbooks for a single course or to spend considerable time in libraries. A single volume that covers the entire life span should ease the burden.

This book is intended for students who have already had courses in basic nutrition, biochemistry, and physiology: for example, graduate or upper level undergraduate students of nutrition, dietetics, nursing, or medicine; and students of human development, public health, or other allied fields. This book can also serve as a source of comprehensive and updated information for workers in nutrition and other health professions.

In this book I have chosen to concentrate primarily on normal growth, development, and nutrition for all ages except the elderly, for whom nutrition and degenerative diseases are inextricably intertwined. Little of the text is devoted to the nutrition of the young adult because most basic nutrition courses tend to focus on that age group. Each reader may also identify other areas of concern that are not included in this book or are given only passing mention. This is inevitable, since a single volume cannot include details of all aspects of nutrition in the life span.

For example, several aspects of metabolic abnormalities and deficiency diseases are not discussed in detail in this book. Only brief references are made to inborn errors of metabolism, failure to thrive, growth abnormalities, protein-energy malnutrition, and other topics in therapeutic nutrition. These problems require extensive and detailed study, and the reader can readily find excellent books written by specialists with practical experience in each of these specific conditions.

As the science of nutrition grows and understanding of nutrient metabolism increases, controversy accompanies most new discoveries. Such controversy stimulates further research, and eventually initial theories are either confirmed or disproved. In the interim, the student of nutrition is often faced with opposing points of view, either of which may be correct.

Therefore, I have tried to indicate in this book where differences of opinion exist. The bibliography at the end of each chapter not only provides sources of the data presented, but also lists reviews and controversial publications on many specific topics. As a teacher, I hope that some students will be stimulated to go into research to supply answers.

Illustrations have been taken from many sources, primarily books and journals in nutrition and medicine. In addition, I have used serial data from growth studies at the Child Research Council and the Harvard School of Public Health; I participated in both studies and am familiar with their concepts and findings. They make the data more comprehensive.

The footnote in Chapter 5 explains the use of masculine pronouns when applied to the embryo, fetus, infant, and young child of either sex. This is deliberate, to differentiate the child (he, him) from the mother (she, her) without constantly diverting the reader's attention from the meaning of the text by the awkward use of methods to eliminate sexist references.

References to the most recent Recommended Dietary Allowances may be confusing. This manuscript was prepared before the Food and Nutrition Board had made a final decision on the values to be included in the ninth edition. As a result, references to the rationale of the allowances are based on the 1974 text, and that reference is given in the bibliography of each chapter. When the new tables (but not the text) became available in September 1979, this manuscript was revised; the new tables are included in Appendix 1. However, the rationale for changes between 1974 and 1979 must await publication of the ninth edition of the RDA text.

Several people have contributed to the writing of this book, including many who did not realize it. The children and parents enrolled in the two longitudinal studies with which I have been associated provided observations of children, how and what they eat, and how they grow. The staff of the Child Research Council continuously shared knowledge of their own specialties and expanded my understanding of the interfaces of nutrition with other sciences. The late Dr. Alfred H. Washburn, as Director of the Child Research Council until 1960, imparted to all his staff a deep respect for individual variation. Students have helped me to refine methods of presentation and content of the course that became the subject of this text. The generous and conscientious reviewers of this manuscript improved it by new ideas and by new approaches to old ideas. To all of them and to others from whom I have learned, I am grateful.

Virginia A. Beal

Contents

CHAPTER 1. NUTRITION, GROWTH, AND BODY COMPOSITION

CHAPTER 3. PREGNANCY

NUTRIENT REQUIREMENTS AND DIETARY ALLOWANCES   149

CONTENTS

CHAPTER 7. MIDDLE CHILDHOOD

CHAPTER 8. PUBESCENCE AND ADOLESCENCE

CHAPTER 9. THE ADULT AND THE ELDERLY

1

NUTRITION, GROWTH, AND BODY COMPOSITION

Each person is a biological unit different from every other person. The individual is the product of unique ontogeny and ecology. Each person's life history, development, and interrelationship with and adaptation to a specific environment are not identical to any other individual's. As an infant, an adolescent, a young adult, or an elderly person, one's state of physical and mental health at the present is always conditioned by the biological remembrance of the past. Status at any age in the life span rests upon the accumulated events and influences earlier in life. To understand or evaluate an individual, one must have knowledge of that person's past life and experiences.

The ability of a woman to foster and nourish a fetus and to survive delivery of a live baby is determined in part by her health and nutritional status not only during pregnancy but throughout her life prior to conception. The fetus is the product of the genetic potential supplied by both parents and is influenced by the intrauterine environment and the transplacental passage of the materials needed for development. If genes are abnormal or if there is a limitation or interruption in the supply of nutrients, hormones, enzymes, and other biological compounds necessary for cell differentiation and growth, embryonic or fetal development may be imperfect. If the fetus survives, newborn health may be comprised and the infant may start life with handicaps. The neonate may be large or small, healthy or defective, vigorous or lethargic.

The success of the mother in breast-feeding her infant depends on a complex of physiological, psychological, and social influences. The groundwork for each of these influences was laid long before she conceived and reflects

1

her own life history but may be altered by events during her pregnancy and delivery. The quantity and nutrient values of her milk are affected by her dietary intake, her physiological capabilities, and her response to her environment during the lactation period. These affect the growth rate and health of the young infant. When all conditions for lactation are satisfactory, the healthy infant thrives. In many areas of the world where food supplies are minimal and of low biological value, breast milk is essential to the infant's survival. However, if breast milk is meager in volume or deficient in nutrients, infant growth is slow and deficiency diseases, such as infantile beriberi, may ensue.

In technologically advanced countries the availability of alternative foods for infant feeding makes breast-feeding a matter of choice for the mother. Health supervision and sanitation have improved the quality of life, and environmental factors are conducive to the promotion of growth and development of the infant in an acceptable pattern. However, in developing countries the cessation or lack of breast feeding in conjunction with unsanitary conditions have too often been followed by energy-protein malnutrition with a high mortality rate. The infant who survives early deficiency may have retardation of skeletal growth or brain development which may affect abilities and performance throughout life.

Physical growth and psychosocial development during all of childhood influence the adult's ability to adapt to his society. The child who is healthy, well-nourished and loved is likely to become a strong, happy, and well-adjusted adult. On the other hand, if severe illness, malnutrition, or physical or emotional deprivation interfere with normal growth and maturation, the health status of the adult may be compromised. If adverse factors operate for only a short period of time, it may be possible to catch up in either physical growth or mental development, depending on the timing of the adversity and the degree of environmental improvement that follows. Nature provided to humans, but not to animals lower in the evolutionary scale, a second period of rapid growth during puberty and adolescence. When conditions during childhood are not optimal, prepubertal growth may be extended and adolescent growth and maturation delayed, providing a longer period of growth before maturity is reached. There is some evidence that the observed secular increase in height is due at least partially to earlier maturation and attainment of adult size that have resulted from improvements in health care, nutrition, and other environmental influences.

At no time during the life span is the effect of earlier experiences more clearly seen than in the elderly. Survival to old age is a selective process. Individual differences become more pronounced as life is extended because of the longer period of diverse experiences. Each elderly person has a unique history of all circumstances in life—living conditions, activity, diet, disease, surgical procedures, medications, and mental and emotional patterns.

Therefore the physiological capabilities and needs of one elderly person are unlike those of any other. We have just begun to investigate some of the processes of aging. Degeneration is inevitable since the human body is not programmed to live forever, but early life experiences may speed or retard the process. The quality of life in the older years is the culmination of all that has happened in the life span.

Overt disease and malnutrition as well as gross abnormalities in development can readily be recognized. However, despite rapid progress in biological and social sciences, we are not yet wise enough to identify the significance of small gradations in health and development or the relative importance of each of the etiological factors as they operate within the individual. It is difficult to evaluate the effects of subtle variations of health within a range that allows the individual to function with some degree of success within his society. Even more elusive is the identification of specific physiological and environmental influences on the health, development, and function of the individual when there is a delay in the appearance of symptoms.

Growth of the child determines adult size, and growth can be measured with relative ease. However, the influences on growth are more difficult to measure. Genetic inheritance is one determinant of size, but in a population that is not inbred or of uniform body size, the genetic potential of the individual cannot be measured. The severity and duration of illnesses, especially during periods of rapid bone formation, may alter the rate of growth, but their influence varies from one child to another. Dietary intake may be measured with some accuracy, but the efficiency of utilization of nutrients cannot be readily assessed. Adaptation of the body to stress, whether physical, physiological, or nutritional, varies from one individual to another; a given type or degree of stress may be detrimental to one person but easily handled or compensated for by another. Therefore, although growth is a parameter that can be readily evaluated and the influences on growth may be identified in general, it is difficult or impossible at our present level of knowledge to measure the relative impact of each of those factors in a given child.

Health, on the other hand, is in itself difficult to measure. In some overt disease states, such as bacterial infections or specific nutrient deficiencies, a direct link between cause and effect may be identified. However, it has long been recognized that individuals differ in their response to the same exposure, for reasons not always clear. In chronic disease states, such as arteriosclerosis, there is no single causative factor but, instead, a complex and ill-defined etiology related to long-term influences that are difficult both to identify and to evaluate; the multiplicity of such factors requires study, and input from a wide range of biological and social scientists is needed.

Freedom from disease is only one aspect of health. More subtle aspects are variations in the degree of vitality, ability to cope with both everyday demands and unusual stresses, adaptation to constant environmental changes, and resistance to disease. Although progress has been made in the identification of some risk factors that may ultimately lead to chronic disease, individual susceptibility and the critical ages when etiological factors may be operative are still unclear. At present there is no way to differentiate between passable health and optimal health in an individual or to be sure that practices that do not jeopardize present health will not compromise health at a later age.

The effects of malnutrition on health are clearly evident in areas of the world where total food supplies are inadequate, especially the expensive protective foods that supply high quality proteins and more readily absorbable micronutrients. However, in countries where the standard of living is high, health services universally available, and food supply plentiful, the health and growth of the population are superior to those in less privileged countries. Differences within a population in Westernized countries tend to be smaller in nutrient intake, in growth rates, and in health status. Therefore the effects of improvement in nutrient intake are less dramatic and may be difficult to identify.

METHODS OF STUDY OF NUTRITION

The history of the burgeoning science of nutrition has shown the interdependence of animal and human studies. For a true understanding of human growth, health, and aging, humans must be their own models. However, human studies are not always possible. Most metabolic balance studies intended to investigate the physiological and biochemical functions of nutrients have been performed on adult males. The moral implications of experimentation during periods of growth or potential growth have restricted study between conception and maturity and in women during the reproductive years. Intervention studies carried out during these periods have been aimed toward observing results that would improve nutritional status rather than toward the lowering of intake that might jeopardize it. The danger of creating permanent damage by placing women and children on deficient diets has precluded studies of such experimental nature. Until recently, few studies have been done on the elderly. However, with lower birth rates and greater longevity, a larger proportion of the population each year is in the elderly category, and this has stimulated studies on the processes of aging.

As a result, knowledge of the nutrient requirements of adult males is far more advanced than for other age or sex categories. A careful reading of the text of the Recommended Dietary Allowances[1] shows very clearly the gaps in knowledge of the nutrient needs of women, children, and the elderly. The RDAs (see Appendix I) for those groups have involved more judgment and assumptions than for the adult male, and the text repeatedly points out the paucity of firm data on which to base those allowances.

Studies of human growth have provided excellent data on external measurements but only limited insights into the physiology and chemistry of growth. Anthropometric measurements have been taken on large numbers of subjects because of the simple methodology. These are noninvasive techniques that can be quickly learned with training. In addition, many studies have included analyses of blood and urine samples and some studies have been done on resting metabolism. X rays taken for measurement and evaluation of bone growth, skeletal age, or chest development, either in large surveys or in longitudinal studies, have given valuable insight into growth parameters, but concern about potential hazards of exposure to radiation now limits x-ray use. Recently techniques of tissue aspiration and analysis have shown promise in contributing to the understanding of changes in body composition and storage, but the difficulties of the procedures preclude widespread use. Methods of differentiating the proportions of bone, muscle, and fat in the body require specialized equipment and are adaptable only to limited centers of study. Therefore, although there is extensive literature on external measurements of growth, less is known about the physiological, hormonal, and biochemical concomitants of human growth.

ANIMAL STUDIES

Historically animal studies have contributed greatly to an understanding of the physiological and biochemical functions of nutrients. Animal experimentation has provided much of our present knowledge of reproduction, lactation, and growth. In the early twentieth century the economic benefits of improved performance of dairy cows and beef cattle led to extensive studies of the effects of nutrients. Continued dependence on animal studies is essential in view of the restrictions placed on human experimentation. However, despite the necessity and advantages of animal studies, caution must be used in the application of findings to humans.

There are many advantages to the use of laboratory animals in the study of nutrition. The methodology of animal studies is much more flexible than is possible with humans. Diet can be controlled, both in total quantity and in specific nutrients, and deficiencies may be deliberately created to observe their results. Genetics and environment may be controlled in ways impossible with humans, permitting evaluation of the effects of specific variables. The animals may be sacrificed for tissue analysis to observe changes within the body. The shorter life of laboratory animals permits the study of the entire life span or of several generations to follow the long-term effects of various levels of nutrient intake. These advantages give much greater freedom in experimentation, greater precision of factor control, and actual observations of physiological and biological alterations than would be possible with humans.

On the other hand, species differences necessitate care in attributing animal findings to humans. The ratio of offspring weight to maternal weight affects the degree to which maternal nutrient deficiencies disturb the growth and development of the fetus. The weight of a litter of guinea pigs is approximately 50 percent of maternal body weight, and for the rat 25 percent. Therefore the nutrient demand on the maternal body is high and a deficiency has a more drastic effect on the offspring. In contrast, the ratio of newborn weight to maternal weight in the human is close to 6 percent, which provides greater leeway for the maternal body to buffer the effects of maternal dietary deficiency on her fetus. Only in severe human deficiencies is it even possible to reproduce the defects in the offspring demonstrated so clearly in animal studies such as the classic experiments of Warkany.[2]

Rates of fetal growth and degree of maturity at birth differ among species. For example, the timing of maximal growth rate of the brain ranges from midgestation in the guinea pig to midlactation in the rat. The peak increment in brain weight in the human occurs late in fetal life.[3] Therefore the timing of deficiencies and their effect on organ development do not permit simple cross-species application of findings.

Postnatal growth rates of the total body differ among species, and the terminology requires clarification. Since linear measurements are rarely done on animals, "growth" usually refers only to increase in body weight. Growth in length as well as growth in weight is measured in the human, and each measurement has a different meaning in regard to body composition. The growth curve is different for humans and higher primates than for lower animals.[4] The latter increase in weight from birth in a single sigmoid curve of acceleration and then deceleration to the end of growth at maturity. In contrast, the distinctly primate pattern, observed in humans, chimpanzees and rhesus monkeys, has a second acceleration of the growth curves for both weight and height in the prepubertal period and a second deceleration to mature size. Therefore, a different evaluation of the effects of early growth retardation must be considered in the human in view of this second acceleration. Undernutrition of lower animals in early life may result in permanent deficits, but this may not necessarily be true for humans. There are indications that in the human the timing, rate, and duration of the adolescent growth spurt may be different in children who were undernourished or suffered other adverse influences during early childhood in contrast to children who were always well-nourished. This suggests that undernutrition during early stages of growth may have somewhat less permanent effects on the child.

Biochemical functions and capabilities also vary among species. Perhaps the best known example to students of nutrition if the absence of L-gulonolactone oxidase, necessary for the conversion of glucose to ascorbic acid, in

NUTRITION, GROWTH, AND BODY COMPOSITION

primates, guinea pigs, one type of bird and bat, and at least two kinds of fish. All other animals thus far tested can synthesize ascorbic acid and do not have a dietary requirement of the vitamin. Physical differences, such as whether the body covering is skin, hair, or feathers, also alter physiological requirements. There are numerous examples of enzyme and hormone differences that affect nutritional requirements and physiological functions among various species.

Psychological responses of the human to food are more complex than those of lower animals. Stress may alter the absorption and utilization of nutrients, and species differences exist in what constitutes stress and what effect it may have on nutrient requirements.

Therefore, although animal studies are indispensable to the clarification of functions and interrelationships at the tissue, cellular, and molecular levels, findings on animals are not always directly applicable to humans.

HUMAN STUDIES

Studies of humans fall into three main categories: balance studies, cross-sectional studies, and longitudinal studies. Each has advantages and limitations. All three have a place in furthering knowledge of events in the life span, and the data gained from all three are complementary.

Balance Studies

These studies require the weighing and analysis of all food consumed and the measurement and analysis of urinary and fecal output, and perhaps also of sweat and nail clippings. The degree of precision required limits this type of study to special centers with necessary facilities, but balance studies have provided the only informative data on the retention of nutrients from varied levels of dietary intake. As previously noted, most of the studies have been carried out on adult men. The most extensive studies of pregnant and lactating women and of children were done by the Children's Fund of Michigan.[5] Other balance studies will be cited in various sections of this book. Balance studies have been used as a major basis for calculating the nutrient requirements of humans.

Many questions have been raised about the interpretation of the results of balance studies, primarily because of the restrictions of the methodology and some as yet unsolvable difficulties. The precision of this type of study necessitates its limitation to small groups of subjects studied for a relatively short period of time, usually 10 to 14 days. Since the absorption of many nutrients is complex, the type of experimental diet selected may alter conditions in the gastrointestinal tract and the results may not be applicable to persons consuming other kinds of diets. The body has the capacity to store some nutrients and draw on these reserves or increase its efficiency in the re-utilization of nutrients when dietary intake is low; it is difficult or impossible to assess the body's adaptation to changes in nutrient supply, especially within a two-week period. Methodological and laboratory errors may distort findings. For example, in nitrogen studies, methodological errors tend to underestimate requirements. For some nutrients, such as nitrogen and calcium, increased retention is observed with intakes that are increased to relatively high levels, with little evidence of a plateau. In a review of several nitrogen balance studies on adults, pregnant women and preadolescent girls, Hegsted estimated that, above a zero balance of 5 g N/day, retention remained at approximately 20 percent of intake even as intake increased. He concluded that results of balance studies must be viewed with caution and skepticism with present methodology.[6]

Cross-Sectional Studies.
In these studies each subject is examined or measured only once. If successive ages are investigated, a different population is used for each age group. The data may be compiled in a table or graph to show the distribution of findings for each age group. The primary advantage of the cross-sectional study is that a great mass of data may be obtained in a relatively short time on a large number of subjects. Major cross-sectional surveys in the past decade or two have included the Ten-State Nutrition Survey[7] and the Preschool Nutrition Survey,[8] both of which were completed between 1968 and 1970. The Health and Nutrition Examination Survey[9,10] has also used cross-sectional methods, but in conjunction with a plan for repeating the procedures on different subjects after an interval of time in order to monitor continuously dietary intakes and the health status of the population.

One example of the value of large surveys is the development of growth standards representative of the entire U.S. population of children. For many years the tables most commonly used to evaluate physical growth were based on relatively small numbers of children measured in longitudinal studies in Boston and Iowa City.[11] In 1976, the National Center for Health Statistics[12] published tables of the distributions of body measurements of children examined throughout the country (see Appendix II).

The aim of each of the national surveys has determined the selection of the population samples. Since the Ten-State Nutrition Survey was intended to estimate the prevalence and type of malnutrition in the United States, its studies concentrated on geographical areas where average income was in the lowest quartile in the 1960 census. The other national surveys cited here used sampling techniques to obtain data typical of the population as a whole. Thousands of subjects were included in each survey, providing a wider distribution of values for each of the factors investigated than was available from earlier studies of more limited population groups.

One example of the value of large surveys is the development of growth standards representative of the entire U.S. population of children. For many years the tables most commonly used to evaluate physical growth were based on relatively small numbers of children measured in longitudinal studies in Boston and Iowa City.[11] In 1976, the National Center for Health Statistics[12] published tables of the distributions of body measurements of children examined throughout the country (see Appendix II).

NUTRITION, GROWTH, AND BODY COMPOSITION

Most of the currently available data on the elderly segment of the population are also cross-sectional. With this group there are special limitations on the interpretation of trends with advancing age. Subjects at older ages are elite in that they have survived. Therefore, while distributions of physical, physiological, or biochemical findings on a group of 40-year-old subjects are likely to be more representative of the general population, with each added decade of age the group becomes more selective. The characteristics that may be associated with earlier mortality take their toll, leaving survivors with the characteristics consistent with longevity. For example, cross-sectional studies have shown lower average body weights and triceps skinfold measurements after 50 years of age;[13] this may, at least in part, be due to death of the obese and survival of the lean. Cross-sectional data do not include the previous history of the subject group; therefore one cannot conclude from these data that individuals get thinner as they increase in age, but only that the subjects examined at 60 or 70 years of age weighed less and had less subcutaneous fat than the subjects examined at 50 years.

Another limitation of cross-sectional and other studies of the elderly is that those who are included in most surveys are physically mobile and mentally alert. The need for cooperation of the subjects is a factor in the selective process. Not only are the elderly an elite group of survivors, but those included in surveys are likely to be in better physical and mental health than the bedridden or mentally incompetent who are unable to participate.

Longitudinal Studies

In longitudinal studies individual subjects are followed over an extended period of time. Although practicality unfortunately limits the duration of most longitudinal studies, the continuum of the life span makes it obvious that the status of the adult is dependent on his or her entire life history. For example, it is becoming increasingly clear that arteriosclerosis in the elderly may have its origin in earlier arterial changes, perhaps in the late teen years. If obesity in the adult began in chilhood, it is essential to determine the events in childhood that led to the excess deposition of adipose tissue. Animal experiments have shown that the restriction of food intake in the young leads to greater longevity; we do not know whether this is also true of humans. Many of the health deficits of the adult and elderly are of chronic, long-term etiology. Therefore, it is impossible to understand the problems of the adult without far greater knowledge than we now have of the origin and development of aberrations in physiological and biochemical function.

During the White House Conferences on Children in 1925 and 1930,[14] the need for long-term studies of children became obvious. There were extensive data on cross-sectional standards for height and weight that showed the status of children at any given age, but there was little evidence to indicate the patterns by which individual children actually grew. Unfortunately, mass data obscure individual patterns. During adolescence, when the timing of the growth spurt has wide variation, the use of average or percentile curves broadens the time span and minimizes maximum velocity of growth in both height and weight, so that the average curves do not reliably depict the actual growth rates of individual children. But further questions were raised even about the age periods when growth is not so dramatic. For example, if two seven-year-old boys had heights that approximated the fifth percentile, how could the examiner determine whether their growth was following a healthy pattern? Only by longitudinal study, with repeated measurements of the same children could patterns of growth be established. In the example of the two boys, one might have been small from birth with annual increments acceptable for his age. The other boy may have been tall until the age of four, and then grown progressively more slowly so that his height steadily dropped in percentile rank; such a curve would provide a danger signal to investigate possible causes of growth retardation. The White House Conferences, therefore, clearly demonstrated the need to observe how individual children grew, what patterns of growth were demonstrated at progressive age levels, and how one might identify the child whose growth was aberrant.

Following the Conferences, several growth studies were established throughout the United States. Programs that followed individuals from birth to maturity included the Oakland-Berkeley studies in California, the Child Research Council in Colorado, the Fels Research Institute in Ohio, and the Harvard School of Public Health Growth Study in Massachusetts. The history of these studies has been reviewed elsewhere.[15] These were followed by studies in other countries. As a result, patterns of physical growth and many of the factors that influence growth have been extensively studied. Unfortunately many of the studies were terminated, either by design or by lack of funding, some at maturity of the subjects and some at later ages. With the present increasing interest in the health of adults and the elderly, and awareness of the significance of occurrences early in life on the later development of disease, the need for longitudinal study is again emphasized. Studies that had originally been established to observe the growth and health of children would have provided invaluable data on the origin and development of later chronic conditions.

Human longitudinal studies are lengthy undertakings and are therefore expensive to conduct. They are limited to relatively few subjects; with one exception, each of the major longitudinal growth studies in the United States had enrolled fewer than 350 subjects. However, the intensity of the study provides a careful evaluation of the health of each subject and a record of illnesses. Although the protocol varied from study to study, most have included biochemical and physiological evaluations, and some have investigated dietary intake, psychological development, and a variety of environmental influences on growth and development.

The cross-sectional surveys provide data on a large number of subjects, each at a single age, to reflect the population as a whole at the time of the survey. Covering a very wide range of economic, ethnic and geographic groups, they represent findings on a widely diversified group. On the other hand, longitudinal studies make the unique contribution of the how and why of development of a small group of individuals. One study methodology is concerned primarily with status at a given age, and the other is designed to trace the changes of each individual over time. The findings from both cross-sectional and longitudinal studies, combined with the biochemical findings from balance studies and, more recently, tissue studies, have provided several different levels of understanding of the mechanisms of the human body and the interrelationships of multiple variables on growth, development, health, and aging. Each type of research, despite limitations, makes its own contribution to the gradual accumulation of knowledge of how the body functions at different stages of development, under differing environmental conditions, and at various levels of biological organization.

CELL AND TISSUE GROWTH, MATURITY, AND AGING

All of life depends upon the cell. From conception, when the union of two cells forms the beginning of the organism, to the final degeneration of cell function at the end of the life span, cellular structure and function determine the quality of life. The role of nutrition is to supply to each cell the materials it needs for growth, maintenance, repair, and metabolic activities. The requirements of the cell for nutrients, oxygen, and water must be met for life to exist, and the degree to which the needs of cells are supplied determines the level of somatic growth and the ability of the cells to perform their specific metabolic activities. Therefore, nutritional adequacy is essential for optimal body formation and for all aspects of health throughout the life span.

Nutrition, however, must be viewed in its broadest sense. The science of nutrition is concerned not only with nutrients but also with the many factors that influence the availability of food, individual food selection, ingestion, efficiency of digestive and absorptive processes, transport, utilization of nutrients by cells, and elimination of waste products. While the biochemistry and physiology of nutrition are, in the final analysis, the processes of utmost importance to the cells, the complexity of food supply and the availability of food to the gastrointestinal tract must also be considered. Factors that have an impact on the nutritional status of an individual range from the global food supply to the intensely personal food choices. Agriculture and world politics, food technology and transportation, economics and education, sociology and cultural anthropology all impinge on the availability of food to the individual and to the selection of the foods he consumes. The nutrition of the individual is as much the product of his physical and cultural environment as it is of his psychological and physiological acceptance of food. Furthermore, since the individual is not static but is constantly in a state of dynamic change, both environmental influences and physiological requirements vary from age to age and even from day to day. Therefore, as we trace the influence of nutrition on the organism through growth, maturity, and aging, the focus on the cells and tissues of the body must always be viewed in the context of the larger environment and the body's continual need for adaptation.

Growth and development are interdependent processes associated with the period from the fertilization of the ovum to maturity. The terms are used in tandem and sometimes even interchangeably, although they are different processes. Growth can be measured quantitatively. It is the increase in size of the body and, therefore, of any part of the body. Increase in size results from both cell multiplication and expansion of cell cytoplasm. In the initial phases of cell division in the embryo, cells differentiate for structure and function, controlled in some remarkable way by chromosomes, with the formation of different organs of the body. After completion of the differentiation phase, cells reproduce themselves and grow in size. Therefore, growth is the result of assimilation of nutrient materials into protoplasm.

Development is a complex process of integrating structure and function, with the gradual acquisition of physiologic competence.[16] It is the maturation of function of the organs. Development is a broad term; it includes such diverse processes as the increase in neuromuscular coordination that leads to control of hand and finger motion and the physiologic and hormonal changes of sexual maturation. Development leads to the highly organized and specialized functional capacity of body organs.

Cells and tissues must be formed in the process of growth before development is initiated. Thereafter the two processes continue at the same time. Even as tissues are growing, their structure and functions are maturing. The developmental process itself influences growth. The molding and reshaping of bone occur in response to body movement and changes in stress. The development of organs in early puberty results in the production of sex hormones that stimulate adolescent growth.

Winick[17] has developed a theoretical scheme of cell growth based on the content of deoxyribonucleic acid (DNA) and protein (Figure 1.1). DNA, which is responsible for genetic transmission, appears primarily in the cell nucleus, although trace amounts may be in smaller organelles. Each human diploid cell, a cell with normal double chromosome count, contains 6.0 pg

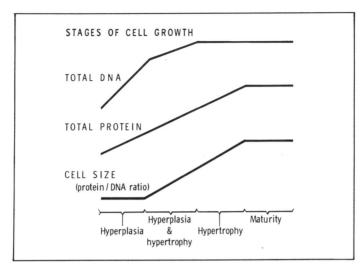

Figure 1.1 Theoretical scheme of cell growth. (Reprinted from Winick, M. Cellular Changes during Early Malnutrition. Ross Laboratories, Columbus, Ohio, 1971.)

of DNA. The number of cells in a given weight of tissue may be calculated by measuring its DNA content. Protein, on the other hand, is a basic component of cell structure and increases in the tissue when cells either multiply or grow in size. Therefore, the changes in DNA and protein content of the tissue may be used to differentiate the kind of growth occurring within the tissue. During the initial period, which Winick termed hyperplasia, both DNA and protein increase proportionately and their ratio remains constant, indicating cell multiplication. This is followed by a period of slower cell division, with a decelerating increase in DNA, concomitant with increase in cell size, indicated by the continuing rise in protein content and a higher protein/DNA ratio. In the final period, hypertrophy, the tissue has its full complement of cells, with no further increase in DNA, and growth is entirely the result of increase in size, as shown by the continued rise in protein content. Once the tissue has reached the mature stage and growth has ceased, there is no further accretion of protein. Although the DNA method of counting cells is not used with adipose cells, the sequence of increase in number and size of cells seems to occur in all tissues, each with its specific timing.

Growth proceeds in an orderly and continuous sequence, but not at a uniform rate. Although there are no real chronological boundaries in the flow of the growth process, each stage has distinguishing characteristics that make it different from all other stages. The simplest method of depicting growth is by the measurement of height and weight. The Stuart–Meredith percentiles of length or height and weight of girls from birth to 18 years of age[11] are shown in Figure 1.2. The continuous increase in body size is evident, but the slope of the curve is steeper during infancy and puberty, the

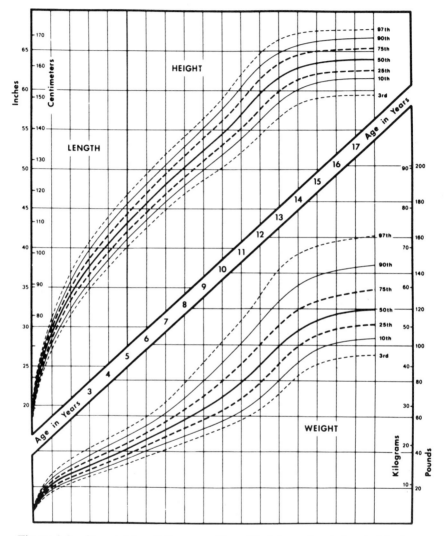

Figure 1.2   *Stuart-Meredith percentiles of height and weight of girls from birth to 18 years. (Reprinted from Valadian, I. and Porter, D. Physical Growth and Development from Conception to Maturity. Little, Brown, Boston, 1977.)*

NUTRITION, GROWTH, AND BODY COMPOSITION

two periods of postnatal growth when the rate of increment is greatest. Boys and girls differ in the timing and amount of growth, and the differences are especially wide during the pubertal spurt. Therefore sex differentiation is essential in the assessment of growth.

However, the use of measurements for total weight and height, taken for the simplicity of the procedures, masks the fact that each organ and segment of the body is growing at a rate that is uniquely its own. Body proportions change in a pattern that is not always appreciated. For example, many of the early paintings of infants show them with the proportions of an adult. By the simple technique of holding height constant, Scammon[18] in 1929 presented his classic outlines of the human body from the fetal stage to the adult (Figure 1.3). During fetal life, growth tends to follow a cephalocaudal direction, and the head and upper body grow at a more rapid rate than the lower body. At birth, head length constitutes approximately one-fourth and leg length three-eighths of total body length. Postnatally there is proportionally less growth of the head and more of the lower part of the body, so that head length comprises only one eighth and leg length nearly one half of total length by the time mature height is attained. Body proportions change considerably because of the differential growth of body segments.

In a further analysis of the variability in timing in different parts of the body, Scammon[19] also depicted the growth of lymphoid, neural, and genital tissues in contrast to general body growth (Figure 1.4). The pattern of general growth (solid line) is typical of the body as a whole, musculature, skele-

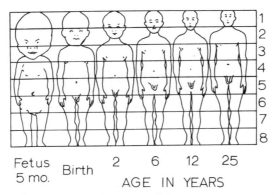

Fetus 5 mo.   Birth   2   6   12   25

AGE IN YEARS

Figure 1.3 Changes in body proportions during growth, keeping height constant. (Adapted from The Development and Growth of the External Dimensions of the Human Body in the Fetal Period by Scammon, R. E., and L. A. Calkins. Copyright 1929 by the University of Minnesota. University of Minnesota Press, Minneapolis.

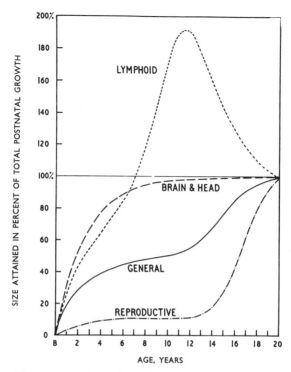

Figure 1.4   Growth of four types of body tissue as percent of adult size. (Adapted from Scammon, R. E. Measurement of the Body in Childhood. In: The Measurement of Man. University of Minnesota Press, Minneapolis, 1930.

ton, blood volume, and respiratory and digestive organs. In contrast, neural tissue, including the brain, grows rapidly in utero and in early postnatal life, reaching 90 percent of adult brain weight by 6 years of age. Lymphoid tissue, including the thymus, grows rapidly until puberty, then actually decreases to adult size. Growth of genital tissue is slow postnatally until puberty when sexual maturation occurs. Therefore, body growth is the sum of many tissues growing at different rates at different ages.

When Winick's schematic order of cell growth is applied it is apparent that the time sequence of hyperplasia and hypertrophy for each tissue or body segment has particular significance to nutrition in several respects. Since cell growth is dependent on nutrient supply, the rate of body growth may be factored into estimation of nutrient requirements during any period of growth. The requirement includes the amount of the nutrient required for maintenance of body tissue plus an allowance for new tissue to be

NUTRITION, GROWTH, AND BODY COMPOSITION

formed. This allowance for growth may even be adjusted for specific tissues, as in the estimation of the iron requirement of adolescent males who have a marked increase in muscle mass, requiring both myoglobin for muscle fibers and hemoglobin for increased blood supply.[20]

The vulnerability of the growing organism to any interruption or inadequacy of nutrient supply is greatest in organs undergoing most rapid growth at the time of the shortage. In his animal experiments, Warkany[2] produced defects in development of specific organs of the offspring by the careful timing of maternal dietary deficiencies. Another example of the limitation of cell replication during the critical period of hyperplasia was shown by Winick et al.[21] in their study of the number of brain cells in infants who died of severe malnutrition during the first year of life, when brain growth normally is rapid. Abnormal development of a single organ, then, can sometimes be demonstrated when the timing of the major growth of that organ has been identified to coincide with a period of severe malnutrition.

Growth of the total body is a composite of many growth rates and, therefore, the effects of malnutrition on total growth are more complex. There is ample evidence that retardation of linear growth may result from malnutrition during childhood. In developing countries, cessation or slowing of growth in length is used as one of the earliest indices of poor nutritional status. Even with lesser degrees of environmental inadequacy, a variety of factors are capable of influencing both the velocity of growth and the chronological ages at which developmental changes occur. Dreizen et al.[22] observed retardation in skeletal maturation, later menarche, and a longer growth period in undernourished girls. This suggests a slowing of many of the processes of growth, both directly on tissue increase that can be measured, and indirectly on organ growth or hormone production that cause a delay in the normal sequence of sexual maturation.

Understanding the processes of growth and development is vital to understanding the aging process. Changes that occur early in life can be correlated with those occurring late in life, and the study of aging can be considered as a corollary to the study of development.[16] As developmental changes occur gradually, so do the decline and degeneration of functional competence. Just as growth is multifaceted and occurs at several levels of biological integration, aging also is not a single independent phenomenon but a complex of related component processes that occur at different times as the result of a variety of influences. Growth, in its strictest sense of increase in size, occurs only between conception and maturity. Development is a term to describe the maturation of function. There is no comparably simple terminology to encompass the maintenance and eventual decline of function at the levels of molecules, cells, tissues, and the organism as a whole. However, there are few biological boundaries that subdivide the life span, with the exceptions of conception, birth, and death. Life is a continuum of gradual changes and constant adaptation and readaptation to internal and environmental influences. In this book, for purposes of convenience, the life span is divided into categories of age or biological characteristics, but these are arbitrary and false divisions, especially when applied to individuals.

MEASUREMENT OF THE BODY

In evaluating growth, a distinction must be made between the two most common measurements, height and weight. Height is a measure of linear growth and reflects primarily increase in length of the skeleton, with small contributions from tissues between the vertebrae and between long bones. It is, therefore, a simple direct measure of increase in one dimension of a single component tissue of the body. Weight, on the other hand, varies with all body tissues, including adipose tissue, and with body water. Edema and excessive fat deposition, both undesirable conditions, contribute to an increase in body weight and must be taken into account when this measurement is used to evaluate growth.

LINEAR GROWTH

Linear growth is measured as crown-heel length in the fetus, infant, and young child and, thereafter, usually as standing height. Fetal growth data have been derived primarily from measurements of abortuses and prematurely born infants since the coiled position of the fetus makes accurate assessment of length impossible by other means. The increase in crown-heel length of the fetus, as shown in Figure 1.5, is close to a straight line after the initial acceleration in the first eight weeks. Postnatal increase in height was shown in Figure 1.2, based on the Stuart-Meredith percentiles. Supine length is measured on infants and young children until they can stand still and straight for accurate measurement of erect height. The age for transition from length to height in tables and graphs used for growth standards has varied from two to six years. Length tends to be slightly greater than erect height, and erect height is somewhat less at the end of the day than in the morning. Measurements of length or height are based on the actual size of individuals or groups related to age and may be derived from either cross-sectional or longitudinal studies.

Measurement of the velocity of growth, however, is possible only when individuals have been measured at successive ages, and it is in the evaluation of growth velocity that longitudinal studies have made a major contrbution. Velocity, or rate, is the amount of growth achieved within a stated period of time, usually six months or one year. The velocity curve[23] shows clearly the periods of relatively fast or relatively slow growth, as seen diagramatically in Figure 1.6. The very rapid rate of increase in the size of the fetus is

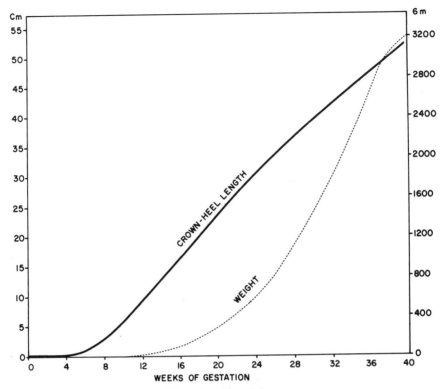

Figure 1.5   Increase in fetal length and weight.

followed by a diminishing rate in infancy and early childhood, a relatively stable rate of increment in the years until the start of pubescent growth, a second acceleration of the rate, and then a decline to maturity. The sex differences in adolescent growth rates are obvious. The rate curve has particular significance to nutrient requirements of the body. During periods of rapid growth, a steady supply of nutrients is needed for cell multiplication and increase in cytoplasm and for the extracellular materials essential to body function. The vulnerability of the body to limitation of nutrients is greater during rapid growth phases than during the period of slow but steady increase in body size.

WEIGHT

As an index of growth, weight is subject to greater variation than height, both between individuals and within a single individual over time. Weight gain of the infant and child has often been used as a criterion for the adequacy of growth, and for many years parents, physicians, and school health personnel used various standards of weight and weight gain as "norms" or

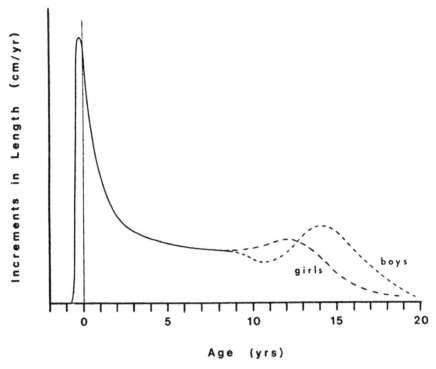

Figure 1.6   Schematic rate of growth in length, fetal and postnatal. (Reprinted from Valadian, I., and D. Porter. Physical Growth and Development from Conception to Maturity. Little, Brown, Boston, 1977.)

"ideals" to be attained. A reevaluation of this viewpoint has become necessary. Bone, muscle, and some body organs are likely to be proportional to stature and show relatively little variations between individuals per unit of height. Fat, however, is the most variable component and has a large influence on weight. Recent concern about obesity in infants and young children has raised questions about the wisdom of using weight gain as an index of satisfactory growth. A child who is "growing well" by a weight index may actually be adding excessive fat tissue. In severe undernutrition, such as the kwashiorkor form of protein-energy malnutrition, edema often masks the loss of weight of both lean body mass and fat. Therefore, while weight is a useful measure of body size, its meaning should be subjected to more qualifications than in the past.

The fetal weight curve presents a very different pattern from the length curve. As shown in Figure 1.5, length increases early in intrauterine life and from eight weeks to term follows essentially a straight line. In contrast, the average weight of the embryo is less than 50 g by the end of the first trimes-

NUTRITION, GROWTH, AND BODY COMPOSITION

ter. Acceleration of weight gain in the second trimester results in an increase of nearly 1 kg. In the final trimester the fetus nearly triples in weight, largely because of the deposition of fat tissue. The initial weight loss after delivery is usually regained by the tenth day, and thereafter the postnatal weight curve more nearly resembles the height curve (Figure 1.2). A rapid increase in weight during the first year is followed by a relatively slower gain in the preschool and early school years, with a second acceleration in the pubescent period, with gradual deceleration to maturity. However, since there is no further increase in height after mature stature has been reached, height can be used as an index to the termination of the growth period. Weight has a different pattern with less clear demarcation between childhood and adulthood.

Changes in height and weight during adult years have been studied less intensively than during childhood. Longitudinal data over long time spans in adults are unavailable. Cross-sectional data have been obtained on military, industrial, and consumer groups, but the longest age span of cross-sectional data on the United States population are those of the Ten-State Nutrition Survey[7] and the National Center for Health Statistics[24] surveys. Different age groupings were used, and percentiles were calculated in the former and means in the latter survey, so that the data are not directly comparable. However, in both surveys male subjects measured at 75 to 80 years of age were 7.0 to 8.1 cm shorter and female subjects 6.4 to 7.2 cm shorter than other subjects measured in early adulthood when stature was at its peak. This may reflect a true decrease with age, a secular change in height, a chance selection of subjects at different ages, or a combination of these factors. The median or mean weight, however, continued to increase to a peak between 35 and 54 years in men and between 50 and 64 years in women before declining.

Dissatisfaction with the inadequacy of height and weight as sole indices of growth has led to many attempts to devise more meaningful measurements. Height is a simple and informative measurement, expecially when it is repeated on the same child. Weight, however, is a complex of many body components and requires further clarifications. However, most other measurements that differentiate the components of weight require either specialized equipment or training of the examiner to minimize errors. A number of techniques have evolved using height and weight to give a better index of body proportions and to incorporate heredity and maturational levels in their interpretation.

DEVELOPMENT OF GROWTH CURVES

Early standards for height and weight were based on mean values of populations at given ages. It soon became obvious that using one or two standard deviations above and below the mean to establish a "normal" range was satisfactory for height but not for weight. For measurements with normal, or Gaussian, distributions, the use of means and standard deviations is justified. Height distributions are essentially normally distributed. However, distributions of weight are skewed to the right. Many values cluster below the mean, but there is a wide range of values above the mean. The degree of overweight may be much greater than the degree of underweight. The standard deviation falsely equalizes distribution about the mean.

In order to identify underweight and overweight children, many authorities arbitrarily selected a percentage deviation from the mean to establish a central channel of acceptable weights. A deviation of 6, 7, or 10 percent below the mean was used as the lower acceptable limit for young children. For adolescents, whose individual variation is greater, the most common standard for classifying underweight was a level of 15 percent or more below the mean. There was greater agreement that the overweight individual was 20 percent or more above the mean. Although this eliminated the problem of the inequity of standard deviations, the elevation of the mean was still a problem because it included very high values in its calculation.

Percentiles had been introduced by Galton in 1891, but were generally ignored until they were once again applied to body measurements by Burgess[25] in 1937. Percentiles have been in general use since that time. They depend more on the distribution of observations than on magnitude and provide a better description of the frequency with which a given level of weight may be found in a population. The 50th percentile (median) is the central value when all observed measurements have been arranged by order of magnitude. An equal number of observations fall above and below the median, regardless of their distance from the median. Other centiles may be selected as desired. For example, 25 percent of observations fall below the 25th percentile or above the 75th percentile. The 3rd or 5th percentile is usually the lowest level calculated and the 95th or 97th the highest.

Some variations in percentile standards are to be expected because of the populations on which they were based and because of possible secular changes in growth. The two standards most widely used are the Stuart-Meredith tables (1946)[11] and those of the National Center for Health Statistics (1978).[12] The former were composite tables based on two longitudinal studies of children between birth and 18 years of age. The health and economic status of the children was known. They probably represent how children grow under generally good environmental conditions. Some children were thin, some heavy, but all were healthy and without the extreme degrees of thinness or obesity found in larger and more diverse populations. The NCHS data from 2 to 17 years were derived from large populations throughout the United States by a stratified probability sample design to represent the national population. This group, therefore, could be expected to have a wider distribution of values. An example of the NCHS graphs is shown in Figure 1.7, with the range of percentiles from the 5th to the 95th for weight of boys from 2 to 18 years. This graph shows clearly the skewness of the distribution; the distance from the 95th to the 50th percentile is at all ages greater than the distance between the 5th and 50th percentiles, and the

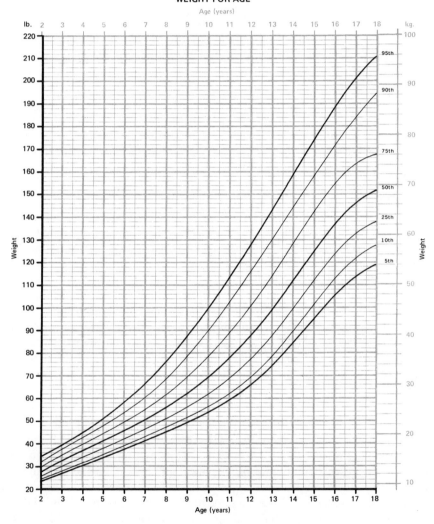

Figure 1.7   NCHS percentile curves of weight for age of boys from 2 to 18 years.

dispersion becomes greater with increasing age. Similarly skewed distributions are found for many physiological measurements, and percentiles are now widely accepted in the computation and presentation of data.

WEIGHT-TO-HEIGHT RELATIONSHIP

The relationship of weight to height is difficult to evaluate if they are graphed separately, except by comparison of the percentile level of the child on each graph. In 1941 Wetzel[26] devised a grid "for evaluating physical fitness in terms of physique (body build), developmental level and basal metabolism." His first grid was for use in plotting weight against height, without regard to age, for children from 5 through 18 years of age, followed 5 years later by a grid for children under 3 years of age. The grid (Figure 1.8) was based on the principles that in healthy growth development proceeds along a channel of a given body type on an age schedule specific for the subject, and that each child should be his or her own standard of comparison. The grid is divided into two connected graphs. On the left, weight is plotted against height, and the child falls within one of nine "physique channels" ranging from very thin to very fat. Crossing the channel markers are "isodevelopmental level lines," to be reached in a given time span. The child is not expected to shift more than one-half channel width within 10 isodevelopmental lines; any greater deviation from the child's own physique channel should alert the examiner to investigate further. The isodevelopmental lines cross to the second graph to plot the child's level against chronological age, to evaluate "auxodromic" progress or developmental age with sex differences indicated. The combination of both graphs identifies shifts in weight for height and in developmental progress. Two columns on the far right of the grid identify caloric needs for basal metabolism according to the child's isodevelopmental level and estimate dietary energy needs as twice the basal calorie needs. The Wetzel grid is complex, allows little deviation in channel position, and implies that weight for height is synonymous with maturity. The overweight child appears on the grid to be further toward maturity than the average or slender child. These inadequacies may result because the grid was not based on serial data.

The most recent graphic presentations of weight for height without regard to age were derived from the NCHS growth data.[12] Figure 1.9 shows the graph for prepubertal girls from 2 to 10 years of age. With inadequate data on the presence or absence of prepubescent changes, including growth acceleration, the committee decided that the tallest children might have entered puberty and therefore eliminated from the calculations girls whose height was above the 95th percentile by 8 years. The NCHS graph for boys extends to 11½ years, eliminating those over the 95th percentile for height after 9½ years, allowing for the later maturation of boys.

NUTRITION, GROWTH, AND BODY COMPOSITION

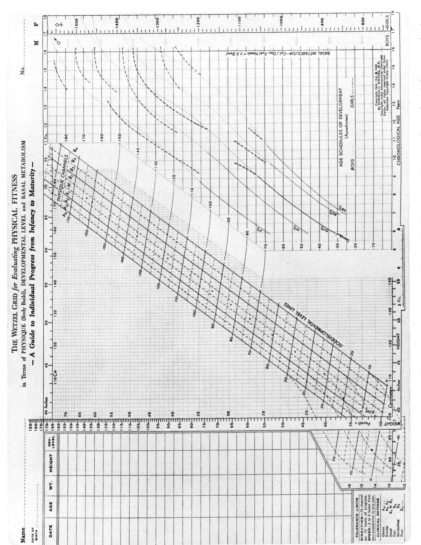

Figure 1.8   The Wetzel grid for evaluating physical fitness. (Reproduced with permission from N.E.A. Service, Inc., Cleveland, 1948.)

25

PRE-PUBERTAL GIRLS FROM 2 TO 10 YEARS

WEIGHT FOR STATURE

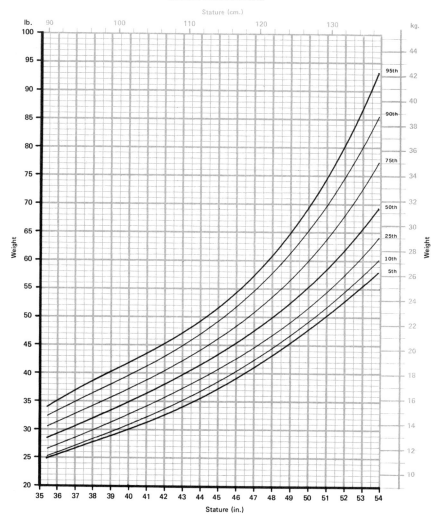

Figure 1.9 NCHS percentile curves of weight for stature in prepubertal girls from 2 to 10 years.

A number of techniques have been developed to relate weight to height, primarily in attempts to assess adiposity. Most of the data pertain to adults, and there has been little agreement about which indices are most effective in identifying excessive fatness. Sargent[27] used measurements of 160,000 U.S. college students to establish six classifications ranging from underweight (15 percent or more below mean weight) to obese (30 percent or more above

NUTRITION, GROWTH, AND BODY COMPOSITION

mean weight) for men aged 21 to 29 years and for women aged 17 to 29 years, without reference to skeletal size, muscle mass, or adipose tissue. The National Center for Health Statistics reported weight for height data from the Health Examination Survey[28] of 1960–1962 for adults aged 17 to 79 years and from the Health and Nutrition Examination Survey[29] of 1971–1974. These values were computed from the regression equation of weight on height by age, expressed as means and standard error values to represent percentiles of the population.

Of greater complexity are several weight-to-height indices that have been developed. Even with adults there is little agreement about which index is most meaningful. Billewicz et al.[30] suggested two criteria: (1) The index must be highly correlated with weight and other measurements of fatness, and (2) it must be independent of height in that the numerical index should be the same for persons of standard weight at different heights. Since body weight and height in adults are linearly related, a standard weight for height may be calculated by a regression equation, and deviations from the standard weight may be identified. Among the indices that have been applied are the following:

Relative Weight: The ratio between the observed weight of an individual and the "standard" weight for sex and height. This index has been widely used and has led to tables of "desirable" weight for height.

Weight/Height (W/H): This simple ratio appears to underestimate obesity.[31]

Weight/Height^2 (W/H^2): This index, sometimes called the Quetelet index, takes into account the fact that height is a linear measurement and weight reflects body mass or volume. Several investigators[31-33] have concluded that W/H^2 applied to adults most nearly meets the criteria. Thomas et al.[34] developed a nomogram to simplify the calculation of W/H^2.

Weight/Height^3 (W/H^3): This index has been suggested as more applicable to children.[35] Adult indices do not readily apply to children because of the difference in complexity of the relationship of weight to height. There is now a great deal of evidence that obese children tend to be taller than thin children and that during growth weight is not independent of height, although statistical analyses of weight–height relationships in children have seldom progressed beyond simple correlations.

Height/Cube Root of Weight $(H/W^{1/3})$: Sometimes called the ponderal index. This ratio tends to overestimate the incidence of obesity in short individuals.[31] It also creates confusion since a higher value indicates thinness and a lower value fatness.

Other indices of body composition and obesity standards require more extensive types of measurements. One source of dissatisfaction with weight-height ratios is their failure to distinguish between adipose tissue and lean body mass as components of weight. A heavily muscled individual may be overweight but not overfat. Other factors in individual growth that have not been taken into account in weight–height standards are genetic influences and degree of maturity. It has long been recognized that heredity has a major influence on the size of an individual and that children vary in maturational level, especially during puberty and adolescence.

By using growth data from the Fels Research Institute, Garn[36] developed a table that introduced the heights of parents into the evaluation of heights of their children. The heights of the mother and the father were averaged to give a midparent stature, and three midparent stature groups were identified. The mean heights of children of each sex at yearly age levels were calculated according to parental size. The height of a child being measured could then be evaluated according to potential genetic size. Table 1.1 pre-

Table 1.1 Fels Parent-Specific Standards for Height: Children's Stature by Age and Midparent Stature in Inches[a]

| | Midparent Stature | | | | | |
| | 64.0 inches | | 66.5 inches | | 69.0 inches | |
Age	Boys	Girls	Boys	Girls	Boys	Girls
1–0	29.0	29.0	29.5	29.0	30.5	29.5
2–0	33.6	33.0	34.5	33.5	35.0	34.5
3–0	36.5	35.5	37.5	37.0	39.0	38.0
4–0	39.0	38.0	40.5	41.0	42.0	41.0
5–0	41.5	40.5	43.5	43.0	44.5	43.5
6–0	43.5	43.5	45.5	45.5	47.0	46.0
7–0	45.7	46.0	48.0	47.5	49.0	49.0
8–0	48.0	48.0	50.0	49.5	51.5	51.0
9–0	50.0	50.5	52.0	52.0	53.5	54.0
10–0	52.0	53.0	54.0	54.0	55.5	56.5
11–0	54.5	55.5	56.0	56.5	58.0	59.0
12–0	57.0	58.0	58.5	59.0	60.0	61.5
13–0	59.5	60.5	61.0	62.0	63.0	63.5
14–0	62.5	62.5	63.5	63.0	66.0	65.5
15–0	65.5	63.0	66.0	64.0	69.0	66.5
16–0	66.5	63.0	68.0	64.0	69.5	67.0
17–0	67.5	63.5	69.0	64.5	70.0	67.5

[a]Age-size tables for Ohio white children whose midparent stature (or parental midpoint) is the average of the statures of the two parents. All values rounded off to the nearest half inch.

Source: S. M. Garn, The applicability of North American growth standards in developing countries. Can. Med. Assoc. J. 93:914–919, 1965.

NUTRITION, GROWTH, AND BODY COMPOSITION

sents these values from 1 through 17 years of age. The categories of parental size were later expanded.

Bayley[37] presented a series of growth curves for boys and for girls that included an evaluation of maturity. Since the maturity rating was based on skeletal age determined from X rays of the hand and knee, these graphs are not comparable to the height and weight curves that we have thus far discussed, but they illustrate the problem of identifying patterns of maturation that has persistently frustrated both the originators and the users of growth charts. Children differ in size at a given age because of several factors, and the deviations become more pronounced during adolescence. It is a truism among researchers on growth and development that no child is "average"; the need is for a tool to differentiaite healthy growth from aberrant growth, to allow for individual variation but to be able to detect deviations that signal abnormality.

Bayley differentiated four patterns of growth compared to the average, all based on skeletal age. Figure 1.10 presents the curves for growth in the height of girls from birth to 21 years. The central curve is the average. Adjacent curves, one above and one below the average, show slightly higher or lower growth patterns until puberty; the higher curve represents girls who were accelerated in maturity and had an early adolescent spurt, and the lower curve represents later maturation. In sharp contrast are the two outlying curves. The top curve was the mean for girls who were "constitutionally" large from an early age, with rapid growth and accelerated bone age, who had an early adolescence, and who became tall adults. The lowest curve was the mean for girls who were small from an early age, grew and matured slowly, and were still short as adults. Since skeletal age is an indicator of the individual child's timetable of growth in height, Bayley recommended evaluation of skeletal age in children whose growth did not approximate the three central curves.

Standards of height for age, weight for age, or weight for height are useful screening tools. They identify the position of the child within the distribution of that measure for the population. They can be more easily interpreted for adults who have completed growth in stature than for children who are constantly changing. Their value in childhood increases if repeated measurements are taken at successive ages so that the consistency of the child in maintaining a channel of growth can be monitored. Increment curves, or growth rates, are more informative. However, the child who grows at a pace faster or slower than the average is not necessarily abnormal, and standards of any sort tend to incorporate a rigidity that looks for conformity and make little allowance for individual variation. Some children grow slowly and always remain small. Some grow rapidly and always remain large. However, many small children mature later than the average; they have a longer total period of growth that may result in greater adult

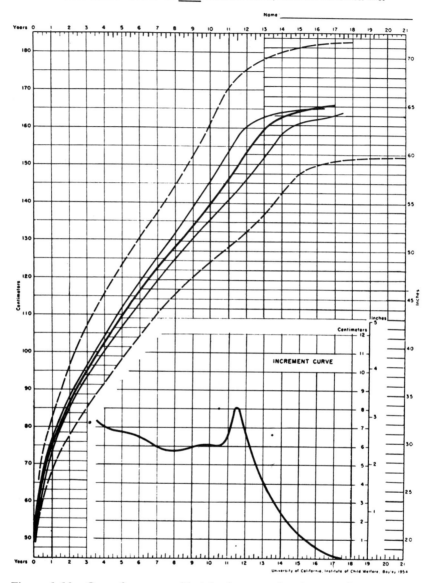

Figure 1.10   Growth curves of height for age of girls related to skeletal maturity. (Reprinted from Bayley, N. Growth curves of height and weight by age for boys and girls, scaled according to physical maturity. J. Pediat. 48:187–194, 1956.)

30   NUTRITION, GROWTH, AND BODY COMPOSITION

PERCENTS OF
MATURE HEIGHT

Age Years	Average	Accel- erated	Retarded
Birth	30.9		
1.0	44.7	48.0	42.2
2.0	52.8	54.7	50.0
3.0	57.0	60.0	55.0
4.0	61.8	64.9	59.8
5.0	66.2	69.3	63.9
6.0	79.3	73.4	67.8
7.0	74.0	76.0	71.5
8.0	77.5	79.5	74.5
9.0	80.7	83.5	77.7
10.0	84.4	87.9	81.0
11.0	88.4	92.9	84.9
12.0	92.9	96.5	88.2
13.0	96.5	98.2	91.1
14.0	98.3	99.1	95.2
15.0	99.1	99.5	97.8
16.0	99.6	99.9	98.9
16.5		100.0	
17.0	100.0		99.6
18.0			100.0

Case Number_____ Birth Date _____

RECORD OF MEASURES

Date	Age Year	Month	Stature Inches	Cent	Annual Gain	Skeletal	Rating Age Eq	Predict. of Adult Height

Figure 1.10 (Continued)

stature than might have been expected. On the other hand, large children tend to be advanced in physiological development and to mature early, thus shortening the period of growth and limiting adult stature.[38]

The pattern of human physical growth in height or weight has been well established for both sexes and the variations from the central trend determined by measurements of several population groups. However, the evaluation of the individual must take into account that overall growth is a composite of differing rates of tissue growth, each unique to the individual. The tendency to use judgmental terms, such as retarded and advanced, suggests that children should follow the central trend and that deviation, especially on the negative side, implies abnormality. Percentile standards based on longitudinal studies of children known to be healthy include small or slowly growing children as well as tall children; it is difficult to label the extremes as unhealthy. On the other hand, percentiles based on large population groups whose health status has not been screened probably include at the upper and lower levels subjects whose growth is clinically abnormal. The difficult decision is the identification of cutoff points in the distribution of a measurement to signify abnormality. For example, there is little concensus on the dividing line between overweight, which may be physiologically harmless, and pathological obesity, which increases the risk of some disease states. From the nutritional point of view, weight deviation is a subject of concern both for the very fat and the very thin. However, deviation in height is of greater concern with the small child than with the tall; true retardation of growth in stature may result from nutritional deficiencies. A child whose height measurement is at the fifth percentile of standards based on a large population group should be of greater concern than one whose height is at the fifth percentile of standards based on healthy children.

A number of formulas have been devised to predict adult height from measurements in childhood. These formulas are based on group observations and represent averages; therefore, they have a high degree of error when applied to the individual. In early childhood it is impossible to predict accurately the magnitude and duration of the individual's adolescent growth spurt, which will have a large influence on ultimate size. The predictive error obviously decreases once the adolescent pattern has been established and the individual approaches maturity. Using longitudinal data from the Aberdeen and California studies, Tanner[39] correlated adult heights and weights with heights and weights of the same individuals during childhood. Graphs of these correlation coefficients are shown in Figure 1.11. The relationship of adult height to length in the newborn period was very low, but the coefficients rose rapidly during the first two years and maintained a level of approximately 0.7 to 0.8 until prepubescence. The correlation dropped during the early pubescent period, reflecting individual variation in the timing of height acceleration, then rose as the subjects approached maturity. In contrast, correlation coefficients of adult weight with childhood weights, equally low at birth, rose with age in nearly a straight line but had less decrease at puberty than the height correlations. The prediction for stature was better than for weight.

SECULAR INCREASE IN HEIGHT

For the past century or more an increase in body size has been documented in several populations. Although it is impossible to identify causative factors, speculation has centered primarily on improvements in the environment. Better nutrition, advances in medicine, improved health care, elimination of child labor, and improved housing have been suggested as contributing factors. It has even been postulated that greater mobility of people has widened the genetic pool with less inbreeding. Whatever the causes may be, the reports from the United States and several other countries in the northern hemisphere are consistent. Concomitant with the secular increase in height has been earlier maturation, resulting in faster growth over a shorter time span. A century ago maximum adult height was reached at approximately 26 years of age; at the present time in technologically advanced countries adult height is reached in females at an average of 17 to 18 years and in males at an average of 19 to 21 years. Therefore, in the com-

NUTRITION, GROWTH, AND BODY COMPOSITION

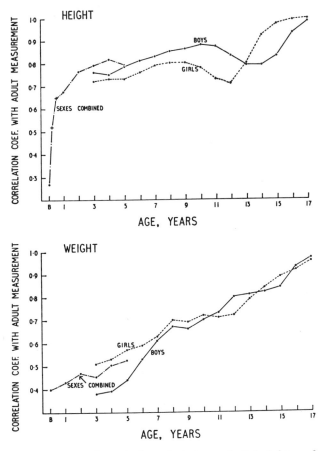

Figure 1.11 Correlations between adult height and weight and the heights and weights of the same individuals as children. (Reprinted from Tanner, J. M. Growth at Adolescence. Blackwell Scientific Publishers, Oxford, England, 1962.)

parison of heights of college students and army inductees, on whom the most extensive data are available, the earlier maturation and attainment of adult height must be taken into account.

Meredith[40] compiled measurements of heights of children from 1870 to 1960. When the NCHS data were added (Figure 1.12)[41] the calculated regression line indicated that 10-year-old boys had a height increase of 0.13 cm/year, which represented an increase of 10 percent in height over the 90-year period.[42] For contrast, the NCHS mean heights of boys in the low and

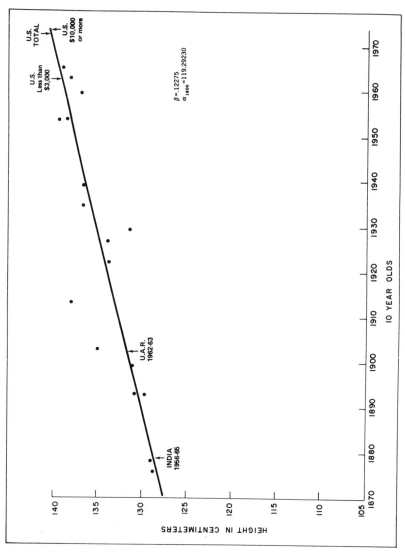

Figure 1.12 Secular increase in height of 10-year-old boys in the United States, 1870 to 1970. Indicated are average heights of boys from families with incomes below $3000 and above $10,000 in the 1963–1965 Health Examination Survey and average heights of boys in India and the United Arab Republic. (Reprinted from Hamill, P. V. V., F. E. Johnston, and S. Lemeshow. Height and Weight of Children: Socioeconomic Status, United States. DHEW Publ. No. (HSM) 73-1601. U. S. Government Printing Office, Washington, D.C., 1972.)

34

high income families in the 1963–1965 survey and heights of boys in India and the United Arab Republic were indicated on the graph. The data, aside from showing the secular change, "strongly suggest that more of the factors conducive to greater size of children are available to the lowest socioeconomic groups in the United States than to all but the most highly favored few in India and to no classes at all in the underdeveloped countries such as Burma and Ethiopia."[41]

The average heights of inductees into the United States Army increased 3 cm and average weights increased 8 kg from 1918–1919 to 1957–1958.[41] Data on the heights and weights of college students in the United States, compiled by Hathaway and Foard,[43] showed that those born in 1951 were, on the average, 7.5 cm taller and 4 kg heavier than those born in 1836. Bakwin and McLaughlin,[44] however, suggest that the secular increase in height may have ceased in the 1930s in the upper socioeconomic group in the United States. Among schoolchildren in New York City, those in private schools showed no increase in height after that period, while children in public schools continued to grow. Students entering two New England colleges from public schools continued to be taller and heavier, but those entering from private schools showed no increase in height between the 1930s and 1958–1959. Middle and upper-middle class subjects in three U.S. longitudinal studies also showed no secular increase in height over the period of time. Evidence from Sweden, too, indicates that for some groups the secular increase in height has ceased. It may be speculated that in the upper socioeconomic groups maximum height has been achieved within the past 40 years and that continued increase in height may be expected only in lower socioeconomic groups of children, at least in some technologically advanced countries.

BODY PHYSIQUE

Estimations of body physique have been attempted since Hippocrates, who described two types: habitus phthisicus, who was tall, thin, and susceptible to tuberculosis, and habitus apoplecticus, who was stocky, obese, and inclined to vascular disease. The early attempts at classification were related primarily to the susceptibility to certain diseases by different body types. Temperament was later introduced into the evaluation as some specialists in mental health used a combination of physical and mental traits in classifications.

Sheldon[45] introduced his somatotyping procedure in 1940. Although earlier indices separated people into distinct groups with little allowance for intermediate individuals, Sheldon recognized that there were few discrete types, but that individuals were distributed along a continuum of grading of the components of physique. Somatotyping depended more on body shape than height, although he applied the $H/W^{1/3}$ formula to his types. Using nude photographs of males 20 to 25 years of age, he assigned ratings for body contours, prominence of bony structures, fat covering, musculature, size of body segments, and other defined characteristics. His three types were based on the three embryonic germ layers and were labeled endomorphy, mesomorphy, and ectomorphy. Each individual was given a rating from 1 to 7 in each category. Endomorphy rates elements of softness and roundness, with a predominance of abdominal mass and soft tissue. Although obesity is not a necessary component, the extreme endomorph (7–1–1) is usually obese. Bone and muscle predominate in the mesomorph, who has a large head, broad shoulders and chest, and heavily muscled arms and legs. The ectomorph tends to linearity, with thin face, chest, and extremities, delicate bone structure, and little muscle or subcutaneous fat. Extreme ratings, 7–1–1, 1–7–1, and 1–1–7, are rare, and the most common somatotypes are 3–4–4, 4–3–3, and 3–5–2. The typing is theoretically constant throughout life. Criticisms of the somatotypes have centered around the subjectivity of rating, inapplicability to women and children, and the need for adjustment to changes in body composition beyond the young adult years.

Attempts to classify body physique by observation have been largely replaced by anthropometric measurement of external dimensions of the body. More than 100 measurements have been used by various investigators in cross-sectional or longitudinal studies, but the list of meaningful measurements is much smaller. These will be discussed more fully in Chapter 2. The measurements of greatest value vary with age of the subject. For example, head circumference is usually taken on small children, but makes negligible contribution to evaluations after six years. The measurements most commonly used are selected from the following list:

Weight
Height or crown-heel length
Sitting height or crown-rump length
Circumferences: Head, chest, waist, hip, biceps, maximum forearm, wrist, thigh, knee, calf, ankle, foot
Widths: Head, chest, hip, elbow, hand, knee, ankle, foot
Lengths: Head, arm, leg, hand, foot
Depth: Chest
Skinfold thicknesses: Triceps, subscapular, chest
No attempt will be made here to discuss the techniques of measurement. However, each measurement should be taken using a standard methodology. Personnel taking measurements should be trained in careful techniques, and efforts should be made to minimize interexaminer errors.

External measurements are the most easily obtainable index to changes in body size, conformation, and components. The ratio of one measurement to another, such as weight to height, or head circumference to chest circumference, provides information on the relative rates of growth of various body tissues. They are indirect measures of body composition. Other methods of attempts to measure the amounts of bone, muscle, and fat in the intact body will be discussed in Chapter 2.

CHANGES IN BODY TISSUE WITH AGE

BONES AND TEETH

Bone is a specialized tissue that supports the body mechanically, allows motion, and protects vital organs. It also manufactures red and white blood cells and platelets, and serves as a reservoir of calcium to maintain homeostasis of that mineral in blood. Ossification begins at approximate eight weeks of gestation in the occiput and mandible and by 12 weeks in the humerus.[16,46] It continues until maturity, at the completion of growth. The body contains different kinds of bones. The flat bones of the skull, for example, consist of two layers of compact bone separated by a layer of spongy tissue and are formed directly from embryonic tissue. As was shown in Figure 1.3, growth of the head is most rapid in utero and is nearly completed in the first six years postpartum although growth of the face continues to maturity. Growth of other segments of the body have different time schedules. Sitting height (crown–rump length) is a measure of growth of the head and vertebrae. Figure 1.13, from the longitudinal data of the Child Research Council,[47] shows the changing proportions of sitting height in relation to stature from birth to maturity. In the first six months crown–rump length constitutes approximately two-thirds of total body length. Thereafter increment in leg length exceeds increment in trunk and head, so that by early adolescence sitting height contributes slightly more than one-half of total stature. The continued growth of the trunk for a period of time after legs have ceased to grow results in a slight increase in relative sitting height in late adolescence. Growth of the extremities and appearance and size of centers of ossification have been of particular interest in longitudinal growth studies.

Endochondral bone is formed by the replacement of cartilage by a calcified bone matrix, due to the action of osteoblasts, which are highly specialized cells. Long bones of the extremities have a central cylindric compact portion, the diaphysis. At each end of the diaphysis is an area of metaphysis, which contains columns of spongy tissue with a cartilagenous plate where most of the active growth in length occurs. The epiphysis, or secondary ossification center, at each end of the long bone, is separated from the

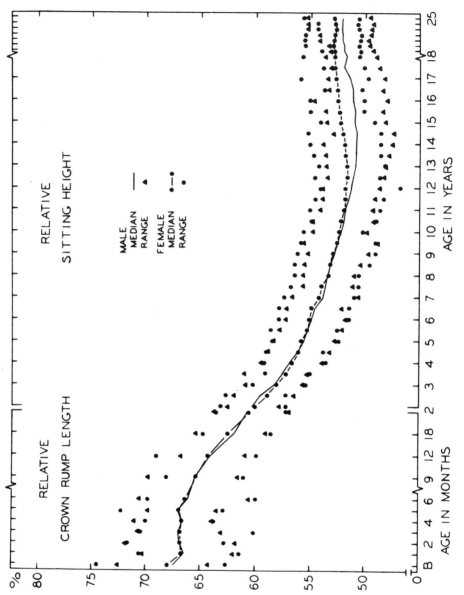

Figure 1.13 Crown-rump length and sitting height as percent of total height. (Reprinted from Hansman, C. Anthropometry and Related Data. In: McCammon, R. W., Ed. Human Growth and Development. Charles C Thomas Co., Springfield, Ill., 1970.

38

diaphysis by the cartilagenous plate. Increase in bone length occurs as the cartilage proliferates and is gradually replaced by calcified osseous tissue, increasing the length of the diaphysis (Figure 1.14). Toward the end of adolescence, the cartilage diminishes and the epiphysis becomes fused to the end of the diaphysis, eliminating further increase in length of the bone,

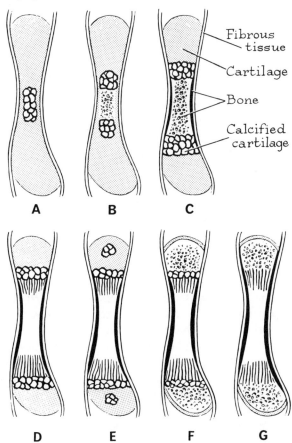

Figure 1.14 Diagrammatic representation of the maturation of a long bone. The approximate age scale is: A, 6 weeks prenatal; B, 7 weeks prenatal; C, 8 weeks prenatal; D, 10 weeks prenatal to 2 years; E, 2 to 6 years; F, 6 to 16 years; G, adulthood. (Reprinted from Roche, A. F. The elongation of the mandible. Am. J. Orthodontics 53:79–94, 1967.)

leaving only articular cartilage.[48] The timing of fusion varies with different bones within an individual; there is wider variation in timing between individuals.

The bone shaft increases in width by the formation of new osseous tissue under the periosteum, the membrane surrounding the bone. The periosteum retains the ability to form new bone even after maturity, permitting early desposition of bone in the healing of a fracture. Even while new bone is being formed, bone already formed undergoes changes. Osteoclasts absorb some of the matrix of the diaphysis, creating a cavity in the center of the bone. This cavity becomes filled with marrow, which has the ability to form blood cells. Marrow in the long bones loses this ability during childhood, probably around six years, but hematopoietic ability is retained in the bones of the skull, face, vertebrae, ribs, and pelvis. The shape of the bone changes with age because of resorption of mineral and remodeling in response to stress. The quality of bone and its mineral density depend on the supply of protein, minerals, and vitamins essential to bone formation and maintenance, as well as on the hormones that control mineralization and growth. The sex difference in bone width is evident throughout childhood, as shown in Figure 1.15 from X-ray data of the Child Research Council. The sum of measurements of widths of bones in the forearm, thigh, and calf show that the mean values of boys are increasingly greater than the mean values of girls as age progresses, and that the differences are accentuated during adolescence.[49]

The small bones of the wrist and foot are covered partly by periosteum and partly by cartilage. They continue to grow until they abut contiguous bone or until all the cartilage has been ossified. The appearance and size of these centers of ossification follow a pattern of progression that has been extensively studied from X rays of the wrist. Norms have been developed for each age from birth to maturity and for both sexes.[50, 51] By comparison with the norms, a skeletal age may be assigned to an individual child from his wrist X ray. Because there is a high correlation between skeletal maturity, sexual maturity, and total body maturity, skeletal age is often used as an index of maturation. In the early-maturing child, skeletal age is greater than chronological age, and in the late-maturing child skeletal age is less than chronological age. The comparison of skeletal age with chronological age assists in the evaluation of the height measurement of a child. For example, a short 12-year old boy with the skeletal age of a 10-year-old has greater

Figure 1.15   Sum of widths of bone, muscle, and fat from xrays of the forearm, thigh, and calf. (Courtesy of Marion M. Maresh, M.D.)

NUTRITION, GROWTH, AND BODY COMPOSITION

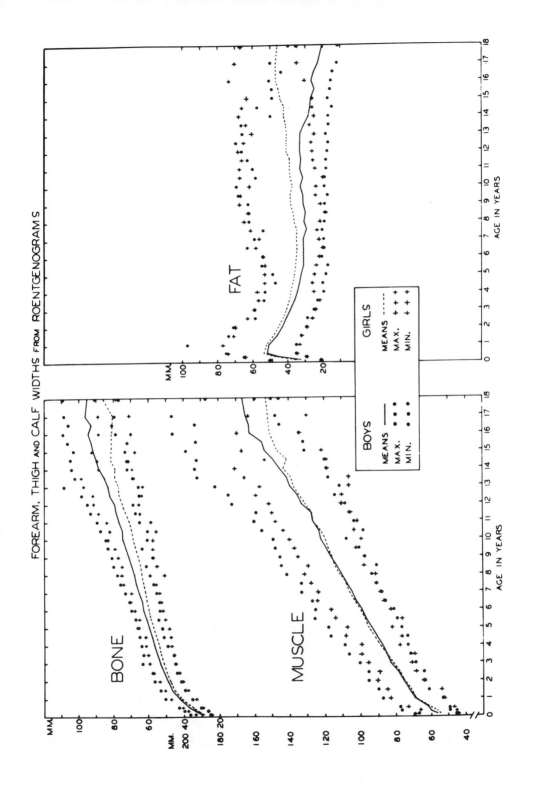

FOREARM, THIGH and CALF WIDTHS FROM ROENTGENOGRAMS

FAT

BONE

MUSCLE

BOYS
MEANS ———
MAX. ● ● ●
MIN. ● ● ●

GIRLS
MEANS ┈┈┈┈
MAX. + + +
MIN. + + +

AGE IN YEARS

growth potential than if his skeletal age were commensurate with his chronological age, since it can be assumed that he can anticipate a longer period of growth.

Illness, nutritional deficiency, or other stress may interfere with growth, especially during periods when the rate of growth should be most rapid. Skeletal maturation is less likely to be affected unless the adverse condition persists for a period of time. When the problem is corrected and conditions for growth improved, growth may be much faster than normal for some time since the body has an impetus to reestablish the previous pattern of growth. If skeletal maturation has been slowed, its rate may also increase during recovery. This phenomenon is known as catch-up growth. When adverse conditions are severe or long-lasting, the spurt of catch-up growth may not occur, but the whole time sequence of maturation may be delayed, allowing a longer period for both growth and development.

Decrement of bone is a characteristic of aging. Head size remains relatively constant, but there is a decrease in stature and in sitting height.[24] Cross-sectional studies of heights of the elderly must be interpreted in view of the secular increase in height previously discussed. However, breadth of shoulders and depth of chest also tend to decrease. The density of long bones and vertebrae declines as they lose calcium. Osteoporosis, characterized by a decrease in bone density and increased susceptibility to fractures, is more common in women than in men. Estimates of some degree of osteoporosis in the elderly range as high as 50 percent of the population. Like many other changes with age, the etiology of osteoporosis is not clear, but multiple factors are suspected. Changes in parathyroid hormone or estrogens and deterioration of the ability to synthesize collagen have been suggested. Long-term inadequacy of calcium intake, diminished absorption of calcium or reduced ability to limit calcium excretion, and cumulative losses of the mineral with pregnancy and lactation have all been implicated in the development of osteoporosis. There is some evidence that fluorine, in altering the crystallization of bone mineral, may be protective against osteoporosis.

Tooth development begins about the sixth week of embryonic life with the differentiation and growth of specialized epithelial cells. Development starts at the crown, or occlusal surface, and proceeds toward the root. The formation of the organic matrix is followed by calcification. The incisors are the first of the deciduous teeth to calcify, starting in the second trimester. At birth all 20 deciduous teeth are present in the jaws, as well as the first permanent molars, which start to calcify before birth. The lower permanent incisors and cuspids begin to calcify shortly after birth. The chronological development of deciduous and permanent teeth is shown in Figure 1.16,

NUTRITION, GROWTH, AND BODY COMPOSITION

which indicates the average ages when calcification begins and when it is completed in each tooth; it also shows the age of eruption.[52]

There is wide individual variation in the age of tooth eruption. For example, the lower central incisors are usually the first teeth to erupt, at an average age of 6 to 7 months, but the variation may be from 3 months to 1 year. As with other maturational developments, girls tend to be earlier than boys in tooth eruption. Most of the permanent teeth have erupted by the age of 12 years with the exception of the third molar, which is not included in Figure 1.16. Calcification of the third molars begins usually between 7 and 10 years of age and may continue until 18 to 25 years, with eruption between 17 and 22 years. Individual variation in the age of eruption is greater than variation in the order of appearance of both deciduous and permanent teeth.

Dental development tends to parallel other maturational patterns in the individual in that children with advanced skeletal development are likely also to have early eruption of teeth. However, dental development is not as good an index of maturity as skeletal age.

MUSCLE

There are three types of muscle in the body.[16,23] Skeletal striated muscle constitutes the bulk of body musculature and is under voluntary control. It influences body shape, posture, and locomotion. Smooth muscle, which is controlled by the autonomic nervous system, includes the muscles of the stomach and intestines; the smooth muscle cell has a single nucleus. Heart muscle is similar in structure to skeletal cells.

Muscle development begins early in fetal life. With the first heart beat at about the fourth week of gestation, circulatory function is initiated. Muscle cells are of mesodermal origin. Muscle fibers increase rapidly in both number and size throughout fetal life. The innervation of muscle occurs as early as the fifth or sixth week. By the eighth week muscles of the trunk, limbs, and head begin to develop. By 15 to 16 weeks the nerve endings are developed and in contact with the muscle fibers, which are then capable of sustained contraction. By midpregnancy musculature accounts for approximately 16 percent of fetal weight and by birth 20 to 25 percent of weight.[23]

Skeletal muscle is composed of muscle fibers in addition to connective tissue that carries blood vessels, nerves, and lymphatics essential for nourishing and controlling the muscles. Muscle fibers are elongated cells filled with myofibrils that are transversely striated and, in the adult form, contain many nuclei. During growth the increase in the number of myofibrils increases the cell diameter. During infancy, muscles continue to grow rapidly, then the rate of growth is slower until adolescence, when the rate increases,

Chronologic development of primary teeth.

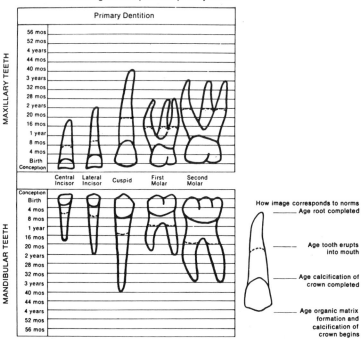

How image corresponds to norms
— Age root completed

— Age tooth erupts into mouth

— Age calcification of crown completed

— Age organic matrix formation and calcification of crown begins

Chronologic development of the permanent teeth.

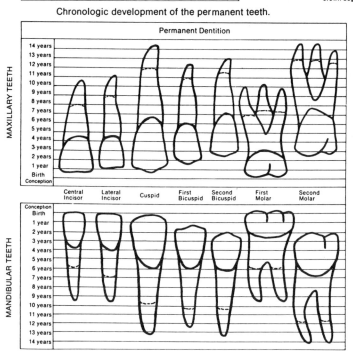

Figure 1.16 Chronological development of deciduous and permanent teeth from initial calcification of crown to completion of root. (Reprinted from Bowers, D. F. Tooth Development and Abnormalities of Appearance. In: Johnson, T. R., W. M. Moore, and J. E. Jeffries. Children Are Different: Developmental Physiology, Second Edition. Ross Laboratories, Columbus, Ohio, 1978.).

especially in males. By maturity muscle may comprise as much as 40 percent of body weight.

Factors in the growth of muscle are complex, and include metabolic function of the body, supply of nutrients, and physical activity. During childhood muscle growth is believed to be under the control of pituitary growth hormone, thyroid hormones, and insulin. With the onset of puberty, adrenal androgens are thought to be responsible for increased muscle growth in both sexes, with testosterone in males causing even greater muscle growth. There is relatively little difference between boys and girls in muscle width as measured from X rays of the extremities (Figure 1.15) until adolescence, when the acceleration of muscle growth in males is greater than in females.

Muscle strength increases with age, reaching its maximum between 20 and 30 years of age, after muscle mass has reached maturity. During adolescence, males have greater strength, as measured by grip strength, as well as greater muscle mass. Physical training and exercise affect muscle mass, and there is wide individual variation both in size of muscles and in their efficiency of oxygen uptake during physical activity.

Changes with aging include decline in physical strength and in muscle tone.[16] The changes are probably due to biochemical changes in the muscle fibers and to alterations in myoneural junctions as part of body degeneration, along with decreased skeletal density and regressive changes in cartilage. There is a decrease in functional cellular mass, but there may be an increase in connective tissue. It is not known how great an influence reduced physical activity has on muscle degeneration.

ADIPOSE TISSUE

Adipose tissue is the most variable of the major body constituents. Adipose cells store fat when there is an excess of caloric intake over body needs. Adipose tissue contains 68 to 88 percent fat[53] and therefore acts as a reserve supply of convertible energy. A layer of subcutaneous fat covers most of the body and protects against extremes of environmental temperature. Deep body fat cushions organs and protects them from injury. Total body fat is difficult to measure, so there are conflicting data in the literature on its assessment as well as on the proportion of total fat found under the skin. Methods for measurement are indirect and based on a number of assumptions, as will be discussed in Chapter 2. Subcutaneous fat may be measured by calipers applied to a skinfold pinch and has been measured from X rays in longitudinal studies (Figure 1.15). However, the total volume of subcutaneous adipose tissue cannot be extrapolated from either measurement.

Early in pregnancy there is little fat deposition in the fetus. It has been estimated that by midgestation fat constitutes only 0.5 percent of fetal weight. Fat increases to 6 percent during the fifth fetal month, and then acceleration of fat deposition is rapid, with the major amount accumulated during the last two months. At birth fat is approximately 16 percent of body weight. From the curves of fetal length and weight in Figure 1.5, the prematurely born infant can be expected to have a greater deficit in weight than in length, and inadequate body fat is characteristic of the premature infant.

The rapid deposition of fat in late intrauterine life continues for the first six to twelve months postnatally and then tapers off. During the preschool years fat deposition lags behind skeletal growth so the child appears thinner. Sex differences in amounts and sites of body fat are evident throughout childhood. After six years there is a steady accumulation of subcutaneous fat in the female, continuing through adolescence and sometimes into adult life. In contrast, the male has a smaller increase after six years; he is likely to have a slight acceleration at the beginning of the pubertal spurt, but the average male has a decrease in fat widths during the period of greatest increase in stature. The male's increase in weight during adolescence is primarily from bone and muscle. It should be noted that both skinfold and X-ray measurements reflect the thickness of the subcutaneous fat layer and not the total volume of subcutaneous fat. The linear extension of the fat layer parallels bone growth.

The amount and distribution of subcutaneous fat during adulthood continue to show marked sex differences. In the Ten-State Nutrition Survey and in the National Center for Health Statistics survey, obesity was more common among women than among men. However, income and ethnicity have a stronger relationship to weight and skinfold measurements in adults than in children, as will be discussed in Chapter 2. After the peak in thicknesses during the adult years, there is a progressive decline in skinfold measurements with aging.[13]

MEASUREMENT OF BODY COMPOSITION
DIRECT MEASUREMENT OF BODY COMPOSITION

The only direct method of determining body composition is by chemical analysis of the whole body. As Widdowson[53] stated in her summary of available data, chemical analysis "has obvious limitations, for it can be applied only after a person is dead, and healthy people do not die except as a result of accident, suicide or murder." The legal and practical difficulties of acquiring a body after sudden death and the chemical manipulation of anything so large and complex as an adult human body have limited accumulation of direct data on body composition. Between 1859 and 1881, analyses of several bodies were reported, but the chemical methods at that time cast doubt on their current validity. Between 1945 and 1956, analyses of seven adult bodies were reported. A number of analyses have been done on fetuses and stillborn infants, but none on older children.

In the five adult bodies without edema, body weights ranged from 84 to 110 percent of standard weight, and fat ranged from 4 to 24 percent of body weight. No data are available on the direct measurement of fat content of obese bodies. Fat is the constituent with the greatest individual variation. The percent of water in the body varied inversely with the fat, but in the fat-free part of the body water comprised approximately 72 percent (range 69.4 to 73.2 percent). Therefore other body components are often expressed in terms of the fat-free body. Widdowson[53] has summarized data on composition of fetuses and stillborn premature and full-term infants for comparison with the average values of the five adult males, as shown in Table 1.2. From fetal life to adulthood there is an increase per kilogram of fat-free body weight in nitrogen, potassium, calcium, magnesium, phosphorus, and zinc. Water, sodium, and chloride decrease. Iron and copper increase during fetal life but are less concentrated in the adult than in the newborn.

INDIRECT MEASUREMENT OF BODY COMPOSITION

Attempts to compartmentalize the body have been aimed toward the separation of fat from nonfat tissue, or toward the distinction between tissue with low metabolic rates and tissue with high metabolic requirements. The traditional classifications of bone, muscle, fat, and other organs have been discussed in the previous section. The physical and chemical procedures in this section result in measurement of somewhat different body compartments, and the terminology has sometimes led to confusion.

The "fat-free body" is the remainder after ether extraction of fat in whole body analysis. However, some body fat is essential to life. Widdowson[53] estimated that even the most undernourished adult body contains about 4 percent fat. Behnke[54] proposed differentiation by "lean body mass" and fat; his definition of lean body mass included the least amount of fat compatible with health, at first estimated as 10 percent and later as 2 percent. Therefore, fat-free body and lean body mass are somewhat different concepts. The distinction of adipose tissue from other body tissues also requires qualification. Adipose tissue is not pure fat, but contains connec-

Table 1.2   Effect of Development on the Chemical Composition of the Human Body

	Foetus, 20–25 Weeks' Gestation	Premature Baby	Full-Term Baby	Adult Man
Body weight, kg	0.3	1.5	3.5	70
Fat, g/kg whole body	5	35	160	160
Water, g/kg whole body	880	830	690	600
Composition of fat-free body tissue				
Water, g/kg	880	850	820	720
Total N, g/kg	15	19	23	34
Na, m-equiv./kg	100	100	82	80
K, m-equiv./kg	43	50	53	69
Cl, m-equiv./kg	76	—	55	44
Ca, g/kg	4.2	7.0	9.6	22.4
Mg, g/kg	0.18	0.24	0.26	0.50
P, g/kg	3.0	3.8	5.6	12.0
Fe, mg/kg	58	74	94	74
Cu, mg/kg	3	4	5	2
Zn, mg/kg	20	20	20	30

Source: E. M. Widdowson, Chemical Analysis of the Body. In J. Brozek (Ed.) *Human Body Composition: Approaches and Applications,* Pergamon Press, New York, 1965.

tive tissue, blood vessels, and cell walls. Its water content has been variously estimated as 12 to 20 percent. Fat constitutes only approximately three-fourths of adipose tissue (68 to 88 percent).

Keys and Grande[55] suggested that body tissues should be differentiated by their energy metabolism. The relatively nonactive part of the body includes fat, extracellular fluid, the mineral portion of the bony skeleton, nails, and hair. The remainder, which is active tissue or "cell-residue", represents 30 to 65 percent of total body weight but accounts for virtually all of the energy metabolism of the body. Cheek[56] estimated that visceral organs account for 80 percent and muscle for 17 percent of resting metabolism.

Because of the lack of valid data on the actual body composition of healthy individuals and because there are wide individual variations in content, the interpretation and calculation of findings are based on the best judgment of the examiners and change with new knowledge and new approaches to reasoning. Most studies have been done on adults. Children present additional difficulties in the estimation of body composition because of changes with age. There is a progressive decrease in extracellular fluid volume with age, and increases in intracellular fluids, cell solids, muscle mass, and potassium concentration in muscle, all of which are included in some of the formulas for computing body composition. In elderly individuals there are alterations in the concentration of tissue constituents. Therefore age and the maturation of body tissue must be factored into the calculations. Most of the following discussion refers to studies of young adults.

Densitometry

This method is based on the fact that body fat has a different density from nonfat tissue. Human fat, extracted by ether from surgically removed adipose tissue, has a density of 0.9000 gm/ml at 37 °C, with little variation between sexes, individuals, or body locations. The density of the nonfat portion of the body is in the vicinity of 1.10 gm/ml at 37 °C, but with wide variations. In the healthy 25-year-old male with weight and height at the U.S. average ("standard average body"), studies have shown a density of 1.064 gm/ml at 37 °C, and the fat content of the "standard body" was estimated at 15.3 percent.[55] As weight and body fat increase, density decreases. Body density is measured as the ratio of body volume to body weight. Body volume is measured by water displacement on immersion in a calibrated tank with correction for residual air in the lungs. From the calculated body density, the amounts of fat and water may be computed as follows:[57]

Body fat (kg) = 4.834 × body volume (liters) − 4.366 × body weight (kg)
Body fat (%) = body fat (kg)/body weight (kg) × 100
Body water (kg) = 73.0% × fat-free mass (kg)
Body water (%) = body water (kg)/body weight (kg) × 100

Total Body Water

This may be measured by dilution techniques. After intravenous injection or an oral dose of a known amount of a substance that dissolves in all body water and is not rapidly metabolized, time is allowed for uniform distribution and then the concentration in blood or urine is measured. From this concentration, total body water may be estimated. Assuming that water constitutes 73 percent of fat-free mass the percent of body fat can be calculated:[57]

> Fat-free mass (kg) = total body water (kg)/0.73
> Fat (kg) = body weight (kg) − fat-free mass (kg)
> Fat (%) = fat (kg)/body weight (kg) × 100

The substances most commonly used for dilution are deuterium or tritium, although antipyrine, N-acetyl-4-aminopyrine, and urea have also been used.

Extracellular water may be measured by a similar dilution technique, using administration of thiocyanate or inulin, which become distributed in extracellular fluids but do not cross the cell membrane. Intracellular water may be calculated as the difference between total body water and extracellular water.

Body Potassium

Since potassium is primarily intracellular, the measurement of potassium in the body provides an estimate of cell mass. The amount of potassium in various body tissues varies; it is especially high in muscle. Therefore the potassium content of the body per unit of weight depends on the relative amounts of various tissues. Forbes and Lewis[58] found that in four adult male cadavers the average potassium content of the fat-free body mass was 68.1 mEq/kg, and this figure is commonly used. However, a value of 73 mEq/kg has also been used for computation of lean body mass.[55]

Body potassium may be measured by either of two methods. In one method the gamma radiation emitted by naturally occurring ^{40}K in the body is measured by means of a sodium iodide crystal in a total body counter. Since ^{40}K occurs in a constant proportion of 0.0118 percent of the total potassium in the body, the ^{40}K count provides for the calculation of total body potassium. Potassium occurs primarily in nonfat tissue, so the lean body weight may be calculated as follows:[57]

> K (g) ÷ 39.0 (g atomic weight) = mEq K
> mEq K ÷ 68.1 = fat-free mass (kg)
> Fat (kg) = body weight (kg) − fat-free mass (kg)
> Fat (%) = fat (kg) ÷ body weight (kg) x 100

Alternatively, ^{42}K may be administered intravenously as an isotopic tracer and its dilution will provide an estimate of total exchangeable potassium.

Allowance must be made for age and sex in potassium determinations. The concentration of potassium in the body increases during childhood. Women have been reported to have a lower concentration of potassium per kilogram of cell mass than men, and the concentration in both sexes decreases with advancing age.

NUTRITION, GROWTH, AND BODY COMPOSITION

Creatinine Excretion

This is an index of muscle mass during growth. Creatinine in the urine is derived almost exclusively from the phosphocreatine of muscle. It has been estimated that 1 g of urinary creatinine per day is equivalent to 20 kg of muscle mass.[59] There is, however, evidence that both diurnal and daily variations in creatinine excretion must be considered in using this metabolite as an index. A 24-hour urinary excretion sample is more meaningful than a single random sample obtained at any time of the day.

Anthropometric Measurements

In the evaluation of body composition, anthropometric measurements have included various circumferences, widths, depths, and lengths, as previously noted. Skinfold, or more properly fatfold, thicknesses measured by calipers at specified body sites will be discussed more fully in Chapter 2. There is little direct knowledge about what proportion of total body fat is subcutaneous or how age and sex affect the proportion. Therefore, estimations of total body fat from skinfold measurements have a high degree of error. However, standards for the measurements themselves have been established for several population groups.

When measurements of arm circumference and triceps skinfold measurements are available on the same individual, formulas have been derived for estimating the diameter, circumference, and mass of muscle in the arm.[60] A nomogram has also been constructed for the rapid conversion of measurements of arm circumference and triceps fatfold to the three muscle estimations.[61] These formulas do not allow for the compression of fat by calipers or for the double thickness of skin.

X-ray Studies

In X-ray studies the shadows of bone, muscle, and fat are measured. Figure 1.15 is based on the summation of widths of these tissues in the forearm, thigh, and calf. Some attempts have been made to convert width measurements to volumetric measurements, but the changing conformation of body segments makes this conversion difficult. X rays have also been used to estimate skeletal weight and bone mineralization, although the soft tissue overlying the bone complicates the evaluation of bone mineralization.

All of the indirect measurements of body composition at any age have limitations.[62] For some the equipment needed is not readily accessible, as for ^{40}K counting or underwater weighing. Laboratory procedures for estimating body water compartments do not always result in comparable findings. X-ray studies involve body radiation. Even skinfold measurements, which are practical in almost all examining situations, are subject to the errors of tissue compressibility and individual differences in body fat distribution. All methods depend on assumptions based on inadequate data from direct body analyses and require further verification of interpretation.

REFERENCES

1. *Recommended Dietary Allowances*, Eight Edition. National Academy of Sciences, Washington, D. C., 1974.
2. Warkany, J. Disturbances of embryonic development by maternal vitamin deficiencies. *J. Cellular Comp. Physiol. 43*: (Suppl. 1) 207–236, 1954.
3. Dobbing, J. Effects of experimental undernutrition on development of the nervous system. In: Scrimshaw, N. E., and J. E. Gordon. *Malnutrition, Learning, and Behavior*. MIT Press, Cambridge, Mass., 1968.
4. Laird, A. K. The evolution of the human growth curve. *Growth 31*: 345–355, 1967.
5. Macy, I. G. *Nutrition and Chemical Growth in Childhood*. Vols. I-III, 1942-1951. Charles C Thomas, Springfield, Ill.
6. Hegsted, D. M. Balance Studies:Editorial paper. *J. Nutr. 106*:307–311, 1976.
7. U.S. Department of Health, Education, and Welfare. *Ten-State Nutrition Survey, 1968–1970*. DHEW Publications No. (HSM) 72-8130, 72-8131, 72-8132, and 72-8133. Supt. of Documents, U.S. Government Printing Office, Washington, D. C., 1972.
8. Owen, G. M., K. M. Kram, P. J. Garry, J. E. Lowe, and A. H. Lubin. A study of nutritional status of preschool children in the United States, 1968-1970. *Pediat. 53* (Suppl., Part 2): 597–646, 1974.
9. Abraham, S., F. W. Lowenstein, and C. L. Johnson. *Preliminary Findings of the First Health and Nutrition Examination Survey, United States, 1971–1972: Dietary Intake and Biochemical Findings*. DHEW Publication No. (HRA) 74-1219-1. Supt. of Documents, U.S. Government Printing Office, Washington, D. C., 1974.
10. Abraham, S., M. D. Carroll, C. M. Dresser, and C. L. Johnson. *Dietary Intake Findings, United States, 1971–1974*. DHEW Publication No. (HRA) 77-1647. Supt. of Documents, U.S. Government Printing Office, Washington, D. C., 1977.
11. Stuart, H. C., and H. V. Meredith. Use of body measurements in the school health program. *Am. J. Pub. Health 36*:1365–1386, 1946.
12. Hamill, P. V. V., T. A. Drizd, C. L. Johnson, R. B. Reed and A. F. Roche. NCHS Growth Curves for Children Birth—18 Years. DHEW Publ. No. (PHS) 78-1650. Supt. of Documents, U.S. Government Printing Office, Washington, D. C., 1978.

NUTRITION, GROWTH, AND BODY COMPOSITION

13. Garn, S. M., and D. C. Clark. Trends in fatness and the origins of obesity. *Pediat. 57*: 443–456, 1976.
14. White House Conference on Child Health and Protection. *Growth and Development of the Child.* Vols. I-IV. The Century Co., New York, 1932.
15. Martin, E. A., and V. A. Beal. *Roberts' Nutrition Work with Children,* Fourth Edition. University of Chicago Press, Chicago, Ill., 1978.
16. Timiras, P. S. *Developmental Physiology and Aging.* Macmillan, New York, 1972.
17. Winick, M. *Cellular Changes during Early Malnutrition.* Ross Laboratories, Columbus, Ohio, 1971.
18. Scammon, R. E., and L. A. Calkins. *The Development and Growth of the Human Body in the Fetal Period.* University of Minnesota Press, Minneapolis, 1929.
19. Scammon, R. E. Measurement of the Body in Childhood. In: Harris, J. A., C. M. Jackson, D. G. Patterson, and R. E. Scammon: *The Measurement of Man.* University of Minnesota Press, Minneapolis, 1930.
20. Hepner, R. Discussion on iron requirements. In: McKigney, J. I., and H. N. Munro (Eds.) *Nutrient Requirements in Adolescence.* MIT Press, Cambridge, Mass., 1976.
21. Winick, M., J. A. Brasel, and P. Rosso. Nutrition and cell growth. In: Winick, M. (Ed.) *Nutrition and Development.* John Wiley and Sons, New York, 1972.
22. Dreizen, S., C. N. Spirakis, and R. E. Stone. A comparison of skeletal growth and maturation in undernourished and well-nourished girls before and after menarche. *J. Pediat. 70*:256–263, 1967.
23. Valadian, I., and D. Porter. *Physical Growth and Development from Conception to Maturity.* Little, Brown, Boston, 1977.
24. Stroudt, H. W., A. Damon, and R. McFarland. *Weight, Height, and Selected Body Dimensions of Adults, United States, 1960–1962.* Public Health Service Publ. No. 1000—Series 11—No. 8. Supt. of Documents, U.S. Government Printing Office, Washington, D.C., 1965.
25. Burgess, M. A. The construction of two height charts. *J. Am. Stat. Assoc. 32*:290–310, 1937.
26. Wetzel, N. C. Physical fitness in terms of physique, development and basal metabolism. *JAMA 116*:1187–1195, 1941.
27. Sargent, D. W. Weight-height relationship of young men and women. *Am. J. Clin. Nutr. 13*:318–325, 1963.
28. Roberts, J. *Weight by Height and Age of Adults, United States, 1960–1962.* Public Health Service Publ. No. 1000—Series 11—No. 14. U.S. Department of Health, Education, and Welfare, Public Health Service, Washington, D. C., 1966.

29. Abraham, S., C. L. Johnson, and M. F. Najjar. *Weight by Height and Age of Adults 18-74 Years: United States, 1971-74.* Advance Data from Vital and Health Statistics of the National Center for Health Statistics, No. 14, Nov. 30, 1977. U.S. Department of Health, Education, and Welfare, Washington, D.C.

30. Billewicz, W. Z., W. F. F. Kemsley, and A. M. Thomson. Indices of adiposity. *Brit. J. Prev. Soc. Med. 16*:183-188, 1962.

31. Khosla, T., and C. R. Lowe. Indices of obesity derived from body weight and height. *Brit. J. Prev. Soc. Med. 21*:122-128, 1967.

32. Keys, A., F. Fidanza, M. J. Karvonen, N. Kimura, and H. L. Taylor. Indices of relative weight and obesity. *J. Chron. Dis. 25*:329-343, 1972.

33. Benn, R. T. Some mathematical properties of weight-for-height indices used as measures of adiposity. *Brit. J. Prev. Soc. Med. 25*:42-50, 1971.

34. Thomas, A. E., D. A. McKay, and M. B. Cutlip. A nomograph method for assessing body weight. *Am. J. Clin. Nutr. 29*:302-304, 1976.

35. Bardeen, C. R. The height-weight index of build in relation to linear and volumetric proportions and surface area of the body during postnatal development. *Contributions to Embryology. No. 46. Carnegie Institution of Washington Bulletin 9*:483-554, 1920.

36. Garn, S. The applicability of North American growth standards in developing countries. *Can. Med. Assoc. J. 93*:914-919, 1965.

37. Bayley, N. Growth curves of height and weight by age for boys and girls, scaled according to physical maturity. *J. Pediat. 48*:187-194, 1956.

38. Garn, S. M., D. C. Clark, and K. E. Guire. Growth, Body Composition, and Development of Obese and Lean Children. In: Winick, M. (Ed.) *Childhood Obesity.* John Wiley and Sons, New York, 1975.

39. Tanner, J. M. *Growth at Adolescence,* Second Edition. Blackwell Scientific Publications, Oxford, 1962.

40. Meredith, H. V. Change in stature and body weight of North American boys during the last 80 years. In: Lipsitt, L., and C. Spiker (Eds.) *Advances in Child Development and Behavior,* Vol. 1. Academic Press, New York, 1963.

41. Hamill, P. V. V., F. E. Johnston, and S. Lemeshow. *Height and Weight of Children: Socioeconomic Status, United States.* DHEW Publ. No. (HSM) 73-1601. U. S. Department of Health, Education, and Welfare, Public Health Service, National Center for Health Statistics, Rockville, Md., 1972.

42. Hamill, P. V. V., F. E. Johnston, and W. Grams. *Height and Weight of Children, United States.* Public Health Service Publ. No. 1000—Series 11—No. 104. U. S. Department of Health, Education, and Wel-

fare, Public Health Service, National Center for Health Statistics, Rockville, Md., 1970.

43. Hathaway, M. L., and E. D. Foard. *Heights and Weights of Adults in the United States.* Home Econ. Res. Report No. 10, Human Nutrition Research Division, U.S. Department of Agriculture, Washington, D.C., 1960.

44. Bakwin, H., and S. M. McLaughlin. Secular increase in height. Is the end in sight? *Lancet 2*:1195–1196, 1964.

45. Sheldon, W. H. *The Varieties of Human Physique.* Harper and Brothers, New York, 1940.

46. Vaughn, V. C. III. Developmental Pediatrics. In: Vaughn, V. C. III, R. J. McKay, and W. E. Nelson (Eds.) *Nelson Textbook of Pediatrics,* Tenth Edition, W. B. Saunders, Philadelphia, 1975.

47. Hansman, C. Anthropometry and Related Data. In: McCammon, R. W. (Ed.) *Human Growth and Development.* Charles C Thomas, Springfield, Ill., 1970.

48. Roche, A. F. The elongation of the mandible. *Am. J. Orthodontics 53*: 79–94, 1967.

49. Maresh, M. M., and V. A. Beal. A longitudinal survey of nutrition intake, body size, and tissue measurements in healthy subjects during growth. *Monographs Soc. Res. Child Dev.: Physical Growth and Body Composition,* Serial No. 140, *35*:33–39, 1970.

50. Pyle, S. I., A. M. Waterhouse, and W. W. Greulich. *A Radiographic Standard of Reference for the Growing Hand and Wrist.* Case Western Reserve University Press, Cleveland, Ohio, 1971.

51. Tanner, J. M., R. H. Whitehouse, W. A. Marshall, M. J. R. Heady, and H. Goldstein. *Assessment of Skeletal Maturity and Prediction of Adult Health.* Academic Press, New York, 1975.

52. Bowers, D. F. Tooth Development and Abnormalities of Appearance. In: Johnson, T. R., W. M. Moore, and J. E. Jeffries (Eds.) *Children are Different: Developmental Physiology,* Second Edition. Ross Laboratories, Columbus, Ohio, 1978.

53. Widdowson, E. M. Chemical Analysis of the Body. In: Brozek, J. (Ed.) *Human Body Composition: Approaches and Applications.* Pergamon Press, New York, 1965.

54. Behnke, A. R. Fat content and composition of the body. *Harvey Lect. 37*:198–226, 1941.

55. Keys, A., and F. Grande. Body Weight, Body Composition and Calorie Status. In: Goodhart, R. S., and M. E. Shils (Eds.) *Modern Nutrition in Health and Disease.* Lea and Febiger, Philadelphia, 1975.

56. Cheek, D. B. Growth and Body Composition. In: Cheek, D. B. (Ed.) *Fetal and Postnatal Cellular Growth.* John Wiley and Sons, New York, 1975.

57. Krzywicki, H. J., G. M. Ward, D. P. Rahman, R. A. Nelson, and C. F. Consolazio. A comparison of methods for estimating human body composition. *Am. J. Clin. Nutr. 27*:1380–1385, 1974.

58. Forbes, G. B., and A. M. Lewis. Total sodium, potassium and chloride in adult man. *J. Clin. Invest. 35*:596–600, 1956.

59. Graystone, J. E. Creatinine Excretion during Growth. In: Cheek, D. B. (Ed.) *Human Growth: Body Composition, Cell Growth, Energy and Intelligence.* Lea and Febiger, Philadelphia, 1968.

60. Frisancho, A. R. Triceps skin fold and upper arm muscle size norms for assessment of nutritional status. *Am. J. Clin. Nutr. 27*:1052–1058, 1974.

61. Gurney, J. M., and D. B. Jelliffe. Arm anthropometry in nutritional assessment: Nomogram for rapid calculation of muscle circumference and cross-sectional muscle and fat areas. *Am. J. Clin. Nutr. 26*:912–915, 1973.

62. Owen, G. M., and J. Brozek. Influence of Age, Sex, and Nutrition on Body Composition during Childhood and Adolescence. In: Falkner, F. (Ed.) *Human Development.* W. B. Saunders, Philadelphia, 1966.

NUTRITION, GROWTH, AND BODY COMPOSITION

2

ASSESSMENT OF NUTRITIONAL STATUS

The concept of nutrition is both simple and complex. The body is dependent upon caloric intake for energy and metabolic activities, and upon nutrients, oxygen, and water for cell and fluid formation, growth, and function. Therefore, in simple terms, the health of the individual depends upon the adequacy with which dietary intake meets the needs of the body for growth, development, and maintenance. The lack of some nutrients may lead to specific recognizable symptoms or physiological states that can be identified by clinical, biochemical or cytological examinations. In the early period of the development of the science of nutrition, many of the studies that led to gradual appreciation of the effects of diet were based on the cure of specific deficiency diseases. Scurvy could be cured by the administration of foods containing ascorbic acid. Beriberi could be prevented by a diet adequate in thiamin. A simple cause and effect were evident.

With the virtual elimination of single-nutrient deficiency diseases in many parts of the world, the concept of nutrition has become more complex. Simple and direct links of nutrients to growth and health are often difficult to evaluate because of the enormous complexity of the human organism. A diet deficient in one nutrient is probably deficient in many nutrients. Even when a deficiency state is labeled as protein-energy malnutrition, with the implication that the shortage is only in protein and calories, it is obvious that such a diet is also deficient in other nutrients. In addition, the metabolic interdependence of nutrients may create a domino effect when a deficiency of one nutrient interferes with the absorption and utilization of other nutrients. At a level of intake that does not lead to a clearly identifiable deficiency state, it is difficult to evaluate the effects of varying levels of intake above the physiological minimum. Differences in growth, health, and performance as a result of intakes ranging from marginal to generous may be small, may require long periods of observation or large numbers of subjects, or may not be measurable by present technologies. To understand some of the complexities and to realize why cause and effect are not always clear, we need first to explore some of the reasons why simple correlations between nutritional intake and physical status are not always possible.

Nutrition is a relatively new science, and our understanding of the metabolism and functions of nutrients is far from complete. Lavoisier is usually given credit for initiating the science of nutrition with his studies of energy in the eighteenth century. Except for isolated studies, like Lind's, which identified the role of citrus fruits in the prevention and cure of scurvy, most early work was devoted to furthering knowledge about energy in respiration and metabolism. In the nineteenth century, separation of food into its macronutrient components (carbohydrate, lipid, and protein) became possible with methods for determining carbon, hydrogen, and nitrogen. This was followed by identification of some of the minerals in ash. By the end of the nineteenth century, when feeding of purified diets containing the components then known to be essential resulted in poor growth or in death of experimental animals, the concept of "accessory food factors" was developed and led to a period of intensive research on vitamins in the twentieth century. Recently the development of microtechniques has focused attention on trace minerals. For example, research is currently being done on the role of zinc in growth and of selenium as a component of glutathione peroxidase. To date, approximately 50 nutrients have been identified which are essential to human growth and health.

However, lack of precise knowledge about the metabolic functions of some nutrients and about the interdependence of macronutrients, vitamins, and minerals has led to a state of constant change in scientific thinking. Concepts are continually being expanded, refined, altered, or rejected. As a result, the association of nutritional intake with clinical and metabolic findings is always subject to new interpretations in view of each additional bit of knowledge. This has been clearly demonstrated in the past 30 years by the search for clarification of the role of diet in cardiovascular disease and more recently in the study of fiber as an essential food component involved in the etiology of gastrointestinal diseases. Gaps in information create controversy; controversy stimulates formulation of new theories and further research to validate them. Each new bit of information must be verified and then put into its proper place as in a jigsaw puzzle to form the final picture.

As the science of nutrition has passed from its initial concentration on the identification and cure of single-nutrient deficiency diseases to the present appreciation of the multiplicity of factors in the etiology of diseases, espe-

ASSESSMENT OF NUTRITIONAL STATUS

cially those involving degenerative processes, complexity has increased. Early nutrition studies were done primarily by physiologists and biochemists, then gradually involved all of the physical and biological sciences, and now increasingly nutrition has become dependent on the contributions of sociologists, psychologists, and other related specialists. The initial focus on the body and its metabolic functions has expanded to encompass the wide range of social, economic, and political influences on the relationship of nutrition to health.

NUTRITIONAL ASSESSMENT, MONITORING, AND SURVEILLANCE

Nutrition affects the individual, but when large numbers of persons within a population are found to have similar nutritional problems, the emphasis shifts from individual health to public health. Screening procedures performed in a physician's office or in a clinic are basically clinical functions to identify the individual in need of therapy. When a nutritional problem is widely prevalent, indicating the need for governmental intervention by public health programs with a focus on nutrition, basic data on the extent and causes of the problem are essential. Habicht et al.,[1] in discussing a program for national nutritional surveillance, distinguished between nutritional assessment, nutritional monitoring, and nutritional surveillance. Their thoughtful analysis of past surveys, present status, and future needs will be briefly summarized here.

"Nutritional assessment includes the measurement and description of the nutritional status of a population in relation to those economic, sociodemographic and physiologic variables that can affect the nutrition of that population."[1] One purpose of assessment is to identify and establish the validity of indicators of nutritional status. "The usefulness of any indicator of malnutrition or of toxicity that is not clearly related to a symptomatic health risk is open to question." A large number of nutritional and nonnutritional variables should be included in the assessment program. For example, the finding of low hemoglobin levels in many of the U.S. population has not resolved the question of the extent to which those low levels are due to iron deficiency. Additional variables, including other nutrients, lead, and diseases such as hookworm or malaria infestation, should be included in the assessment program. Socioeconomic differences in the prevalence of obesity among subjects in the Health and Nutrition Examination Survey (HANES) suggested that "exercise must be considered a nutritional variable in the United States." Serum protein is a sensitive indicator of severe protein deficiency but is not a useful measure of mild protein deficiency. Nutritional assessment, then, is aimed to measure the impact of nutrition on the health, performance, or survival of the population, to identify risk groups within the population, to validate the clinical usefulness of indicators of nutritional status, and to provide leads toward identification of causative factors.

"Nutritional monitoring is the measurement of changes over time in the nutritional status of a population and therefore requires repeated assessments either periodically or continually."[1] It should include all nutritional disorders of present or probable future public health importance, whether or not effective intervention is possible. The sampling and measurement methods must be the same throughout all assessments so that the statistical significance of changes may be determined.

"Surveillance indicates activities directed to the early detection of community nutritional problems so that they can be quickly corrected."[1] This requires monitoring for nutritional changes in the population by sensitive and specific indicators for those nutrients of proven public health significance. Surveillance data should be immediately available to those responsible for delivery of health care services for relevant intervention and therefore should be linked to an ongoing health program.

DEVELOPMENT OF NUTRITIONAL DEFICIENCIES

Pearson[2] outlined the sequence of events in the development of nutritional deficiency symptoms as follows:

1. Initial deficiency, either primary or secondary. A primary deficiency is caused by lack of one or more nutrients in the diet. A secondary deficiency is the result of altered metabolism, caused by impairment of absorption, transport, or utilization of a nutrient, or by increased destruction, excretion, or requirement of a nutrient.
2. Depletion of tissue levels.
3. Development of biochemical lesion, leading to distortion of function of cells or tissues.
4. Clinical lesion as a result of functional impairment.

McLaren[3] presented a similar sequence, but inserted between stages 1 and 2 the immediate but temporary adaptive changes in the body.

This sequence of events illustrates the contribution of specialists in many fields to the total picture of nutritional status. Combined team efforts are essential, and each member is dependent on all others. When the focus is on a single individual, a nutritionist or dietitian may obtain dietary intake data by one of several investigative tools. However, the individual's selection and consumption of food are influenced by socioeconomic, cultural, educational, and psychological characteristics. Calculation of the nutrient content of the diet is based on the chemists' analyses of foods, either directly for an individual's diet or indirectly by contributions to food value tables, which are compiled usually by governmental agencies. When the focus is on a population group, food availability or food disappearance figures may be used to judge dietary adequacy on a regional or national level, requiring input from specialists in agriculture, transportation, economics, and politics.

Metabolic aspects of deficiencies fall within the realm of the biochemist and the cytologist. Clinical evaluation includes examinations by physicians and dentists and body measurements by anthropometrists and roentgenologists. Nutritional assessment, then, requires a team approach. Each member contributes a specialized area of knowledge, but it is the sum of diverse data that establishes the presence of malnutrition and validates the association of the physical state with the causative factors.

Despite the logic of sequential events proposed by Pearson, it has been difficult or impossible in the national surveys that have been done to validate statistically that clinical symptoms or low biochemical levels in blood or urine resulted from dietary deficiencies. With current methodology, the component parts of the surveys have measured events with differing time elements, and valid data on all four stages of the sequence are not available for any individual or any population group. As a result, correlation coefficients between dietary intake levels and either biochemical or clinical findings are likely to be low.

Except for longitudinal studies in which repeated dietary histories are taken at stated time intervals on individuals, most dietary data are limited to one or two days prior to the examination. In large surveys, this has been standard methodology. Although it is possible to obtain historical data on food intake of an individual, retrospective data are often unreliable and merely descriptive rather than quantitative; they do not lend themselves to nutrient calculation. Intake in the previous 24 hours may not be typical of long-term intake and therefore can be expected to have little correlation to levels of substances measured in blood. Clinical symptoms appear only after an extended period of dietary inadequacy and have even less relationship to intake in the previous 24 hours. Despite the different time elements combined into the usual assessment protocol, many workers have had unreasonably high expectations of correlations from nutritional assessment surveys.

McLaren[3] recognized that assessment of all factors that underline and determine nutritional status, that is, a causal analysis, has not been carried out and therefore erroneous conclusions have been made. Nutritional assessment is the evaluation of the nutriture or status of an individual at a given moment in time. On the other hand, nutrition is a process that leads to nutritional status. Therefore he suggested that the assessment of nutritional status and the assessment of the process of nutrition should be separate units within the evaluation program.

NUTRITIONAL ASSESSMENT

The nutritional status of individuals is initially evaluated by examination, measurement, and questioning. This is a screening device to identify persons who should be evaluated by more extensive testing that would determine whether they would benefit from nutritional or other therapy. The term "nutritional assessment" has been increasingly applied to public as well as personal health. The aggregate of information from selected geographic, ethnic, or income population groups has become a focus of concern in planning health programs. In this section, nutritional assessment of population groups will be emphasized, but one must remember that individuals make up the population, and it is the health of each individual that is important.

In recent years several national surveys have assessed the nutritional state of various groups. The Ten-State Nutrition Survey (TSNS)[4] was conducted between 1968 and 1970 with the express charge of investigating the type and degree of malnutrition in the United States. Impetus for this survey had come from a number of reports to the United States Senate and in the popular press that severe malnutrition could be found in the country. On the assumption that malnutrition occurs more often in people with restricted incomes, geographical areas with average incomes in the lowest quartile of the 1960 census were chosen for TSNS, which was not designed to be typical of the U.S. population. On the other hand, the Preschool Nutrition Survey (PNS)[5] of 1968–1970 and the Health and Nutrition Examination Survey (HANES)[6-8] of 1971–1974 were based on selected stratified random samples that included all ethnic, geographic, and income groups assumed to be representative of the general population. PNS surveyed children between 1 and 6 years of age, and HANES included noninstitutionalized persons between 1 and 74 years of age. The Nutrition Canada National Survey (NCNS)[9,10] of 1970-1972 was designed to sample three population groups (general, Indian, and Eskimo) at different income levels and at two seasons of the year. The types of data obtained in the four surveys were similar, but the population base and the standards of evaluation differed.

The protocol of each of the surveys included four areas of investigation: (1) community assessment or demographic data; (2) clinical examination with emphasis on physical signs associated with malnutrition, dental examination, and anthropometric measurements; (3) laboratory assessment of blood and urine samples; and (4) dietary intake studies. The methods of surveying populations in technologically advanced nations are basically similar to those in developing countries, although adaptations must be made for the use of central examining facilities or traveling field facilities. In developing countries a higher prevalence and more severe degree of malnutrition are found, especially in young children. The reader is referred to other sources, primarily the extensive publications of the World Health Organization (WHO), for more detailed practical application of methods for study in developing countries. In contrast, nutritional deficiency diseases occur with lower prevalence in technologically advanced countries, and the clinical symptoms found are more likely to be nonspecific and to correlate poorly with dietary and biochemical findings.

COMMUNITY EVALUATION

A description of the demographic, epidemiologic, geographic, and cultural characteristics and facilities of the community to be studied provides a basis for identifying problems that may exist. Since malnutrition is more often found in areas where the income and educational level are low and health facilities either inadequate or poorly used, a description of the area will supply leads to the probability of finding malnutrition. It will help to identify high risk groups, to determine the extent of risk, and to indicate the most critical needs of the community. Sources of data include census and vital statistics tabulations, hospital and clinic records, welfare and public health agencies, schools, and private health-related organizations.

Income levels and socioeconomic stratification within the community are closely related to problems of housing and sanitation. Educational attainment gives an index of literacy rates. Racial or ethnic concentrations suggest the influence of food patterns, beliefs, prejudices, and nutritional practices. Local grocery stores reflect the availability of different types of foods and the cost and quality of foods.

Census and vital statistics records of the city, town, or county provide a variety of descriptive information. The age distribution of the population indicates whether problems may be concentrated in children or in the elderly. Occupations and levels of unemployment may indicate pockets of poverty. Mortality rates may be examined for infant and maternal death rates, which are often used as an index of nutritional health. The causes of death such as coronary heart disease, hypertension, diabetes, alcoholism, parasitism, and tuberculosis, may be nutrition-related. Birth records provide clues to the number of home deliveries, illegitimate births, birth weights, and the number of mothers under 18 years of age.

Schools in the community can supply information on whether they provide feeding programs, whether health education is included in the curriculum, and whether they have screening programs for medical and dental health. Many schools routinely weigh and measure children, although some make little use of the data obtained. School records on absenteeism may indicate health or social problems of the children.

The availability of health services takes into account the number of physicians, dentists, hospitals, clinics, nursing homes, and extended care facilities in the community. Of greater value is the number of people who use the facilities. The nutrition and dietetic components of the health facilities should also be investigated. Gaps and overlaps in services, both professional and voluntary, may be identified. Hospital records provide a profile of disease rates, which may be searched for nutrition-related conditions. Birth weight data may be examined to determine the prevalence of weights under 2500 g, and maternal–infant records for evidence of malnutrition. The availability of dental programs, public or private, should be checked, especially in regard to the care of persons in the lower socioeconomic groups. Fluoridation may be included in the local water supply or in local dental programs or may not be adequately provided to some segments of the population.

These sources of data vary in reliability. However, they may provide a broad picture of the nutritional health of a community and form a basis for identifying environmental factors associated with findings from other components of nutritional assessment. They can be used as a baseline for action programs by establishing the priority needs of the community.

CLINICAL ASSESSMENT

The clinical segments of nutritional assessment include a physical examination and health history, a dental examination, and anthropometry, with the possible addition of a hand-wrist X ray to estimate skeletal age in children. The age of the individual determines which procedures should be done. A detailed listing of procedures adapted to each stage of the life span and to the facilities available has been developed by a committee of the American Public Health Association and published in *Nutritional Assessment in Health Programs*.[11] It is an excellent guide to the protocol of studies in technologically advanced countries, similar to those WHO has prepared for developing countries.

Physical Examination and History

These are the basic components of clinical assessment. Although history of previous and current health of the individual has sometimes been omitted from survey protocols, partially because of the time involved in obtaining the information, it is essential for understanding present findings, and becomes even more necessary in the examination of elderly subjects.

The general appearance of the subject often presents a clue to the state of health. Visual evaluations of the size and degree of fatness or leanness can be readily made, although they should be validated by measurements. The behavior of the individual during the examination should be noted. Apathy, passivity, and lack of energy suggest that health is not optimal and may be symptomatic of malnutrition. Alertness, facial expressivity, and social interaction with the examiner may represent merely individual behavioral characteristics but may also be indicative of nutritional status. The child who slumps with indifferent submission to examination procedures provides different clues from the child who is bright-eyed, alert, and interested.

In addition to the usual procedures in a physical examination, special attention should be given to signs that may indicate malnutrition. Table 2.1 was adapted from a WHO classification that distinguished between signs often associated with nutritional deficiency and those possibly related to malnutrition. Their value in clinical screening is subject to qualifications. Many of the signs are nonspecific in that they may be due to nonnutritional factors. They have differing degrees of reliability for diagnosis. Unless the team of examiners are carefully trained in observation and techniques, and unless definitions and descriptive recording are standardized, interexaminer differences in prevalence of findings may be high. Since single-nutrient deficiencies are relatively uncommon, symptoms of more than one deficiency may occur simultaneously. The combination of symptoms observed may vary from one population to another, in part becuase of differences in basic dietaries.

Table 2.1 is focused on areas of the body where deficiency signs may be found. A different basis of classification was suggested by WHO,[12] related to specific nutrients, from which the following list was adapted:

Dietary obesity: Excessive weight–height ratio, excessive skinfolds, excessive ratio of abdominal girth to chest girth.
Undernutrition: Mental and physical lethargy, low weight–height ratio, diminished skinfolds, exaggerated skeletal prominences, loss of skin elasticity.
Protein-calorie deficiency diseases: Edema, muscle wasting, low body weight, psychomotor changes, hair changes (dyspigmentation, easy pluckability, thinness, sparseness), flaky paint dermatosis, diffuse skin pigmentation.
Vitamin A deficiency: Xerosis of skin and conjunctiva, follicular hyperkeratosis, kermatomalacia, Bitot's spots.

Table 2.1   Physical Signs Indicative or Suggestive of Malnutrition

Body Area	Normal Appearance	Signs Associated with Malnutrition
Hair	Shiny; firm; not easily plucked	Lack of natural shine; hair dull and dry, thin and sparse; hair fine, silky and straight; color changes (flag sign); can be easily plucked
Face	Skin color uniform; smooth, pink, healthy appearance; not swollen	Skin color loss (depigmentation); skin dark over cheeks and under eyes (malar and supra-orbital pigmentation); lumpiness or flakiness of skin of nose and mouth; swollen face; enlarged parotid glands; scaling of skin around nostrils (nasolabial seborrhea)
Eyes	Bright, clear, shiny; no sores at corners of eyelids; membranes a healthy pink and are moist. No prominent blood vessels or mound of tissue or sclera	Eye membranes are pale (pale conjunctivae); redness of membranes (conjunctival injection); Bitot's spots; redness and fissuring of eyelid corners (angular palpebritis); dryness of eye membranes (conjunctival xerosis); cornea has dull appearance (corneal xerosis); cornea is soft (keratomalacia); scar on cornea; ring of fine blood vessels around corner (circumcorneal injection)
Lips	Smooth, not chapped or swollen	Redness and swelling of mouth or lips (cheilosis), especially at corners of mouth (angular fissures and scars)
Tongue	Deep red in appearance; not swollen or smooth	Swelling; scarlet and raw tongue; magenta (purplish color) of tongue; smooth tongue; swollen sores; hyperemic and hypertrophic papillae; and atrophic papillae
Teeth	No cavities; no pain; bright	May be missing or erupting abnormally; gray or black spots (fluorosis); cavities (caries)
Gums	Healthy; red; do not bleed; not swollen	"Spongy" and bleed easily; recession of gums *Continued*

Glands	Face not swollen	Thyroid enlargement (front of neck); parotid enlargement (cheeks become swollen)
Skin	No signs of rashes, swellings, dark or light spots	Dryness of skin (xerosis); sandpaper feel of skin (follicular hyperkeratosis); flakiness of skin; skin swollen and dark; red swollen pigmentation of exposed areas (pellagrous dermatosis); excessive lightness or darkness of skin (dyspigmentation); black and blue marks due to skin bleeding (petechiae); lack of fat under skin
Nails	Firm, pink	Nails are spoon-shape (koilonychia); brittle, ridged nails
Muscular and skeletal systems	Good muscle tone; some fat under skin; can walk or run without pain	Muscles have "wasted" appearance; baby's skull bones are thin and soft (craniotabes); round swelling of front and side of head (frontal and parietal bossing); swelling of ends of bones (epiphyseal enlargement); small bumps on both sides of chest wall (on ribs)—beading of ribs; baby's soft spot on head does not harden at proper time (persistently open anterior fontanelle); knock-knees or bowlegs; bleeding into muscle (musculoskeletal hemorrhages); person cannot get up or walk properly

Continued

Body Area	Normal Appearance	Signs Associated with Malnutrition
Internal Systems:		
Cardio-vascular	Normal heart rate and rhythm; no murmurs or abnormal rhythms; normal blood pressure for age	Rapid heart rate (above 100 tachycardia); enlarged heart; abnormal rhythm; elevated blood pressure
Gastroin-testinal	No palpable organs or masses (in children, however, liver edge may be palpable)	Liver enlargement; enlargement of spleen (usually indicates other associated diseases)
Nervous	Psychological stability; normal reflexes	Mental irritability and confusion; burning and tingling of hands and feet (paresthesia); loss of position and vibratory sense; weakness and tenderness of muscles (may result in inability to walk); decrease and loss of ankle and knee reflexes

Source: Christakis, G. (Ed.) Nutritional Assessment in Health Programs. *Am. J. Public Health 63* Suppl., November, 1973.

Riboflavin deficiency: Angular stomatitis, magenta tongue, atrophy of tongue papillae, nasolabial seborrhea, inflammation of angles of eyelids, corneal vascularization.

Thiamine deficiency: Loss of knee and/or ankle jerks, sensory loss, motor weakness, calf muscle tenderness, cardiovascular dysfunction, edema.

Niacin deficiency: Pellagrous dermatosis, scarlet or raw tongue, fissure or atrophy of tongue papillae, skin pigmentation.

Ascorbic acid deficiency: Spongy and bleeding gums, petechiae, echymoses, intramuscular or subperiosteal hematoma, painful enlargement of epiphyses.

Vitamin D deficiency: Epiphyseal enlargement, beading of ribs, craniotabes, muscular hypotonia, frontal and parietal bossing, knock-knees or bowed legs, thorax deformities.

Iron deficiency: Pallor of mucous membranes, koilonychia, atrophy of tongue papillae.

Iodine deficiency: Thyroid enlargement.

This list is helpful in identifying signs and symptoms that may be associated with malnutrition, but the final diagnosis depends on confirmation from other areas of investigation. Dietary intake levels and biochemical concentrations in blood or urine, when applicable, may add confirmation. A trial of therapy with the deficient nutrient would confirm diagnosis if it resulted in cure of signs that are reversible. However, nonnutritional factors may be involved in etiology of many of the symptoms. "The parts of the body which most commonly exhibit abnormalities consistent with malnutrition include the integument, eyes, mouth, skeleton and nervous system. Almost all of the abnormalities which occur are non-specific. Trauma, exposure to the elements, and allergies may produce physical abnormalities which closely resemble the adverse effects of deficiencies."[13]

The difficulty in identifying a specific nutrient deficiency is shown by the fact that changes in the tongue may be caused by deficiency of one or more of the following nutrients: iron, zinc, folic acid, vitamin B_{12}, pyridoxine, and riboflavin.[13] Nasolabial seborrhea is often attributed to riboflavin deficiency, but has been related to pyridoxine deficiency and to defective metabolism of essential fatty acids. In TSNS, thyroid enlargement was unrelated to urinary excretion of iodine, suggesting a cause other than iodine deficiency[4].

Few signs of nutritional deficiencies were identified clinically in the four surveys on the North American continent. "Clinical examinations of malnutrition are most valuable in situations where the deficiency of one or more nutrients has reached the stage of overt disease, i.e., where the health and, in fact, the life of the individual are jeopardized. The value of physical examinations is therefore extremely high for impoverished populations and diminishes in importance as the adequacy of the food supply for a population improves."[9] "Clinical examination proved to be a tool of limited value in the broad assessment of more subtle and inapparent levels of malnutrition."[4] These statements typify conclusions from the clinical components of the surveys. It may be that the techniques of evaluation currently available are not sufficiently sensitive to identify marginal malnutrition. Their value has been well demonstrated in developing countries where the prevalence of acute malnutrition is high, but they fail to differentiate degrees of acceptable to optimal health in economically developed countries.

Dental Examination

This is usually included as part of a nutritional assessment. The state of dental health is an index of nutritional adequacy during tooth development and may reflect fluoride intake and the general effect of diet on tooth decay. In turn, severe dental problems may influence the diet if they result in difficulty in chewing.

The examination may be done by a dentist but, in many situations with limited personnel or facilities, is done by a physician or other trained health worker. Radiographs add considerably to the completeness and accuracy of the examination but are often not feasible. The examination should include obvious dental caries, periodontal disease manifested by hyperemia, edema, ease of bleeding or retraction, calculus deposit, and soft materia alba.[11] Fluorosis should also be noted in relation to excessive fluoride intake.

Indices that may be used are the Decayed-Missing-Filled Index (DMF), the Periodontal Index (PI), and the Oral Hygiene Index (OHI).[4] The use of these indices requires standardization of the techniques of the examiners. The DMF Index requires X rays for a complete count of decayed teeth since not all decay is visible by surface examination. The count of missing teeth includes unerupted, extracted, or replaced teeth. The index is obviously different for deciduous teeth, since the missing teeth may have been shed naturally or may have been extracted. Because the DMF increases with age, evaluation of the index necessitates consideration of the age of the subject. PI quantitates the severity of disease of supporting tissues, such as the gingiva, connecting fibers, and alveolar bone. It is scored by assessment of gingival inflammation, periodontal pockets, and sufficient bone to permit the tooth to function during mastication. OHI measures the amount of plaque and calculus present on selected teeth.

The dental examination has also been used in surveys to record age of tooth eruption. For example, in PNS,[5] the median age in both sexes when all 20 deciduous teeth were present was 2½ years. At the other end of the age scale, loss of teeth was demonstrated by the finding that more than 50 percent of white subjects in TSNS[4] were edentulous in the 65-74 year age group, with somewhat lower rates of tooth loss in black and Spanish-American adults.

The relationship of dietary intake as determined in the surveys to dental state produced few significant correlations. The development of caries depends on the susceptibility of the tooth, availability of fermentable carbohydrate, and the presence of bacteria to ferment the carbohydrate. Tooth susceptibility is related to the integrity of tooth structure; as shown in Chapter 1, tooth formation continues from fetal life well into the period of adolescence. Recent short-term dietary intake is unlikely to affect tooth structure, but the consumption of fermentable carbohydrate, particularly that which adheres to the teeth, may be related to dental health. In the TSNS analysis of data, there was a high association between the DMF ratio of adolescents and consumption of foods containing sugar between meals, but not with sugar-containing foods consumed at meals.

Anthropometric Measurements

These data provide the best index of growth status in children and the degree of leanness or fatness at all ages. They have been used in surveys primarily to identify growth retardation and obesity, both of which may be related to diet.

Of more than 100 body measurements that can be taken, a relatively small number may be selected to provide a meaningful evaluation of either growth or obesity. These measurements should be adapted to the age of the subject. In small children head circumference and its ratio to other body dimensions, such as chest or arm circumference, provide an estimation of nutritional status, but these ratios are of little diagnostic value after the age of 4 to 6 years. For all age groups, measurement of weight, height, selected skinfold thicknesses, and some circumferences or diameters are usually adequate.

The measurement of length in infants or height in older children and adults may be expanded to include crown–rump length or sitting height to differentiate between leg length and trunk length. The circumferences usually obtained are upper arm measurements, primarily because of the ease of obtaining the measurement without asking the subject to undress, but a more complete picture of body dimensions may be obtained by including circumferences of the waist, midthigh, and midcalf. Diameters of the wrist, knee, hips, and shoulder provide an index of skeletal widths. Behnke[14] developed a somatogram or body measurement profile using 11 circumferences and diameters. Skinfold thicknesses have most often been measured at the triceps, subscapula, and chest. The triceps measurement is most commonly taken because of easy accessibility, but individuals vary in location of fat deposited, and measurement at a single site may not be a good index of total body fat. Thicker fat layers tend to have greater compressibility, so caliper measurement of thickness may underestimate fat in the obese. However, for most screening purposes, a small number of measurements is adequate.

McLaren[3] has selected anthropometric measurements that may be used in nutritional assessment, with a concise evaluation of their use and limitations, as well as standards for their interpretation, as shown in Table 2.2. Although they differ somewhat from selections by other workers in the field, they represent six measurements simply obtained for quick assessment. Only the weight and subscapular skinfold measurement require undressing.

The accuracy of measurement depends to a large extent on the skill of the examiner. Weight and height measurements can be well standardized, although care should be taken that the subject wears a minimum amount of light clothing and no shoes. Other measurements require greater training and constant checking to minimize interobserver differences. Infants and very young children are difficult to measure accurately because of crying and resistance to handling. Skinfold measurements vary with compressibility, which is influenced by the thickness and water content of the fat layer and the length of time calipers are applied; these factors may lower the measurement. Calipers most commonly used are either Lange or Harpenden, both of which exert a pressure of 10 g/mm^2, which should be calibrated at intervals to ensure consistency. Equipment and techniques used in surveys have been described in detail,[4,7] and common errors in measurements have been demonstrated.[15]

In cross-sectional data, such as surveys, the single set of measurements obtained may be used to identify the position of the subject in the distribution of that measurement for the population, but give no clue to the process by which the subject reached that position. For example, the child whose height is at the fifth percentile may be growing at a consistent rate or may be growing at a rate slower than would be expected for his age. A single set of measurements provides identification of a short child but is not necessarily a signal of growth retardation. The pattern of growth from a series of measurements is essential for the evaluation of progress of an individual child. The value of single measurements lies primarily in the identification of population groups in which shortness of stature or obesity or some other index of malnutrition is more prevalent than would be expected. The finding of a high percentage of persons with adverse physical characteristics signals the need for further study to determine whether a specific type of public health program should be instituted for that population group.

Table 2.2   Some Anthropometric Measurements Applied in Nutritional Assessment

Measure-ments	Age Groups	Nutritional Indication	Reproduc-ibility	Advantages	Disadvantages	Observer Error	Interpre-tation
1. Weight	All groups	Present nutritional status; under and over	Good	Common in use	Difficult in field, can't tell body composition, need accurate age, height re-lated (insensi-tive)	<100 g in children <250 g in adults	<60% severe 60–80 moderate 80–90 mild 90–110 normal 110–120 over 120 and over obese
2. Height	All groups	Chronic nutritional status (under)	Good	Common in use Simple to do in field	Other factors play a role	<0.5 cm <3.0 cm in adults	<80% dwarf 80–93 short 93–105 normal >105 giant
	7 years child	Chronic under nutrition in early childhood	Good				
3. Head circum-cumference	0–4 years	Intrauterine and childhood nutrition (chronic under nutrition)	Good	Simple	Other factors play a role e.g. brain development	<0.5 cm	

Continued

Measure-ments	Age Groups	Nutritional Indication	Reproduc-ibility	Advantages	Disadvantages	Observer Error	Interpre-tation
4. Mid arm circum-ference	All groups	Present under and over nutrition	Fair	Simple, age independent, child need not be stripped, suitable for rapid survey	No limits for over nutrition, no standard for adult	<0.5 cm	<75% severe 75–80 moderate 80–85 mild >85% normal
5. Skin fold thickness, subscapula or triceps	All groups	Present under and over nutrition	Fair	Measures body composition, detects obesity in adults	Needs expen-sive caliper, difficult with child and in the field, ? eth-nic differences	1.0–1.5 mm	Similar to item (1)

Continued

Method	Age	Detects	Reliability	Advantages	Disadvantages	Classification
6. Weight/ height/ age ratio	All ages	Present under and over nutrition	Good	Index of body build, age independent 1–4 years and adults	Need proper scales, need trained personnel	<75% severe 75–85 moderate 85–90 mild 90–110 normal 110–120 over >120 obese
7. Mid arm/ head ratio	3 months– 48 months	Present under nutrition	Good	Simple, age independent, sex independent, any person can do it in field	No standard for adults	<0.25 severe 0.25–0.28 mod. 0.28–0.31 mild 0.31–0.35 normal >0.35 obese
8. Chest/ head circ. ratio	1–2 years	Present under nutrition	Fair or poor	Simple, age independent	For limited age No classification method	<1 malnourished >1 normal

Source: McLaren, D.S., and D. Burman. Textbook of Paediatric Nutrition. Churchill Livingstone, Edinburgh, 1976.

The anthropometric-clinical component of nutritional assessment may also include a posterior-anterior radiograph of the wrist and hand. The number, calcification, size, and shape of the small bones may be compared to standards for age and sex to evaluate the skeletal age of the child during growth.

The findings from the national surveys on anthropometric measurements were similar.[4,5,7,16] Children in higher income families tended to be taller and heavier, with more advanced skeletal development, than children from low income families. Black children were smaller at birth and in the first 2 to 3 years, then grew more rapidly and tended to be taller than white children through adolescence. However, white children were heavier, with higher subcutaneous fat measurements while black children had greater lean body mass. Despite the ethnic differences, a single set of national reference standards is considered adequate for health and physical growth screening.[17] There are few studies of the growth of other ethnic groups, such as native Americans and those of Latin American or East Asian descent, and interpretation of their size relative to the national reference standard should be made with care.[17]

The relationship of obesity, as measured either by weight to height ratio or by skinfold measurements, to income was not consistent among the surveys. Overnutrition has been increasingly considered a greater problem in the United States than undernutrition, and will be considered in a separate section of this chapter.

Biochemical Assessment

As an index to nutritional status biochemical assessment may vary from only a determination of hemoglobin concentration in the blood to extensive and complex laboratory studies. McLaren[3] has listed laboratory tests in two categories according to their sensitivity, as shown in Table 2.3. The selection of measurements to be used in any study will depend on the type of survey or individual assessment being done, the availability and reliability of laboratory or field facilities and personnel, the probability of finding meaningful levels within a given population, and the significance of variations to the health problems of the study group.

The applicability of the laboratory determinations is partially dependent on the sequence of development of deficiencies. Some determinations reflect current or immediate past dietary intake; some are dependent on depletion of body stores or on deficiencies that have altered tissue function. Therefore the degree of observable change in biochemical levels is influenced by the length and severity of nutrient deficiency, but the influence varies with each determination.

76

Table 2.3   Laboratory Tests for Nutrients and Metabolites

Nutrient	More Sensitive	Less Sensitive
Protein	Plasma amino acids, urinary hydroxyproline, serum albumin, urinary urea/creatinine	Total serum protein
Lipids	Serum cholesterol, triglycerides, lipoproteins	
Vitamin A	Serum vitamin A and carotene	
Vitamin D	Serum 25-OH-cholecalciferol, serum alkaline phosphatase	Serum calcium and phosphorus
Ascorbic acid	Whole blood ascorbic acid	
Thiamine	Urinary thiamine, erythrocyte transketolase activity	Blood pyruvate
Riboflavin	Urinary riboflavin, erythrocyte glutathione reductase	
Nicotinic acid		N_1 methyl nicotinamide and its pyridone in urine
Folic acid	Red cell folate	Serum folate, bone marrow film, thin blood film
Vitamin B_{12}	Serum vitamin B_{12}, serum thymidylate synthetase, urine methylmalonic acid	Bone marrow film, thin blood film, Schilling test
Iron	Iron deposits in bone marrow, serum iron and % saturation of transferrin	Haemoglobin, haematocrit, thin blood film
Iodine		Urinary iodine, tests for thyroid function

Source: McLaren, D. S., and D. Burman. *Textbook of Paediatric Nutrition.* Churchill Livingstone, Edinburgh, 1976.

A direct measure of the concentration in blood or urine is possible for some nutrients. Lipids, protein (total, albumin, or amino acids), calcium, iron, vitamin A, carotene, ascorbic acid, vitamin B_{12}, and folate can be measured directly in blood. Urinary concentrations of thiamin, riboflavin, and N-methyl-nicotinamide can be determined. Urine specimens are more informative if they represent 24-hour collection, but a fasting sample may be used for some determinations, with creatinine used as a reference. Other determinations are indirect measures of function of nutrients, such as hemoglobin, hematocrit, enzymes, or accumulation of substrates. For a limited number of nutrients excessive intakes may be reflected in blood levels, such as in hypervitaminosis A, hypercarotenemia, hypercalcemia, or iron overload, but these represent special situations.

The interpretation of findings varies with each nutrient. Homeostatic mechanisms maintain plasma calcium within a 10 percent range around 10 mg/100 ml, so that measurement of plasma calcium is of limited value in most subjects. Large body reserves of vitamin A must be depleted before there is a significant decrease in plasma level; in adults this may take a year or more. On the other hand, scurvy has been observed in subjects with plasma ascorbic acid levels of 0.2 mg/100 ml or even higher. Fasting blood samples minimize the effect of recent intake and activity on levels of some nutrients. Therefore, the level of a nutrient in circulating blood must be interpreted in the light of the physiological processes of the body, as well as recent intake.

Metabolic functions of vitamins provide the basis for some determinations. The accumulation of pyruvate occurs with incomplete carbohydrate metabolism as a result of thiamin deficiency. Enzyme levels may be an indication of the state of nutrition with respect to some nutrients, such as transketolase in thiamin metabolism and glutathione reductase in riboflavin metabolism. Enzymes involved in metabolism of amino acids, lipids, and carbohydrates have been investigated as indices of protein metabolism, but the significance and direction of change are not yet clear. Urinary concentration of creatinine is an index of muscle mass and hydroxyproline is an index of collagen turnover, but diurnal and daily variations in their excretion necessitate caution in interpretation of these levels.

When laboratory facilities are adequate and extensive studies are indicated, load tests may be used for some nutrients. When a large dose of ascorbic acid is given, a higher percentage of the dose is excreted when tissues are already close to saturation than when tissues are depleted. In a pyridoxine deficiency the feeding of tryptophan results in the excretion of xanthurenic acid because of interruption in the normal conversion of tryptophan to niacin, a process in which pyridoxine plays a vital role. A load test of histidine results in the excretion of formiminoglutamic acid (FIGLU) in folate deficiency. These tests, however, apply more to research purposes than to survey practicality.

Hair analysis has recently been a subject of interest, particularly in zinc and copper metabolism, but methodology and significance are still in the exploratory stages.

"The biochemical measurement of nutrients in the blood (serum or plasma) is at best a crude indicator of the supply of these nutrients. It does not tell us what the nutrient content is in the body stores, such as liver or bone marrow. It is, however, the only feasible method under the circumstances of a field survey."[6] Blood and urine samples are relatively easy to obtain in clinics, physicians' offices, and under survey conditions. Other body tissues require invasive techniques and subject the individual to discomfort or risk, which limits their use to diagnostic purposes primarily. Many of the tests on blood and urine require more specialized equipment or personnel than are commonly available. Reproducibility of tests is often poor, and wide variations have been reported from different laboratories. Techniques for some determinations are not well standardized, and a slight change in procedure in a laboratory may alter the results. The choice of biochemical methods has depended more on the availability of blood and urine, on the simplicity of the analytic procedures, and on the stage of development of laboratory methodology than on the physiological significance of the tests.

Evaluation of the results of biochemical determinations is also subject to difference of opinion, primarily because of the lack of clear criteria on the significance of levels. In the four North American surveys, different standards and terminology have been used. In Appendix 3, the "current" guidelines for evaluation of laboratory findings, developed by the committee of the American Public Health Association,[11] the categories are labeled "acceptable," "marginal," and "deficient." Terminology in the Canadian survey[9] referred to low, moderate, and high risk. However, the four surveys used different cutoff points. Even for a determination as extensively studied as hemoglobin concentration, it is difficult to specify what level of hemoglobin constitutes the dividing line between "normal" and "anemia." In spite of the finding in both TSNS[4] and HANES[6] that mean vitamin A levels increased with age in both sexes and all ethnic groups, a value of 20 ug/100 ml was used for all ages as the lower acceptable level of plasma vitamin A, with the obvious result that infants and young children had a higher frequency of "low" or "deficient" ratings than adults, and that few elderly persons were given low ratings. The percentage of a population deemed to be at risk, based on laboratory assessment, varies with criteria selected.

As more data become available on the factors that affect blood concentration and urinary excretion of nutrients and on the relationship of variations in level with physiological status, the criteria for evaluation may be expected to change. At the present time lack of agreement on cutoff points that signify risk introduces a large element of judgment in the evaluation of biochemical levels.

The surveys done on this continent have shown relatively consistent results. Low hemoglobin and hematocrit values were of greatest concern, and were found in all segments of the populations. In those studies that did additional tests of iron status, the low hemoglobin and hematocrit levels tended to be associated with low serum iron and saturation of transferrin, but observed correlation coefficients were not high. Blacks at all ages and income levels had lower average blood values for iron nutriture than white subjects. As will be discussed later in this chapter, racial differences have been subjected to further analysis and the evidence suggests the need for separate standards.

In TSNS,[4] low serum albumin levels were found in a relatively large proportion of pregnant and lactating women, despite relatively high protein intakes as compared to the standard. Hemodilution during pregnancy and the changing dietary protein recommendations will be considered in greater detail in the chapter on pregnancy. In contrast, in the Canadian survey,[9] protein intakes were low in nearly one-fourth of girls between 10 and 19 years of age despite satisfactory serum protein values.

Serum vitamin A levels were given lower ratings in children than in adults, but there was no supporting evidence of clinical deficiency, and these ratings may have reflected the choice of a standard more than meaningful deficiencies of level. However, in TSNS,[4] Spanish-American subjects in southern states had low plasma vitamin A levels more often than other groups.

In both TSNS[4] and the Canadian study[9] thyroid enlargement in some subjects was unrelated to urinary iodine exretion, suggesting that the goiter was not due to iodine deficiency. The cause was not clear.

Although some segments of the population had low levels of other determinations, the prevalence was relatively small. Indians and Eskimos in Canada tended to have low levels more often than the general population.

Dietary Assessment

Dietary assessment is an integral component of nutritional assessment. The confirmation of the nutritional etiology of clinical and biochemical findings rests with the identification of a dietary deficiency. Unfortunately, methods for obtaining dietary information covering an extended period of time are complex, and those that cover only the immediate past are inadequate. The simplest method is the 24-hour intake, which is the least meaningful and the least productive. Most surveys have used the 24-hour intake as the basis for dietary assessment for practical reasons of ease, time, cost, and personnel. Its major advantage is in showing the distribution of nutrient intakes of a large population of people. Its major disadvantage lies in its application to the individual and therefore to intercorrelation with other data in the survey. A 24-hour intake may not be typical of intake of the individual and may have little relationship to clinical or biochemical status, as was shown in the major surveys conducted between 1968 and 1974.

In an evaluation of nutritional status, the examination of the individual for physical health, size, or biochemical status is done at a single time and represents the state of the individual at that age. In contrast, the effect of nutrition is continuous from conception to the individual's age at the time of the examination. Intake during the previous 24-hour period can be directly related only to those nutrients that are currently in transport in blood or excreted. Efforts to attach greater significance to intake in a single 24-hour period have been generally unsuccessful. Short-term dietary studies tend to overestimate the proportion of inadequate diets in the population and thus to give a falsely high picture of the degree of risk of malnutrition.[19,20]

Daily fluctuations, both in quantity and types of foods consumed, are large, especially in areas where there is a wide variety of food available. Some survey protocols[21] have specified that 24-hour intake should be recorded only between Monday and Friday because many people alter their food consumption on weekends. Although this maintains greater comparability of the data, it gives a false picture of the typical or average consumption by ignoring nearly 30 percent of the week. Variations in appetite, activity or work load, time schedule, temporary illness, and many other factors influence intake on a given day, and it is difficult for many people to determine what is an "average" day. It has been repeatedly observed in studies of low income families that food intake is higher and more varied following receipt of a pay check or welfare check, and lower in the days before receipt of the next check.

In a longitudinal study of children[22] in which intake was recorded on four days at specified time intervals, the median difference between the lowest and highest of the four days ranged from approximately 100 kcal in infants to more than 600 kcal in adolescents. Maximum differences for adolescents were sometimes higher than 1000 kcal. In a study of pregnant women[19] who recorded intakes for six days, one-day deviations were as much as 600 kcal above or below the mean intake, with a few deviations as high as 1000 kcal. The chance selection of a day with very high or very low food consumption gives an erroneous evaluation of usual food intake.

Errors of omission increase when a 24-hour recall is used instead of a 24-hour record. In the recall, the subject is asked to remember what foods were consumed on the previous day. Unless the individual is on a special diet or has another reason to be particularly aware of food consumption, eating is a matter of course and details are quickly forgotten, especially snacks between meals and extra foods at meals. Probing by the interviewer is often necessary to aid completeness of recall. A record of intake kept by the subject as foods are eaten during the 24-hour period minimizes errors of omission, but many subjects are unwilling to take the extra time and thought required, so that often what is assumed to be a 24-hour record is actually a recall.

Basing dietary assessment on a single 24-hour intake is justifiable if the purpose is to show the distribution of intakes of a population group, with the realization that it may overestimate the number at nutritional risk. In some studies the number of days has been increased to five or seven, with comparisons of single days with means of several days.[23-25] In a cooperative study in several northeastern states, 15 days of intake records were required for men and 12 days for women to obtain data within 95 percent confidence limits based on an arbitrarily selected deviation from the RDA, for all nutrients except vitamin A. Daily fluctuations in vitamin A were too great to estimate the number of days required for determining reliability of mean intakes.[23] The variations in nutrient intake from day to day depend to some extent on the distribution of nutrients in foods. Variation is least for nutrients with wide distribution, such as calories, protein, iron, thiamin, and niacin. Daily variation is greater for calcium and riboflavin, which are largely influenced by the presence or absence of milk in the diet. Ascorbic acid is primarily derived from citrus fruit and tomato in the U.S. diet, and the chance selection of a day with or without those foods affects the evaluation of ascorbic acid intake. Extreme differences in vitamin A and especially carotene content of foods result in large daily variations. Even in developing societies with fewer food choices, Flores[26] has considered six days a minimum period of time for adequate evaluation.

Although increasing the number of days provides a better evaluation of food intake of the individual, there is still no assurance that food consumption during the period of observation represents long-time patterns of eating. In addition, alteration of the usual pattern of eating because of participation in a study may be a problem with some individuals or population groups.

Accurate reporting of food intake is affected by a wide range of psychological and social-economic influences. Motivation and cooperation are higher among middle and upper income groups than among low income groups. Persons with higher educational attainment are more capable of giving valid information than those with lower educational levels or problems with literacy or language. Women tend to give better dietary data than men, and young adults better than either children or the elderly. Individuals with relatively stable work situations or life-styles tend also to have more stable food intakes, which are easier to describe, than those with marked shifts in activity, intermittent dieting for weight control, or casual life-styles. There is, therefore, a difference in the reliability of data obtained from various segments of the population.

A variety of other methods have been developed in efforts to determine food intake and to calculate nutrient content of diets. There is, unfortunately, no absolute method of dietary assessment guaranteed to give a picture of usual food intake, either in the present or in the past, since each method is affected by a variety of factors, most of which can be neither identified nor measured. There is also no way of measuring one method against another. "Situations and individuals may be similar, but they can never be exactly the same."[27] As a result, there continues to be controversy about dietary study methodology, with wide variation in viewpoints. Two extensive reviews of methods and their comparisons have been published by Marr[25] and by Becker et al.[27]

Dietary data may be obtained by record or recall of present intake, or by recall of past intake. The forms used may be unstructured, with minimal headings for the time of food consumption, so that no suggestion is offered of what foods might be expected to be consumed, or highly structured forms may be used to remind the subject about the use of cream and sugar in coffee, salad dressings, gravy, butter or margarine on sandwiches, etc. The data may be obtained by a nutritionist or other trained personnel during an interview in a clinic or at home; self-recording of data by the subject may be done, with or without clarification later by the nutritionist; or mailed surveys may be used. The food for consumption may be weighed, measured, or merely estimated. The extent of data obtained may vary from a list of foods limited to the specific interests of the study, such as intake of fats and cholesterol, to comprehensive coverage of all foods consumed.

The objectives of the study must be clearly defined in advance since they determine the choice of method. Even if group evaluations are sought, as in the epidemiological approach of large surveys, the data must be based on information obtained from individuals and therefore the method must be applicable to the population group selected. Detailed descriptions of various methods have been published.[11,28]

A food frequency list may be used to record how often various foods have been consumed in a given period of time. This simple technique may be used with large population groups with a minimum of time involvement by the nutritionist. Since amounts of foods are not recorded, nutrient intake cannot be calculated, but a scoring system may be used for foods or food groups.

A nutrition history of the kinds and amounts of foods consumed during a given period of time is based on recall. If carefully taken from cooperative and highly motivated subjects, calculation of nutrient content of the diet is possible. The validity of this method depends on the skill and experience of the nutritionist, the intelligence and memory of the subject, and the rapport between nutritionist and subject. This method has been used in longitudinal studies [29] and in a variety of short-term nutrition studies.

Weighing of food intake is the most accurate method, but is impractical for extended periods of time except in unusual situations. This method is used in balance studies where precision is essential, and has sometimes been used in studies to verify data obtained by record or history. Weighed intake studies have often been done in Great Britain,[25] where household scales are commonly used in preparing recipes. They are obviously inapplicable to surveys or to most dietary studies.

When dietary intake data, which include both amounts and frequency of foods consumed, have been obtained the nutrient content of the diet may be calculated. Except in rare situations, usually limited to balance study experiments in which aliquot samples of foods consumed may be analyzed directly, the nutritionist is dependent on published food value tables. The level of technological progress in food analysis can expand or limit the reliability of dietary evaluation as a component of nutritional assessment. Complete analyses of foods are slowly becoming a reality, but reliable values for some minerals and vitamins are still unavailable. When analytical techniques are inadequate, food composition tables may be either incomplete or inaccurate. Variations in methodology provide conflicting data from one laboratory to another, compounded by differences in the content of foods grown in various geographical areas or under differing conditions. Reliability also varies with the number of analyses done. For example, far more analyses have been done of milk than of broccoli.

The state of the art of chemical analysis of foods is still in the early stage of development for some trace elements and vitamins, including zinc, copper, manganese, selenium, chromium, folacin, pantothenic acid, and vitamin B_{12}. The recently renewed interest in fiber in the etiology of some gastrointestinal diseases has given rise to conflicting interpretations because of inadequate data on the different components of fiber and the influence of each component on speed of food passage and on biochemical changes in the gastrointestinal tract.[30] The introduction of new food products and changes in food processing methods are followed by a time lag until their nutrient content can be calculated in diets, although the requirements of food labeling by the Food and Drug Administration tend to minimize the time lag. However, despite the best efforts of the U.S. Department of Agriculture, its Nutrient Data Bank cannot keep pace with the changing food supply.

Biological availability of nutrients cannot readily be determined, but is a vital addendum to the analyzed nutrient content of a food. The presence of a nutrient in a food consumed may be calculated from a food value table,

84

but if the nutrient has low availability, a physiological deficiency may occur despite a calculated high intake. With the finding of low hemoglobin and hematocrit levels in many segments of the population in recent surveys, attention has been focused on the biological availability of iron; fortification of food products with iron of low availability provides little benefit to the consumer. Increasing the fiber content of the diet is associated with an increase in phytic acid, which binds many trace elements into insoluble phytates and may substitute one nutritional problem for another.

The many chemical forms of a nutrient complicate dietary intake calculations. The various forms of carotene as precursors of vitamin A have led to the concept of vitamin A activity or retinol equivalents.[31] Similarly, vitamin E activity varies from one tocopherol to another. This concept has been extended to folacin since its calculated dietary level may differ significantly from biological availability of its different forms.[32] The calculation of niacin intake must take into consideration the assumption that 60 mg tryptophan is equivalent to 1 mg niacin[31] although tryptophan has other physiological functions.

Even with a nutrient that has been extensively studied, such as protein, evaluation of dietary intake requires consideration of its components. The major concern with total dietary intake of protein must be tempered by the degree to which amino acids meet physiological needs of the body. Limiting amino acids, such as lysine, threonine, and tryptophan in wheat, or methionine in soybeans, affect the efficiency of the body in using other amino acids in the food. Furthermore, the ratio of one nutrient to another may affect absorption across the gut, increasing or decreasing dietary need to meet physiological requirements. The increased absorption of iron in the presence of ascorbic acid and of calcium in the presence of vitamin D are well-known examples, but the interrelationships among nutrients in determining availability and absorption are extensive.

The problems of evaluating the nutrient content of the diet were summarized by Hunscher and Macy[33] in 1951, and the concepts they presented are still valid. Although practicality demands that food value tables must commonly be used for calculating nutrients, the limitations and errors in their use should temper conclusions drawn from dietary assessment.

Selection of a standard for rating of the calculated nutrient intake, either in a broad survey or in individual studies, has often been arbitrary. While the temptation of most research workers has been to use the Recommended Dietary Allowances or two-thirds of the Allowances in the absence of other acceptable standards, the Food and Nutrition Board have repeatedly cautioned against this use of the RDAs.[31,34,35] Since individual requirements cannot be readily determined, there is no assurance that an intake above the RDA may not be inadequate for a given individual, although it is estimated that only 2.5 percent of the population need more than the RDA. Conversely, an intake below the RDA or even below two-thirds of the RDA may not be deficient for an individual. When adequate data are available, the RDA has been established at two standard deviations above the mean; when data were inadequate, the committee estimated that level. Only the allowance for energy represents average need.

Recommended allowances are based on evaluation of literature available at the time. Gaps in our knowledge of human requirements are gradually lessening, but are still so great that judgment of the committees is essential. Figure 2.1 summarizes degrees of knowledge of human requirements at various ages in 1976.

The uncertainty of established recommended allowances is demonstrated by the contrast of nutrient levels in three sets of "recommended allowances" in the Western Hemisphere. The RDAs of the United States (1974),[31] the Dietary Standard for Canada (1975),[36] and the RDAs for the Caribbean (1976)[37] give similar definitions of their allowances as "the levels of intake of essential nutrients considered to be adequate to meet the known nutritional needs of practically all healthy persons." Although age groupings are not identical, caloric allowances are similar except that the Caribbean values are higher for the female during late adolescence and lactation. Protein allowances at most ages are 1 to 3 g lower in the Canadian standard than in the 1979 United States RDA, although allowances for the adult male are 56 g in both countries. A major difference occurs in the additional protein allowance for pregnancy, which ranges from 13 g in the Caribbean standards to 30 g in the U.S. allowances. The calcium allowance for young children in the United States is 800 mg, in contrast to 500 mg in the other two tables. Calcium allowances in adolescence are generally highest in the United States at 1200 mg, intermediate for Canada, and lowest with a maximum of 700 mg in the Caribbean allowance. The Caribbean allowances for calcium during pregnancy and lactation are 200 mg lower than the other two standards.

Greatest variation among the three standards is shown in iron. The U.S. allowance is twice as high as the Caribbean allowance in the first three years of life and remains higher during early childhood. For the menstruating female, the Canadian allowance is 14 mg, the U.S. allowance is 18 mg, and the Caribbean allowance rises to 19 mg. In the accompanying texts that ex-

Figure 2.1 Knowledge of human nutritional requirements as of 1976. Prepared by the Nutrition Institute, Agricultural Research Service, U.S. Department of Agriculture. (Reprinted from Human Nutrition; Readings from Scientific American, W.H. Freeman and Co., San Francisco, 1978.)

ASSESSMENT OF NUTRITIONAL STATUS

Current Knowledge of Human Nutritional Requirements

	Infants			Children			Adults			
	Premature	0-6 months	6-23 months	Preschool	School Age	Adolescent	Young	Aged	Pregnant	Lactating
Total Energy	O	O	O	O	●	●	●	O	O	O
Carbohydrates:										
Starch										
Sugars	O	O	O	O	O	O	●			
Fibers						O	O			
Total Fat		●								
Essential Fatty Acids		O					O	O		
Protein	●	O	O	O	O	O	●	O	●	O
Amino Acids:										
Arginine		●			O		●			
Histidine	O	●			O		●			
Isoleucine	O	●			O		●			
Leucine	O	●			O		●			
Lysine		●			O		●	O		
Methionine		●			O		●	O		
Phenylalanine		●			O		●			
Threonine		●			O		●	O		
Tryptophan		●			O		●	O		
Valine	O	●			O		●			
Minerals:										
Calcium	●	●	●	O	O	O	●	O	O	O
Magnesium				O	O	O	O			
Iron	●	●	●	●	●	O	●	●	●	●
Phosphorus				O	O				O	O
Sulfur				O	O				O	O
Sodium				O	O		O	O		
Potassium	O	O	O	O	O		O	O		
Copper	O	O		O	O		O			
Molybdenum										
Manganese				O						
Zinc	O	O	O	O	O	O	O		O	O
Chromium				O						
Selenium							O			
Nickel										
Vanadium										
Chlorine										
Fluorine				O	●	O		O		
Iodine				O	O	O	O			
Vitamins:										
Vitamin A	●	●		O	O		●			
Vitamin D	●	●	O	O	O	O				
Vitamin E	O						O			
Vitamin K	O	O						O		
Thiamin	O	O		O	O	O	●	O	O	O
Riboflavin	O	O		O	O	O	●	O	O	O
Niacin							O	O	O	O
Pyridoxine		O					O		O	
Pantothenate							O			
Cobalamin		O					O			
Folic Acid	O	O					O	O	O	
Biotin										
Choline										
Ascorbic Acid	●	●		O	O	O	●	O	O	O

▢ LITTLE OR NO DATA   O FRAGMENTARY DATA   ● SUBSTANTIAL PROGRESS MADE   1976 DATA

plained the derivation of the values, the estimated amount of iron required for daily absorption by the menstruating female ranged from 1.5 mg (U.S.) to 2.8 mg (Caribbean); smaller differences were stipulated for other age groups. Presumably all three committees had access to the same literature sources of data, but different references were cited and obviously judgment differed from one committee to another. These examples selected from the three sets of recommended allowances illustrate the uncertainty among specialists in the nutrition field both in the interpretation of published data and in the establishment of guidelines for nutrient intake.

Not only is there controversy about nutrient needs at a given time in the state of the science, but the changes over time have been relatively large for some nutrients as more data become available. Changes in protein allowances for children are shown in Figure 2.2. The allowances remained constant from 1943 to 1958, decreased markedly in 1963 and again in 1968. Changes between 1974 and 1979 were due to use of different body weights after 7 years of age. With little change in the allowances for energy, the per-

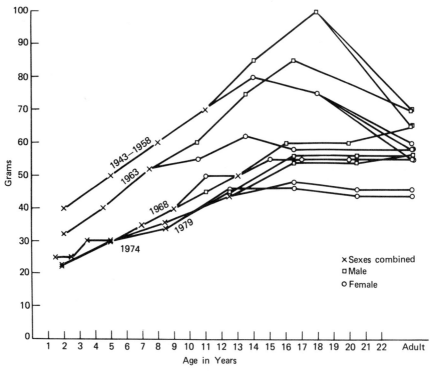

Figure 2.2   Recommended Dietary Allowances for protein, 1943–1979.

ASSESSMENT OF NUTRITIONAL STATUS

cent of calories from protein decreased from 12–13 percent in 1943 to 6–7 percent for preadolescent children and from 10–11 percent to 7–9 percent for adolescents. The allowance for adult males dropped from 70 g protein in 1943 to 56 g in 1979, while the allowance for adult women dropped from 60 to 44 g. One exception to the pattern of decrease was the greater increment of protein for pregnancy in the 1974 edition, an increase that was maintained in the 1979 RDA. Over the same time period, allowances for iron were sharply increased for infants and young children, for women during the reproductive years, and for male adolescents.

Since RDA levels have often been used as the basis for estimating the prevalence of low dietary intakes in various population studies, prevalence estimates vary directly with the changes in RDAs. For example, far more diets were rated inadequate in protein in the 1940s and 1950s than would be given an inadequate rating at the present time. In fact, few diets in the United States do not meet present RDA levels for protein. Conversely, the number of diets given low ratings for iron intake increased sharply following publication of the 1968 RDAs in the three groups for whom allowances were raised. For children under 3 years of age the RDA was nearly doubled, and few diets at that age approach an iron content of 15 mg without fortification. Therefore, in comparing surveys or other studies conducted in the past with those in the present, the prevalence of dietary deficiencies of each nutrient must be reevaluated if the RDA was used as a standard.

The major surveys of nutritional status in the United States and Canada did not use the same criteria for evaluation of dietary risk. Each group developed its own standards and cutoff points. TSNS and HANES differed only in ascorbic acid, but both used calcium and vitamin A values lower than the RDAs, evaluated calories and protein in relation to body weight, and expressed thiamin, riboflavin, and niacin per 1000 kcal. The Canadian survey used standards that differed in many respects from the U.S. surveys. Therefore, the findings of the surveys are not directly comparable but must be interpreted with reference to the specific rating scale of each survey.

Until more definitive data are available on nutrient needs of all subgroups of the population, present allowances and rating standards must be considered tentative and subject to change. This uncertainty is especially acute for the period of growth between infancy and maturity and for pregnancy and lactation.

Despite limitations of standards of evaluation in the surveys, some aspects of nutritional assessment of the U.S. population were shown to merit further attention. In the absence of significant findings of protein or vitamin deficiencies, the major concern in relation to undernutrition was anemia. The primary evidence of overnutrition was obesity.

BIOCHEMICAL IRON DEFICIENCY AND ANEMIA

Some degree of iron deficiency and anemia was found in all population groups in the United States[4-6], but the prevalence was highest for three groups: children under 2 to 3 years of age, menstruating females, and pregnant women. In addition, male adolescents showed a surprisingly high prevalence, but this may be due more to the selection of blood standards than to its clinical significance; iron requirements of the adolescent male will be considered in the chapter on adolescence rather than in the present discussion.

In recent years iron has stimulated more controversy than any other nutrient. The complexity of iron metabolism at all levels has defied easy study and interpretation. The bioavailability of iron, both as it occurs naturally in foods and as it is added in fortification of foods, has recently been subjected to intensive investigation and has led to a reevaluation of the enrichment programs of many countries. Absorption of iron is poorly understood because it is influenced by many unrelated factors. The rate of absorption varies with the chemical form of the iron, the presence or absence of a number of substances in the gastrointestinal tract and in the intestinal mucosal cells, iron storage in the body, rate of growth, and other factors that are difficult to identify and quantify. The prevalence of iron deficiency is uncertain, since the diagnosis is subject to the selection of biochemical determinants. The clinical significance of iron deficiency and its effect on vigor and well-being have been controversial. All of these variables have led to shifts in recommendations of iron intake for various population subgroups.

IRON REQUIREMENTS

Moore[38] has presented a summary of the factorial method of estimating iron requirements (Table 2.4), based on present knowledge of iron metabolism. Iron balance studies are difficult and are subject to a high degree of error. As with other nutrients, adult males have been studied more intensively than other persons, and much of the data have been interpolated from studies of males. Values for adult women were calculated on the assumption that their body content of iron is approximately 35 mg/kg body weight in contrast to 50 mg/kg for men. Iron to replace menstrual losses has been determined in relatively few intensive studies. Moore calculated the additional need for pregnancy based on iron in the fetus, placenta, umbilical cord, and blood lost at delivery; the iron needed for expansion of maternal blood volume was not included in this figure since it was assumed that the mother's blood retains that iron after delivery. However, Moore included iron needs for six months of lactation in the "pregnancy cost." Iron requirements for

Table 2.4 *Estimated Iron Requirements in Mg/Day*

	External Loss[a]	Menses	Pregnancy "Cost"	Growth	Fe Requirement	Daily Food Intake Requirement[b]
Adult males (50–100 kg)	0.65–1.3				0.65–1.3	6.5–13
Nonmenstruating women (45–70 kg)	0.6–0.9				0.6–0.9	6–9
Menstruating women (45–70 kg)	0.6–0.9	0.1–1.4			0.7–2.3	7–23
Pregnancy (50–80 kg)	0.65–1.0		1.0–2.5		1.65–3.5	16.5–35
Adolescent boys (50–100 kg)	0.65–1.3			0.35–0.7	1–2	10–20
Adolescent girls (45–70 kg)	0.6–0.9	0.1–1.4		0.3–0.45	1–2.7	10–27
Children					0.4–1.0	4–10
Infants					0.5–1.5	5–15

[a] 0.013 mg/kg.
[b] Assuming 10 percent absorption.

Source: Moore, C. V. Iron. In: Goodhart, R. S., and M. E. Shils (Eds.) *Modern Nutrition in Health and Disease*, Fifth Edition. Lea and Febiger, Philadelphia, 1973.

91

children were estimated from body growth and its iron content. The male who increases 50 to 100 kg in 20 years, with 50 mg iron per kg body weight, would require 125 to 250 mg iron/year or 0.35 to 0.70 mg/day for growth. The girl's estimated requirement was based on increment of 45 to 70 kg body weight, with a content of 35 mg iron/kg, over a period of 15 years. Absorption was assumed to be 10 percent of dietary iron for all individuals.

Although these estimations make a number of assumptions, they indicate why the risk of iron deficiency is greater for the menstruating woman, the pregnant woman, and the very young child. Physiological factors that increase the need for iron are different for each group, but usual iron intakes may not be adequate, and special attention is necessary to meet requirements.

Loss of iron in menstrual blood varies widely from one woman to another. Hallberg et al.[40] found a range of 1.6 to 199.7 ml of blood lost per period in most women, with much higher losses in women with menorrhagia. Bowering et al.,[41] in a review of balance studies, found average losses reported to range from 8 to 18 mg iron per period, with individual losses ranging from 0.3 to 110 mg iron. Women with infrequent or short periods characterized by small menstrual flow have only a slightly greater iron need than men. However, if the menstrual cycle is short and the flow excessive, either in volume or duration, risk of iron depletion increases. Contraceptive use influences blood loss, which may be less with oral contraceptives and greater with intrauterine devices. The average menstrual loss would represent a daily need of 0.4 to 0.5 mg of absorbed iron in addition to basal body losses, making a total daily need for absorbed iron between 1.0 and 1.5 mg. If iron absorption is assumed to be 10 percent, the diet would need to supply 10 to 15 mg to replace losses for the average woman, and larger amounts for the woman with higher blood loss. Since the usual composite diet supplies approximately 6 mg iron per 1000 kcal, many women may be in marginal iron balance.

During pregnancy the woman will need to supply 200 to 350 mg for a single full-term fetus and 50 to 150 mg for the placenta and other maternal tissues. Increase in her own erythrocyte volume is estimated to require an additional 300 to 500 mg, some of which will be lost in bleeding at delivery and some will be retained. The iron need is somewhat offset by the cessation of menstrual periods. With evidence that body iron in the fetus is independent of maternal blood levels, the pregnant woman must increase her iron intake to avoid depletion of her own body stores.

The child between 6 and 36 months of age has increased risk of iron deficiency because of depletion of fetal storage in a period of rapid growth and expansion of hemoglobin mass. Hemoglobin concentration at birth ranges between 16 and 22 g/100 ml blood in the full-term infant. Since the life span of the fetal red blood cell is estimated to be only 60 to 90 days,[42] hemoglobin concentration decreases to 10–11 g in the second month and then begins to increase again. The iron released from red cells is retained and used in the regeneration of hemoglobin, but this supply is estimated to be sufficient for needs in the first 4 to 6 months, after which a supply of exogenous iron is essential. Milk contains relatively little iron, although the breastfed infant has greater protection against iron deficiency because of the higher absorption of iron from breast milk than from cow's milk.[43] Unless solid foods are added to the diet, iron intake after 6 months may be inadequate. The peak prevalence of nutritional anemia occurs at 18 months. The low birth weight infant, whether premature or small for gestational age, is especially prone to iron deficiency anemia because of low iron storage at birth.

Body iron may be classified into three components.[39] Functional iron includes circulating hemoglobin, muscle myoglobin, and the essential metallo-enzymes, such as cytochromes, peroxidase, and catalase. Transport iron occurs in small amounts in the circulation bound to transferrin or ferritin. Storage iron is found in hepatic parenchymal cells and in the reticuloendothelial cells of bone marrow, liver, and spleen. Aproximately 70 percent of total body iron in the adult male is in the functional component; the full-term newborn has a higher hemoglobin concentration than at any later age and therefore a higher percentage of functional iron.

Storage iron is rarely measured as a routine in nutritional assessment. Aspiration of a sample of bone marrow for evaluation of stainable iron is an unpleasant procedure usually done only for diagnostic purposes. Recent studies suggest that the level of serum ferritin may reflect body stores with sufficient accuracy to become a useful index.[44,45] Methodology for enzyme measurement is difficult and is not a common procedure. Therefore, assessment of iron nutriture is usually based on blood components.

Hemoglobin and hematocrit (packed red cell volume expressed as percent) have been standard procedures for many years and until recently were usually the sole determinations of iron status in surveys. Serum iron and the saturation of transferrin with iron have been increasingly recognized as possible indicators of early iron deficiency. Moore's[38] schematic representation of the development of iron deficiency anemia (Figure 2.3) follows a pattern similar to Pearson's description of the progress of nutrient deficiencies.[2] When iron balance becomes negative, storage supplies of ferritin and hemosiderin will be drawn upon to meet current needs. Although total body iron storage is difficult to measure, it has been estimated that the adult male has 500 to 1500 mg and the adult female 300 to 1000 mg iron in storage. Except in hemorrhage or other blood loss, iron deficiency usually results from small daily deficits in intake, resulting in slow depletion of storage. With small deficits and relatively high storage levels, it may take months or years

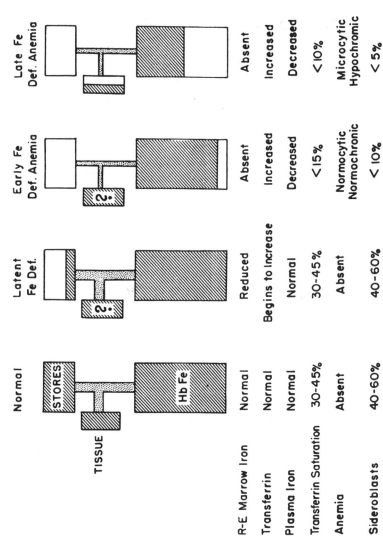

Figure 2.3 Schematic representation of the development of iron-deficiency anemia. The "?" in the tissue blocks indicates uncertainty about when depletion occurs. (Reprinted from Moore, C. V. Iron. In: Goodhart, R.S., and M. E. Shils (Eds.) Modern Nutrition in Health and Disease, Fifth Edition. Lea and Febiger, Philadelphia, 1973.)

before changes in blood levels become evident.[38] Although there has been some speculation that earlier changes may occur in iron-containing enzymes, this has not been clearly documented. In iron deficiency anemia heme synthesis cannot be completed and a relative excess of free protoporphyrin accumulates in the erythrocytes; recent development of microtechniques for measurement of free protoporphyrin may provide another measure of anemia.[46]

The terminology for iron deficiencies has increasingly tended toward a distinction between biochemical iron deficiency and anemia. Biochemical iron deficiency may be diagnosed by a decrease in serum iron concentration and in the percentage saturation of transferrin with iron, thereby increasing total iron-binding capacity of the blood. Levels indicative of iron deficiency have not been standardized and the criteria vary from one medical or research center to another, as does the accuracy of determinations. Transferrin concentration in the blood is usually expressed in physiological terms of its total iron-binding capacity (TIBC), which is normally within the range of 200 to 450 μg/100 ml blood. The amount of plasma iron (90-180 μg/100 ml in adult males and 70-150 μg in women) is sufficient to bind only about one-third of the iron-binding sites on transferrin.[38,47] Therefore, transferrin saturation between 15 and 20 percent has commonly been used as the lower level of normal. Serum iron standards are somewhat more variable and the determination of serum iron is subject to several interpretations. Serum iron shows diurnal variation, with morning levels approximately 30 percent higher than evening levels, as well as increases during the postabsorptive stage and rapid decrease in infections, so it is not a stable measure.[47,48] Standards for serum iron increase with age during childhood.

Changes in the red blood cell are believed to be later developments in iron deficiency. When the supply of iron to the reticuloendothelial cells is insufficient, the red blood cells formed become increasingly hypochromic and microcytic. Both cell volume and mean corpuscular hemoglobin concentration are decreased. At this stage, anemia is diagnosed. Because of the uncertainty about the clinical significance of various levels of hemoglobin concentration, there is little agreement about the cutoff point for dividing marginal or acceptable values from those values indicative of anemia. For example, critical values for the child between 1 and 3 years of age have been considered as 9 g, 10 g, or 11 g/100 ml by different workers. The criteria guidelines for evaluation of laboratory determinations by the committee of the American Public Health Association (Appendix 3) were differentiated for age and sex.[11]

In addition to age, sex, rate of growth, and physiological state, blood levels have been shown to be different for black and white individuals. In the three U.S. surveys, mean hemoglobin levels of black subjects were nearly 1.0 g/100 ml lower than of white subjects in all age, sex, and income groups. Hematocrit levels were similarly lower, but the hemoglobin/hematocrit ratio (mean corpuscular hemoglobin concentration) was not lower; this was interpreted as presumptive evidence that the difference was not due to iron deficiency. Hemoglobinopathy in blacks did not seem to account for differences.[49] In a report of children 5 to 14 years of age without iron deficiency, abnormal hemoglobin, or thalassemia minor, hemoglobin concentrations of black children averaged 0.5 g/100 ml lower than white children, and it was estimated that 10 percent of black children would be mistakenly designated anemic if the same norms were applied for both races.[50]

Figures on the prevalence of iron deficiency, then, depend on the blood factors and standards selected for diagnosis. For example, in the HANES survey,[6] the number of males 12 to 17 years of age with "low" values was 15.5 percent for hematocrit, 7.4 percent for hemoglobin, 2.8 percent for serum iron, and 7.7 percent for transferrin saturation. In contrast, prevalence of "low" values in females of the same age group ranged from 1.1 to 2.4 percent for hemoglobin, hematocrit, and serum iron, and 5.3 percent had "low" levels of transferrin saturation. The standards for males were higher than for females for all determinations. There is general agreement that criteria should be higher for males, but there is little agreement about how great the difference should be.

CLINICAL SIGNIFICANCE

The clinical significance of either biochemical iron deficiency or anemia is not clear. A severe deficiency, with hemoglobin concentration of 7 to 8 g/100 ml or less, may be the result of blood loss or of disease in which the effect on hemoglobin synthesis is secondary. A dietary deficiency of iron severe enough to result in that degree of limitation of hematopoiesis is undoubtedly complicated by other nutrient deficiencies. Severe anemia is most frequent in areas of the world where dietary intakes of energy, protein, and other nutrients are low, where intestinal parasitism is common, and where medical care is inadequate.[38] It is therefore difficult to distinguish the effects of iron deficiency from concomitant problems.

The clinical significance of moderate degrees of biochemical iron deficiency or anemia is equally controversial. It has long been assumed that the individual with anemia is likely to be listless and easily fatigued, with substandard work performance, palpitation on exertion, and increased susceptibility to infection. Each of these symptoms has been subjected to review,[51-53] and the evidence for or against the assumption evaluated; the results are far from definitive. Few precise studies with adequate methodology and controls have been done, the criteria for diagnosis are often poorly defined, and tests of reversal of symptoms with iron repletion have seldom been included. Aside from its function in oxygen transport, iron status is reported to be critical for normal development and integrity of lymphoid tissues that control and mediate immunity. Epithelial changes have been described in iron-deficient individuals; one symptom, koilonychia, is specific for iron deficiency and is not found in any other condition. In addition to epithelial changes that might increase susceptibility to infection, tissue enzymes that contain iron or are influenced by iron-containing cofactors may be depleted in tissues with rapid turnover of cells and result in reduced immunocompetence.

Elwood[51] concluded that there is little evidence of any harmful effects of a low hemoglobin level until the concentration is 7 to 8 g/100 ml or less, below which effects on cardiorespiratory function and fetal survival are clear. Strauss[52] found no conclusive evidence of increased susceptibility to infections involving immunodeficiency or pyogenic bacteria with iron deficiency states. However, the inflammatory response, as measured by skin reaction, was shown to be diminished in iron deficiency and restored in iron repletion, although the precise molecular defect has not been identified.

It has been proposed that a moderate degree of iron deficiency may be protective against infection. Assimilation of iron is a necessary prerequisite for bacterial and fungal growth. Bacteria produce siderophores with powerful iron-chelating properties to extract iron from tightly bound protein-iron complexes, and their synthesis of siderophores is modulated largely by the concentration of iron in the immediate environment. The inhibition of bacterial growth by breast milk may be due to its high lactoferrin content. It has been reported that the antibacterial effect of human milk is lost when iron is added, and that iron injections to malnourished children may increase suspectibility to infection.[53] In a review of the relationship of iron nutriture to infection, Chandra[54] concluded that "it is likely that the outcome of an infective challenge in an iron-deficient organism will depend upon the balance of the effect of iron status on microbial multiplication and on host defense mechanism." At the present time, relationships between iron status and resistance or susceptibility to infection are unclear.

Pica, a craving for unnatural foods or for nonfood items, such as clay, laundry starch, or ice, has been related to iron deficiency, but it is unclear whether it is a cause or effect of anemia or merely a coincidental occurrence. Pica has been most commonly reported among blacks and Spanish-Americans in southeastern or southwestern states and among those who have migrated to northern cities. It is practiced primarily by pregnant women and preschool children, although it has occasionally been observed in men. Geophagia and starch eating may be causes of iron deficiency, either by limiting food intake or interfering with intestinal absorption, and the practice in children has not been eliminated by iron therapy.[55] However, pagophagia (ice craving) has been reported to respond to iron therapy.[56]

The effects of iron deficiency on psychological development and behavior have been studied, but methodological problems have made it impossible to isolate body iron status as a sole or even significant etiological factor.[56] The studies have not been uniformly persuasive nor free of alternative explanations.[57] Most studies of adults have failed to demonstrate psychomotor or behavioral disturbances attributable to iron deficiency. In infants and children, however, some behavioral changes have been reported, primarily a decrease in attentiveness, a short attention span, and random physical behavior. Since the children with low hemoglobin levels have usually been from low income families with less organization and poorer overall function than families of children with higher hemoglobin levels, the factors of motivation and fatigue may affect the testing of intelligence, work endurance, and learning. Nevertheless, "the biochemical ontogeny of some of the neural substrates for these behaviors would lead one to anticipate that the impact of iron deficiency should be most striking when imposed on a developing nervous system."[56] Future studies of young children should utilize more sensitive measures of pyschomotor performance, more complete biochemical assays, and greater control of alternative influences on the testing results.

When severe iron deficiency, by whatever means of diagnosis, has been identified, treatment with iron or other appropriate therapy should be instituted. Therapy should be continued after blood levels have been raised to the normal range so that repletion of tissues and storage is assured. The treatment of severe anemia is a medical problem that must be individualized. The cause may be blood loss due to injury, ulcer, cancer, parasitism, or other illness requiring treatment, and the underlying cause should be identified and treated. Milder degrees of anemia, usually associated with pregnancy, rapid growth, or menstruation, are more widespread among the population, and attention has been focused on prevention as a public health measure. This led to the program of enrichment of bread, cereal, and flour with iron.

BIOAVAILABILITY OF IRON

The enrichment program was begun in 1941. The form of iron to be used was not specified except that it should be "harmless and assimilable." A petition to increase the amount of iron in bread and flour in 1970 stimulated a major reevaluation of the fortification program and its results. Determining the bioavailability of the iron incorporated in food products involves the wide scope of iron absorption and utilization. Just as the identification of iron deficiency is subject to differing interpretations, so also iron absorption is poorly understood and experimental studies performed under differing conditions produce conflicting findings. Unfortunately, species differences in absorption make the application of data from dogs, rats, and mice to humans of doubtful value.[58]

The human body conserves iron to a remarkable degree, recycling iron released from destruction of erythrocytes and other body cells except those that are sloughed from the intestinal mucosa. The body has a limited ability to excrete iron except by bleeding, so normal balance is maintained by the control of absorption. The chemical form of iron as it enters the mucosal cells, the nature of the receptor sites, and the transmucosal transport system are not well understood at the present time. The amount of dietary iron absorbed by adults may be as low as 0.3 percent and is rarely as high as 45 percent.[58] The complexity of factors that increase or decrease absorption have led to inconsistent findings and interpretations.

Gastric acidity aids in releasing iron from complexes in foods, making it soluble and ionized. Reducing agents, such as ascorbic acid, are essential in converting ferric to ferrous iron. Ferrous iron has greater solubility than the ferric form in the neutral to alkaline pH of the duodenum. Chelating agents (ascorbic acid, succinic acid, sugars, or sulfur-containing amino acids) combine with iron to form low molecular chelates and promote absorption. Absorption is increased by a high concentration of iron in the duodenum. Heme iron is presumably absorbed by a different and more efficient process than nonheme iron, and the presence of heme iron may increase absorption of other iron. On the other hand, substances such as phosphates and possibly phytic acid may combine with iron to form insoluble compounds unavailable for absorption. Therefore, absorption of iron from any single food depends not only on the amount and kind of iron in the food itself, but also on the presence in the gastrointestinal tract of other foods in a composite diet.

Physiological factors in the individual also affect iron absorption. When gastric motility is increased, transit time is shortened and absorption lowered. When the body's need for iron is high, absorption is increased; this occurs in anemia and in periods of accelerated hematopoiesis, such as during the latter half of pregnancy and during rapid growth in the child. Iron overload may occur when control of absorption is faulty, in hemochromatosis, or when high iron intakes are prolonged, as observed with the Bantus who consume a beverage fermented in iron pots that contribute large amounts of iron to the beverage.

Absorption from plant sources ranges from 1 to 10 percent and from meat sources 10 to 20 percent.[59] Absorption from mixed diets therefore depends in part on the composition of the diet. For the adult male with normal body iron status, absorption is usually assumed to be 10 percent from mixed diets, and this figure is commonly used in estimating dietary requirements or allowances. However, in the latter half of pregnancy, in infants and children, and in anemic subjects, absorption of iron from mixed diets may average 20 percent or more. The RDAs of the United States[31] were calculated on the premise that 10 percent of dietary iron is absorbed by all age groups. The Caribbean RDAs[37] adopted the estimate of 15 percent used by FAO/WHO. The Dietary Standard for Canada[36] used 10 percent absorption for all except menstruating females for whom 12 percent absorption was used (based on evidence that their absorption is 25 percent higher than for men) and 20 percent absorption in pregnancy and lactation.

The bioavailability of iron in enriched products has intermittently been challenged since the origin of the enrichment program in 1941.[60] However, with lack of specification except that it be "harmless and assimilable," practicality in food processing became a major determinant of the chemical form of the iron.[58] Although it had been recognized in the 1930s that ferrous sulfate was more effective than other iron salts in the treatment of iron-deficiency anemia, it was not commonly used for enrichment purposes because its high reactivity shortens shelf life of the product and it may alter the color of some foods. Reduced iron was shown in some studies to be moderately well absorbed, but, because it has a high density compared to flour, a stable blend was difficult to maintain. Reduced iron, especially the more effective smaller particle size, also affected the color of products to which it was added. Therefore, a large proportion of the iron added to bread, flour, and similar products, was an iron phosphate, either ferric orthophosphate or sodium iron pyrophosphate. The phosphates are chemically inert in flour and inconspicuously white in color. Unfortunately, they also tend to be inert in the gastrointestinal tract.[58] The absorption of these phosphates from enriched infant cereals was found to be less than 1 percent, while absorption of ferrous sulfate from milk- or soy-based formulas was 3.4 to 5.4 percent.[61] Within the past decade there has been a trend toward use of more highly available forms of iron in enrichment. Studies have been done on specially milled iron with particle size of 5 to 10 μm and on encapsulated ferrous sulfate. Bioavailability should obviously be a major criterion in the choice of the form of iron. There is need for official assay methods of assessing bioavailability of iron from different sources.[58] It has also been suggested that it would be prudent to place upper limits on the quantity of iron and other nutrients permitted in enrichment of foods in the United States.[62,63]

OBESITY

"Obesity has become in our time a national problem, if not, indeed, a national obsession."[64] Although it is often thought to be a by-product of affluence, it is found in all areas of the world and, in the United States, in all income groups. Criteria for the definition of obesity are not clearly established for any population group and vary from one group to another. An individual considered obese in one society might not be considered obese in another.[65] Concepts of obesity even within a single society change with time. Not many years ago the "fine figure of a woman" and the "healthy chubby baby" were admired in our culture and are still admired among many subcultures and in many other parts of the world.

Recognition of the medical significance of obesity has caused a shift in attitudes toward excessive weight. The epidemiological evidence of a relationship between obesity and cardiovascular disease, hypertension, and diabetes has caused a reevaluation of the risks of obesity. There is as yet no clear agreement about whether obesity is a causal factor or merely a co-existing condition, but the findings have stimulated extensive research into the physical, metabolic, psychological, and social concomitants of obesity. Many types of therapy have been successful in short-term weight reduction, but their results in the long-term maintenance of lower weight have been disappointing. Therefore attention has increasingly been focused on the etiology of obesity with the hope of developing methods of prevention.

Obesity is the excessive deposition of body fat. When caloric intake exceeds energy output, the surplus is stored in body fat depots with increase in weight. These two statements are generally accepted as true but are deceptively simple. Obesity or, more properly, obesities are multifactorial states with complex genesis. Individual variations in causation, time of development, sites of fat deposition, and clinical significance have defied easy classification of the obesities. Studies of obese individuals have usually been done after the weight gain has occurred, so the information on factors that might have been causative are subject to retrospective error, and the observed physiological or psychological state may have followed rather than preceded development of obesity. As a result, interpretation of reported differences, whether in caloric intake, physical activity, glucose metabolism, or other variables, between obese and nonobese subjects must be undertaken with caution.

ADIPOCYTES AND FAT DEPOTS

Fat is the most variable component of the body, and the difficulties of measurement of total fat preclude direct and precise knowledge. However, it has been estimated that, on the average, fat comprises 12 to 16 percent of body weight at birth in full-term infants. The rapid increase in the first year is evidenced by estimates of 16 percent at one month, 26 percent at four months, and 24 to 30 percent at one year. Estimates then decline to 12 to 14 percent, perhaps by the age of 5 years, with a plateau at that level until the preadolescent increase. Boys are estimated to have an average of 17 percent of weight as fat by age 10 years and decrease to 11 percent by age 16. In contrast, females increase during adolescence to 24 percent by 16 years. Between 20 and 60 years of age, men are estimated to have an increase to 36 percent and women to 40 percent. A body fat content higher than 20 percent of body weight in adult males or 30 percent in females represents obesity.[66]

As analytical techniques have improved, increasing attention has been focused on the fat cell itself, the adipocyte. Obesity may result from either an increase in the number of adipocytes or an increase in the lipid content of cells already present. Adipocytes are assumed to follow the same pattern of cellular development as shown in Figure 1.1. However, the use of DNA as an index of fat cell number is unreliable in adipose tissue since it does not distinguish between the nucleic acid from fat cell nuclei and that from associated fibroblasts.[67] Three methods in use for measuring the size of individual adipocytes are the microscopic measurement of the diameter of the adipocyte in fixed tissue, the optical measurement of the diameter of individual cells isolated by treatment with collagenase, and the electronic count of osmium-fixed fat cells. The first two methods are tedious and measure only diameter. The electronic counting method has the major disadvantage that cells smaller than 25 microns are lost to count.[66]

The electronic counting method, described in 1968 by Hirsch and Gallian,[68] can produce a count of the cells in a given weight of tissue obtained by needle aspiration as well as an estimate of the size of the cells. However, the cell must contain a minimum of 0.01 μg lipid in order to be counted.[69] Therefore, adipocytes may be present, but too small to be counted or too low in lipid to be counted.[70] It is possible, then, by this technique that adipose cells may be present but uncounted in thin individuals or that after weight loss of an obese individual the cell count might appear to drop. In addition, variation in cell size, both in subcutaneous and deep fat depots, is so great between sites in a single individual that estimates of total adipose cell number may vary by as much as 85 percent and that at least three subcutaneous fat sites should be analyzed for a reliable cell count.[71] With these qualifications to the interpretation of current estimates of cell number and cell size, direct studies of adipocytes have already shown differences between obese and nonobese subjects. A more complete view of the changes in individuals before, during, and after the development of obesity can be expected as data from longitudinal observations of individuals are reported.

In obese adult subjects the increase in adipose cell size may be 50 to 100 percent, but the increase in cell number may exceed 200 percent.[67] Therefore, in the grossly obese total body fat seems to be related more to cell number than to cell size. However, further studies have indicated that two types of obesity may be identified.[69,71] Those with hyperplasia have a marked increase in cell number with small to moderate increase in cell size. Those with hypertrophic cells may or may not have an increase in cell number but have cells with higher lipid content. Although there is some evidence that hyperplastic obesity in adults is more likely to have its origin in childhood, it is not yet clear whether all childhood obesity is accompanied by hyperplasia. Weight reduction in adults is accomplished primarily by decrease in cell size as a result of their lower lipid content. It is still controversial whether some degree of decrease in cell number may also occur in weight reduction.[69,72]

BODY MEASUREMENTS OF OBESITY

Overweight and obesity, as well as the converse state of leanness, are not distinct entities but are, instead, differing levels in the continuum of the distribution of body weights. Therefore arbitrary cutoff points must be selected to identify the overweight and the obese, creating some confusion in prevalence based on the points chosen. Definitions also vary with the methods used for measuring or estimating weight, fat, and body composition. As discussed in Chapter 1, usual measurements of body composition are indirect, and the formulas derived are based on assumptions that are difficult to validate in the intact living body. Measurements of fat thickness by calipers have become standard procedure, but individual variations in sites of fat deposition and uncertainty about the percentage of body fat that is subcutaneous leave some questions still unanswered about the interpretation of skinfold measurements.

Body weight per se has repeatedly been shown to be an inappropriate measure of obesity. All obese persons are overweight, but not all overweight persons are obese. The trained athlete with heavy muscles may be overweight due to a large lean body mass rather than fat. It is impossible to make a precise differentiation between body fat and lean body mass, but such a differentiation is critical to the diagnosis of obesity.

Weight for height (relative weight) is a better index than weight alone, but must be specific for age and sex. From early infancy females have more body fat than males. Age changes in body fat are evident from the newborn to the elderly. However, weight is not independent of height during childhood, although it is in the adult. Various indices of weight to height were reviewed in the previous chapter.

Placing an individual into a weight category necessitates the use of a standard for comparison. In the absence of data on what might be considered "ideal" weight, mean or median weights from various sources have been used. For children, initial standards were based on fragmentary measurements taken during health examinations in school. The Stuart-Meredith standards,[73] derived from a longitudinal follow-up of children in Boston and Iowa City, were widely used for many years after their publication. More recently, the cross-sectional growth curves of the National Center for Health Statistics[74] from national representative surveys of children from 2 to 18 years, supplemented by data from birth to 3 years from the longitudinal studies of the Fels Research Institute, have been published. Standards for adults through most of the past century were based on measurements of individuals accepted for life insurance policies; they were measured wearing shoes and indoor clothing. These were refined to include "frame size" and later revised as "desirable" weights based on longevity statistics. The Health Examination Survey of 1960–1962 of the National Center for Health Statistics[75] has provided measurements of a stratified random sample of adults in the United States. These are observed weights and do not represent an "ideal."

Although opinions differ, the most common definitions based on the comparison of weight or weight for height to a standard (mean or median) for age and sex have identified as overweight individuals who are 10 to 20 percent above standard weight and as obese those who are 20 percent or more above the standard. When percentiles have been used rather than percentage deviation, the cutoff point to designate obesity has varied from the 85th to the 95th percentile. Obviously the selection of the criterion for obesity influences its prevalence.

Caliper measurements of fat thickness are directed toward objective estimation of subcutaneous fat itself and are better indices of body fat than either weight alone or weight-to-height ratios. They can be easily obtained without complicated equipment or special laboratory facilities. However, individual, sex, and age variations in patterns of fat deposition affect the degree to which measurement at a specific site reflects total body fat. Validation of various sites as reliable indices has usually been accomplished by comparison with other measures of body fat, such as relative weight, body density, or roentgenography. For example, correlation coefficients of relative weight and skinfold measurements have often been reported in the range of 0.5 to 0.8 in children and adult males, but somewhat lower in women. These correlations are better than with weight alone. Correlations of skinfold measurements with body density are higher.

Age changes in subcutaneous fat measurements were shown in Figure 1.15. There is a marked increase in the first six to nine months, then a de-

104   ASSESSMENT OF NUTRITIONAL STATUS

crease until preadolescence, when subcutaneous fat thickness increases in both sexes. During adolescence the increase continues in girls but boys have a decrease, at least in the extremities, although trunk fat may not show the same decrease. Children tend to have a larger percent of total body fat distributed on the limbs rather than on the trunk, when compared to adults. Adolescent girls and women tend to have greater fat accumulation near the pelvic girdle than men. Therefore, sites for measurement should be chosen to be most representative for age and sex. In a study of infants, Crawford et al.[76] found the suprailiac or triceps skinfold measurements most representative. Triceps and subscapular sites have been found by most observers to reflect body fat best for the adolescent and young adult male. For adolescent and adult females, fat thickness at the iliac crest is a better index of total fatness than measurements on the extremities. Despite increase in body fat and decrease in lean body tissue in the elderly, these changes may not be significantly reflected in subcutaneous fat measurements, although average triceps fatfold measurements decreased in the TSNS subjects.

The fatfold measurement at the triceps has been most commonly used, partially because of the ease of obtaining the measurement quickly without requiring the subject to undress. Standards for defining obesity from the triceps skinfold measurements for American subjects from 5 to 50 years of age have been established by Seltzer and Mayer[77] (Table 2.5). These have been adjusted for skewness of the data and represent one standard deviation above the logarithmic mean.

"CRITICAL AGES" IN DEVELOPMENT OF OBESITY

Several studies have attempted to determine whether there are critical ages during childhood when obesity is more prevalent or when the pattern may be set for later obesity. General somatic growth, as indicated earlier, occurs from conception to maturity, but not in a linear pattern. Growth is most rapid in the fetal period, rapid but decelerating in the first year, slow but relatively steady during early childhood, with a final acceleration in puberty, and cessation at the end of adolescence. Whether adipose cells follow the same pattern has not yet been determined. If adipose cellularity can be increased by overfeeding or restricted by the limitation of intake during infancy or early childhood, the implications for regulating infant feeding are clear insofar as prevention of obesity is concerned, although other aspects of physical and physiological growth must be considered. There is some evidence that hypercellularity may be identified in young children,[78] but to date the range of normal variations has not yet been established and only by long-term studies can the ultimate effects in adulthood be determined. Knittle[78] suggested four questions that need to be answered: (1) At what age in

Table 2.5 Obesity Standards in Caucasian Americans

Age (Years)	Minimum Triceps Skinfold Thickness Indicating Obesity (Millimeters)	
	Males	Females
5	12	14
6	12	15
7	13	16
8	14	17
9	15	18
10	16	20
11	17	21
12	18	22
13	18	23
14	17	23
15	16	24
16	15	25
17	14	26
18	15	27
19	15	27
20	16	28
21	17	28
22	18	28
23	18	28
24	19	28
25	20	29
26	20	29
27	21	29
28	22	29
29	22	29
30–50	23	30

Note: To normalize skewness to the right, longarithmic means rather than arithmetic means were used. The figures represent logarithmic means plus one standard deviation.

Source: Seltzer, C.C., and J. Mayer. A simple criterion of obesity. *Postgrad. Med.* *38*:A101–107, 1965.

man is adult adipose cell number and size achieved? (2) At what age do obese subjects begin to deviate from normal cellular development? (3) At what age do obese subjects exceed normal adult values for size and number? (4) At what age, if any, can cell number be altered by dietary means?

The literature is replete with studies relating weight at birth or during infancy or childhood with weight at some later age. The findings are controversial. "Critical" ages when body weight or weight gain may be setting the pattern for adult obesity or leanness have been concluded by various research workers to be: the last trimester of pregnancy; birth to 6 months or 1 year or 3 years or 4 years; 4 to 7 years; 5 to 8 years; 7 to 11 years; 9 to 13 years; and adolescence. In a review of published studies, Weil[79] concluded that "the likelihood that obesity will progress from infancy to childhood to adult life is still questionable and may be more important in the individual child than as a significant cause of adult obesity." The summary of a workshop on fetal and infant nutrition and susceptibility to obesity[80] contains the statement that "there is still no convincing evidence that the obese child becomes an obese adult; correlations of weight, weight gain, or skinfold measurements at birth or in the first year with comparable measures at ages 7 to 16 years have rarely been found to be as high as 0.25." Not all obese adults were obese as children, and not all obese infants or children become obese adults. The complexity of genetic, nutritional, social, economic, physiological, and psychological factors leads to the realization that the causes and characteristics of obesity are unique to each individual and that generalizations, while useful, are difficult to validate.

In the TSNS findings,[81] the average female had consistently higher triceps fatfold measurements than the average male; in the middle adult years the difference was twofold. After three years of age, white females were fatter than black females only to adolescence; during adulthood black females were heavier than white. When the data were analyzed by income levels, males at all ages from higher income levels were consistently fatter than those from lower income levels. In contrast, women showed an income-related reversal of fatness in late adolescence. Girls from higher income families had thicker fatfold measurements through childhood and early adolescence, but in late adolescence and adulthood women from lower income levels were fatter. These data suggest that if the theory that patterns of obesity may be established by adiposity in early childhood is valid, they may be altered by socioeconomic and cultural factors later in life, related perhaps to differences in energy expenditure and weight control.

REFERENCES

1. Habicht, J.-P., J. M. Lane, and A. J. McDowell. Nutritional national surveillance. *Fed. Proc. 37*:1181-1187, 1978.
2. Pearson, W. N. Biochemical appraisal of the vitamin nutritional status in man. *JAMA 180*: 49-55, 1962
3. McLaren, D. S. Nutritional Assessment. In: McLaren, D. S., and D. Burman (Eds.) *Textbook of Paediatric Nutrition*. Churchill Livingstone, New York, 1976.

4. U.S. Department of Health, Education, and Welfare. *Ten-State Nutrition Survey, 1968-1970.* DHEW Publications No. (HSM) 72-8130, 72-8131, 72-8132, and 72-8133. Supt. of Documents, U.S. Government Printing Office, Washington, D.C., 1972.

5. Owen, G. M., K. M. Kram, P. J. Garry, J. E. Lowe, and A. H. Lubin. A study of nutritional status of preschool children in the United States, 1968-1970. *Pediat. 53* (Suppl., Part 2):597-646, 1974.

6. Abraham, S., F. W. Lowenstein, and C. L. Johnson. *Preliminary Findings of the First Health and Nutrition Examination Survey, United States, 1971-1972: Dietary Intake and Biochemical Findings.* DHEW Publication No. (HRA) 74-1219-1. Supt. of Documents, U.S. Government Printing Office, Washington, D.C., 1974.

7. Abraham, S., F. W. Lowenstein, and D. E. O'Connell. *Preliminary Findings of the First Health and Nutrition Examination Survey, United States, 1971-1972: Anthropometric and Clinical Findings.* DHEW Publication No. (HRA) 75-1229. Supt. of Documents, U.S. Government Printing Office, Washington, D. C., 1975.

8. Abraham, S., M. D. Carroll, C. M. Dresser, and C. L. Johnson. *Dietary Intake Findings, United States, 1971-1974.* DHEW Publication No. (HRA) 77-1647. Supt. of Documents, U.S. Government Printing Office, Washington, D. C., 1977.

9. *Nutrition: A National Priority.* A Report by Nutrition Canada to the Department of National Health and Welfare. Information Canada, Ottawa, 1973.

10. *Food Consumption Patterns Report.* A Report from Nutrition Canada by the Bureau of Nutritional Health Sciences, Health Protection Branch, Department of National Health and Welfare, Ottawa, 1977.

11. Christakis, G. (Ed.) Nutritional Assessment in Health Programs. *Am. J. Public Health 63*: Suppl, November, 1973.

12. Expert Committee on Medical Assessment of Nutritional Status: Report. Tech. Rept. Series No. 528. World Health Organization, Geneva, 1963.

13. Sandstead, H. H., and W. N. Pearson. Clinical Evaluation of Nutritional Status. In: Goodhart, R. S., and M. E. Shils (Eds.) *Modern Nutrition in Health and Disease*, Fifth Edition. Lea and Febiger, Philadelphia, 1973.

14. Huenemann, R. L., M. C. Hampton, A. R. Behnke, L. R. Shapiro, and B. W. Mitchell. *Teenage Nutrition and Physique.* Charles C Thomas, Springfield, Ill., 1974.

15. Zerfas, A. J., I. J. Shorr, and C. G. Neumann. Office assessment of nutritional status. *Pediat. Clin. No. Amer. 24*:253-272, 1977.

16. Roche, A. F., J. Roberts, and P. V. V. Hamill. *Skeletal Maturity of*

Children 6–11 Years: Racial, Geographic Area, and Socioeconomic Differences. DHEW Publ. No. (HRA) 76-1631. Supt. of Documents, U.S. Government Printing Office, Washington, D. C., 1975.

17. McKigney, J. I., and Roche, A. F. Physical growth of ethnic groups comprising the United States population. *Am. J. Clin. Nutr. 28*: 1071-1074, 1975.
18. Owen, G., and G. Lippman. Nutritional status of infants and young children: U.S.A. *Pediat. Clin. No. Amer. 24*:211-227, 1977.
19. Garn, S. M., F. A. Larkin, and P. E. Cole. The problem with one-day dietary intakes. *Ecol. Food Nutr. 5*:245-247, 1976.
20. Hegsted, D. M. Problems in the use and interpretation of the Recommended Dietary Allowances. *Ecol. Food Nutr. 1* :255-265, 1972.
21. Youland, D. M., and A. Engle. Dietary study methodology: Practices and problems in HANES. *J. Am. Dietet. Assoc. 68*:22-25, 1976.
22. Beal, V. A. Nutritional Intake. In: McCammon, R. W. (Ed.) *Human Growth and Development.* Charles C Thomas, Springfield, Ill., 1970.
23. Chalmers, F. W., M. M. Clayton, L. O. Gates, R. E. Tucker, A. W. Wertz, C. M. Young, and W. D. Foster. The dietary record—how many and which days? *J. Am. Dietet. Assoc. 28*:711-717, 1952.
24. Madden, J. P., S. J. Goodman, and H. A. Guthrie. Validity of the 24-hour recall. *J. Am. Dietet. Assoc. 68*:143-147, 1976.
25. Marr, J. W. Individual dietary surveys: Purposes and methods. *World Rev. Nutr. Dietet. 13*:105-164, 1971.
26. Flores, M. Dietary studies for assessment of the nutritional status of populations in nonmodernized societies. *Am. J. Clin. Nutr. 11*:344-355, 1962.
27. Becker, B. G., B. P. Indik, and A. M. Beeuwkes. *Dietary Intake Methodologies. A Review.* Tech. Rept., University of Michigan, Ann Arbor, 1960.
28. *Screening Children for Nutritional Status: Suggestions for Child Health Programs.* U.S. Department of Health, Education and Welfare, Maternal and Child Health Service, Rockville, Md., 1971.
29. Beal, V. A. The nutritional history in longitudinal research. *J. Am. Dietet. Assoc. 51*:426-432, 1967.
30. Kimura, K. K. *The Nutritional Significance of Dietary Fiber.* Life Sciences Research Office, Federation of American Societies for Experimental Biology, Bethesda, Md., 1977.
31. *Recommended Dietary Allowances,* Eighth Edition. National Academy of Sciences, Washington, D.C., 1974.
32. *Folic Acid—Biochemistry and Physiology in Relation to the Human Nutrition Requirement.* National Academy of Sciences, Washington, D.C., 1977.

33. Hunscher, H. A., and I. G. Macy. Dietary study methods. I. Uses and abuses of dietary study methods. *J. Am. Dietet. Assoc. 27*:558-563, 1951.
34. Harper, A. E. Those pesky RDAs. *Nutrition Today 9*:15-22, 27-28, 1974.
35. Hegsted, D. M. On dietary standards. *Nutr. Rev. 36*:33-36, 1978.
36. Dietary Standard for Canada. Printing and Publishing Supply and Services, Ottawa, 1976.
37. Recommended Dietary Allowances for the Caribbean. Caribbean Food and Nutrition Institute, Kingston, Jamaica, 1976.
38. Moore, C. V. Iron. In: Goodhart, R. S., and M. E. Shils (Eds.) *Modern Nutrition in Health and Disease,* Fifth Edition. Lea and Febiger, Philadelphia, 1973.
39. Woodruff, C. W. Iron deficiency in infancy and childhood. *Pediat. Clin. No. Amer. 24*:85-94, 1977.
40. Hallberg, L., A. Högdahl, L. Nilsson, and G. Rybo. Menstrual blood loss: A population study. *Acta Obstet. Gynecol. Scand. 45*:320-351, 1966.
41. Bowering, J., A. M. Sanchez, and M. I. Irwin. A conspectus of research on iron requirements of man. *J. Nutr. 106*:985-1074, 1976.
42. Pearson, H. A. Life-span of the fetal red blood cell. *J. Pediat. 70*:166-171, 1967.
43. Saarinen, U. M., M. A. Siimes, and P. R. Dallman. Iron absorption in infants: High bioavailability of breast milk iron as indicated by the extrinsic tag method of iron absorption and by the concentration of serum ferritin. *J. Pediat. 91*:36-39, 1977.
44. Siimes, M. A., J. R. Addiego, Jr., and P. R. Dallman. Ferritin in serum: Diagnosis of iron deficiency and iron overload in infants and children. *Blood 43*:581-590, 1974.
45. Lipschitz, D. A., J. D. Cook, and C. A. Finch. A clinical evaluation of serum ferritin as an index of iron stores. *N. E. J. Med. 290*:1213-1216, 1974.
46. Piomelli, S., A. Brickman, and E. Carlos. Rapid diagnosis of iron deficiency by measurement of free erythrocyte porphyrins and hemoglobin: the FEP/hemoglobin ratio. *Pediat. 57*:136-141, 1976.
47. Food and Nutrition Board Committee on Iron Nutritional Deficiency. *Workshop on Extent and Meanings of Iron Deficiency in the U.S., March 8-9, 1971. Summary of Proceedings.* National Academy of Sciences, Washington, D. C.
48. Harris, J. W., and R. W. Kellermeyer. *The Red Cell. Production, Metabolism, Destruction: Normal and Abnormal.* Harvard University Press, Cambridge, 1970.
49. Garn, S. M., N. J. Smith, and D. C. Clark. Lifelong differences in

hemoglobin levels between blacks and whites. *J. Nat. Med. Assoc.* *67*:91-96, 1975.

50. Dallman, P. R., G. D. Barr, C. M. Allen, and H. R. Shinefield. Hemoglobin concentration in white, black, and Oriental children: is there a need for separate criteria in screening for anemia? *Am. J. Clin. Nutr. 31*:377-380, 1978.

51. Elwood, P. C. Evaluation of the clinical importance of anemia. *Am. J. Clin. Nutr. 26*:958-964, 1973.

52. Strauss, R. G. Iron deficiency, infections, and immune function: A reassessment. *Am. J. Clin. Nutr. 31*:660-666, 1978.

53. Weinberg, E. D. Iron and susceptibility to infectious disease. *Science 184*:952-956, 1974.

54. Chandra, R. K. Iron and immunocompetence. *Nutr. Rev. 34*:129-132, 1974.

55. Gutelius, M. F., F. K. Millican, E. M. Layman, G. J. Cohen, and C. C. Dublin. Nutritional studies of children with pica. 2. Treatment of pica with iron given intramuscularly. *Pediat. 29*:1012-1023, 1962.

56. Leibel, R. L. Behavioral and chemical correlates of iron deficiency. A review. *J. Am. Dietet. Assoc. 71*:398-404, 1977.

57. Sulzer, J. L. Significance of iron deficiencies. Effects of iron deficiency on psychological tests in children. In: *Food and Nutrition Board Committee on Iron Nutritional Deficiencies. Workshop on Extent and Meanings of Iron Deficiency in the U.S. March 8-9, 1971. Summary of Proceedings.* National Academy of Sciences, Washington, D.C.

58. Waddell, J. *The Bioavailability of Iron Sources and Their Utilization in Food Enrichment.* Life Sciences Research Office, Fed. Am. Soc. Exper. Biol., Bethesda, Md., 1973.

59. Layrisse, M.,and C. Martinez-Torres. Food iron absorption: Iron supplementation of food. *Progr. Hematol. 7*:137-160, 1971.

60. The dietary iron controversy. *Nutrition Today 7*:2-35, 1972.

61. Rios, E., R. E. Hunter, J. D. Cook, N. J. Smith, and C. A. Finch. The absorption of iron as supplements in infant cereal and infant formulas. *Pediat. 55*:686-693, 1975.

62. Crosby, W. H. Editorial—Fortification of food with carbonyl iron. *Am. J. Clin. Nutr. 31*:572-573, 1978.

63. Darby, W. J. and L. Hambraeus. Proposed nutritional guidelines for utilization of industrially produced nutrients. *Nutr. Rev. 36*:65-71, 1978.

64. Mayer, J. *Overweight, Causes, Cost, and Control.* Prentice-Hall, Englewood Cliffs, N.J., 1968.

65. Weil, W. B., Jr. Infantile obesity. In: Winick, M. (Ed.) *Childhood Obesity.* John Wiley and Sons, New York, 1975.

66. Bray. G. A. *The Obese Patient.* W. B. Saunders, Philadelphia, 1976.

67. Garrow, J. S. *Energy Balance and Obesity in Man.* North-Holland/American Elsevier, New York, 1974.
68. Hirsch, J., and E. Gallian. Methods for the determination of adipose cell size in man and animals. *J. Lipid Res. 9*:110-119, 1968.
69. Hirsch, J., and J. Knittle. Cellularity of obese and nonobese human adipose tissue. *Fed. Proc. 29*:1516-1521, 1970.
70. Widdowson, E. M. Cellular growth and function. *Proc. Nutr. Soc. 35*:357-362, 1976.
71. Salans, L. B., S. W. Cushman, and R. E. Weismann. Studies of human adipose tissue. Adipose cell size and number in nonobese and obese patients. *J. Clin. Invest. 52*:929-941, 1973.
72. Hirsch, J. Cell number and size as a determinant of subsequent obesity. In: Winick, M. (Ed.) *Childhood Obesity.* John Wiley and Sons, New York, 1975.
73. Vaughn, V. C., III. Developmental Pediatrics. In: Vaughn, V. C. III, R. J. McKay, and W. E. Nelson (Eds.) *Nelson Textbook of Pediatrics,* Tenth Edition. W. B. Saunders, Philadelphia, 1975.
74. Hamill, P. V. V., T. A. Drizd, C. L. Johnson, R. B. Reed, and A. F. Roche. *NCHS Growth Curves for Children Birth—18 Years,* U. S. DHEW Publ. No. (PHS) 78-1650. Supt. of Documents, U. S. Government Printing Office, Washington, D. C., 1977.
75. Roberts, J. *Weight by Height and Age of Adults, United States, 1960–1962.* Public Health Service Publication No. 1000—Series 11—No. 14, Supt. of Documents, U.S. Government Printing Office, Washington, D. C. 1966.
76. Crawford, B. P., C. A. Keller, M. C. Hampton, F. P. Pacheco, and R. L. Huenemann. An obesity index for six month old infants. *Am. J. Clin. Nutr. 27*:706-711, 1974.
77. Seltzer, C. C., and J. Mayer. A simple criterion of obesity. *Postgrad. Med. 38*:A101-107, 1965.
78. Knittle, J. Obesity in childhood: A problem in adipose tissue cellular development. *J. Pediat. 81*:1048-1059, 1972.
79. Weil, W. B., Jr. Current controversies in childhood obesity. *J. Pediat. 91*:175-187, 1977.
80. Committee on the Nutrition of the Mother and Preschool Child, Food and Nutrition Board. *Fetal and Infant Nutrition and Susceptibility to Obesity.* National Academy of Sciences, Washington, D. C., 1978.
81. Garn, S. M., and D. C. Clark. Trends in fatness and the origins of obesity. *Pediat. 57*:443-456, 1976.

3

PREGNANCY

The union of an ovum and a sperm cell to form a zygote, which becomes an embryo and later a fetus within the uterine environment and finally emerges as an independent neonate, all within a relatively short span of time, involves a wide range of physiological processes in both the mother and her developing offspring. The synchronization of changes in the maternal body, the cooperative formation of the placenta as a link, and the differentiation and growth of tissues in the fetus proceed in a remarkable pattern that we are only beginning to understand, especially in the human.

The importance of nutrition in reproduction is evident from the fact that tissue, whether maternal or fetal, is formed from nutrients that originated in the mother's diet, past or present. A woman who is well-nourished when she conceives and whose diet during pregnancy contains the quantity, quality, and ratio of nutrients to meet her increased requirements is likely to have fewer complications during pregnancy and delivery, to produce a healthier infant, and to be in better physical state after delivery than a woman whose nutritional state is marginal or inadequate. Good nutrition during pregnancy also is the foundation of successful lactation. However, it is difficult to delineate the comparative effects of differing levels of nutrient intake on mother and fetus because of the interdependence of dietary intake with other environmental and physical aspects of socioeconomic status, many of which may also affect the reproductive process.

In addition, the remarkable ability of the body to adjust to changes in the internal milieu and to nutrient supply is especially pronounced during pregnancy. The maternal changes that accompany the pregnant state provide a high degree of protection to the fetus. Increase in the percentage absorption of nutrients results in greater utilization of dietary components. Alterations in hormonal production of the woman during pregnancy are in the direction of increased nitrogen retention, deposition of maternal fat stores that may be mobilized in need, and adequate provision of glucose, amino acids, and other nutrients to the fetus. As a result, the fetus is somewhat sheltered against alterations in the maternal diet, even at the expense of maternal stores. However, evidence is increasing that inadequate maternal diet is closely related to retardation of growth of the fetus and that the drain on the maternal organism of repeated pregnancies without adequate nutritional intake results in long-term detriment to the woman's health.

The nutrition of the woman prior to conception is important to her success in reproduction. The woman who enters pregnancy in good nutritional state with adequate body reserves can provide a margin of safety in the supply of nutrients to the fetus even when her food intake during pregnancy is limited. This was shown by studies emanating from food shortages in World War II. In Holland[1] women who were previously well-nourished but subjected to food shortage only during pregnancy delivered infants who were, on the average, nearly 250 g lighter in weight than would have been expected, but there was no increase in rates of prematurity, stillbirths, or congenital defects. In contrast, average birth weights of the infants of women in Leningrad[2] who were undernourished as a result of a long period of siege were reduced 500 to 600 g, and the rates of prematurity, stillbirths, and neonatal mortality were sharply increased with continued food shortage during pregnancy.

The effects of poor nutritional status prior to pregnancy may be partially offset by improvement of the diet during pregnancy. In a study in Guatemala[3] in which one group of women was given dietary supplements during pregnancy, there was a small but significant increase in the birth weights of infants of the mothers given supplements in comparison to controls in the same villages. The most notable effect was a 40 percent reduction in birth weights less than 2.5 kg.

Concern about the quality and quantity of the diet during pregnancy was stimulated during the 1940s with the findings of several centers[4-8] that the outcome of pregnancy was related to the level of maternal nutrient intake. Women with poor intakes tended to deliver infants who were shorter and lighter in weight, with higher incidence of congenital malformations and higher perinatal mortality than women whose diets were good or those given either food or nutrient supplementation. Interest waned during the 1950s when those study methodologies were questioned and some additional studies did not produce comparable results. In fact, during that decade great emphasis was placed by some physicians on the restriction of weight gain

114

during pregnancy and dietary limitations were advised, usually with supplementation by mineral and/or vitamin preparations.

Since the early 1960s, interest in the adequacy of prenatal diet was again stimulated by realization that fetal growth could be compromised when its supply of nutrients was limited. For some time a birth weight of 2500 g had been used to differentiate between the full-term infant and the "premature" infant. In 1961 Warkany et al.[9] presented case reports of intrauterine growth retardation, and it has become increasingly evident that it is important to differentiate between two groups of infants with birth weights under 2500 g. Infants who are prematurely delivered are small because of insufficient time in utero. The gestational age for defining premature delivery has varied from 36 to 38 weeks, but is now generally accepted as 37 weeks or less. In contrast, a second group of infants with birth weights under 2500 g who have been in utero 37 weeks or more represent retardation of growth. The characteristics of these two groups of infants vary in degree of maturity, in physiological capabilities, and in risks of morbidity and mortality. Extensive studies have been in progress since that time to determine what factors may be operating to restrict growth. The nutritional status of the mother and her dietary intake during pregnancy are among the factors that influence the supply of nutrients to the fetus.

An additional stimulus to a reawakening of concern about maternal diet was the publication of *Maternal Nutrition and the Course of Pregnancy*[10] by the National Academy of Sciences in 1970. A reevaluation of published data on weight gain of the mother during pregnancy and the outcome of that pregnancy showed clearly that best results, both to mother and infant, were seen when weight gain was approximately 10 to 12 kg (24 lb). It was the consensus of the committee that "there is no advantage to be gained by prescribing weight reduction regimens for obese patients during pregnancy either for improving the course of pregnancy or for contributing to the woman's general health." Furthermore, "much greater emphasis should be placed on the value of a good diet during pregnancy, particularly for women entering pregnancy with poor nutritional status and poor dietary habits."

STAGES OF GESTATION

The length of gestation may be measured either by menstrual age or by ovulation age. Since fertilization of the ovum and the start of pregnancy occur after expulsion of the ovum from the ovary, at approximately the fourteenth day after the start of the previous menstrual period, gestation to full term averages about 266 days. However, since the date of the onset of the last menstrual period can usually be determined with more accuracy than the date of conception, menstrual age is more commonly used. In terms of menstrual age, gestation lasts 280 days, or 10 lunar months, or 40 weeks to term.

Since there is a range of variation from the stated expected date of delivery, delivery at or before 37 weeks is usually considered premature, and delivery at 42 weeks or more postmature.

There is no universally accepted time differentiation for various stages of pregnancy. The 9 calendar months may be divided into trimesters. The 40 weeks may be divided into quartiles of 10 weeks each. On the other hand, three or four periods may be identified according to fetal growth. The first period, during which the fertilized ovum travels down the Fallopian tube to the uterus, while cells are dividing to form a blastocyte that is implanted on the uterine wall, is sometimes called the period of blastogenesis, lasting about two weeks. This is followed by the embryonic period, a period of organogenesis, characterized by cell differentiation and formation of organs and structure of the fetus. Organogenesis is essentially completed by 56 to 60 days after conception, but some differentiation continues into the third month. The period from the fourth through the ninth months is considered the fetal period, and may be divided into early fetal (second trimester) and late fetal (third trimester) periods. Since embryonic/fetal development is a continuum and subject to individual variation in timing, such differentiations are not precise but are used for convenience.

FERTILIZATION, IMPLANTATION, AND ORGANOGENESIS

During their maturation before release, both the ovum and the sperm divide by meiosis so that each has the haploid number of chromosomes (23 in the human). Fertilization produces a zygote with the diploid number, half from each parent. The ovum is the largest cell of the female organism, with a diameter of approximately 0.14 mm, and contains a food reserve for the embryo until it begins to feed on exogenous material in the uterus. Between menarche and menopause the woman liberates only a few hundred ova as cells ready for fertilization. In contrast, the sperm is among the smallest of cells, measuring about 50 μ, and the male produces millions of spermatozoa between puberty and old age. Normal sperm content of semen is approximately 100 million/mm, although only a few thousand reach the site of fertilization, and the ovum normally rejects all except one sperm cell.[11-13]

The ovum is expelled from the ovarian follicles into the oviduct, or Fallopian tube, which is lined with ciliated mucosal cells that help to direct the egg toward the uterus and secrete a fluid that increases the fertilizing capaci-

116

ty of the sperm. After penetration of the ovum by the head of the sperm and union of the nuclei of the two cells, the resulting zygote begins to divide by mitosis, with each new cell containing 23 pairs of chromosomes. During this phase of division the cells are small. The cells form a cluster, or morula, which begins about the third day to travel down the oviduct to the uterus.

The early history of the fertilized ovum is characterized not only by cell division but also by cell specialization. Cell differentiation is accomplished by the synthesis of new types of protein, each with specialized characteristics and functions. Although theories have been proposed, the actual mechanism by which cells are differentiated is unknown. After the tissues have been differentiated, cell multiplication is then largely by reproduction of the same types of tissue proteins.

During passage, cells of the morula differentiate into two types. One develops into the blastocyte and will become the embryo. The outer layer forms the trophoblast, a protective and nourishing membrane that will further develop into the placenta and other encircling tissues. The separation of the two layers forms a cavity (blastocele) filled with fluid. By the fifth or sixth day after fertilization, the cluster of cells reaches the site of attachment to the uterus, usually on the posterior wall.

The uterus is an organ with a strong muscular layer, the myometrium, which is lined internally by mucosal cells, the endometrium. After a menstrual period, under the influence of ovarian hormones, first estrogen and then also progesterone, the endometrium thickens and develops a copious blood supply. The blood vessels become increasingly permeable. The effect of progesterone is to prepare the uterus for pregnancy. The process of implantation is a complex but orderly sequence of chemical and physical interactions between the embryonic cells and the uterus, occurring between the seventh and tenth days. It has been estimated that 50 percent of ova do not survive implantation. The trophoblast proliferates and invades the uterine surface by releasing proteolytic enzymes that act on the epithelial and stromal layers of the uterus. Uterine tissues undergo changes to supply a fluid for supplementation of the embryo's own food supply, to form spaces that fill with blood, and to provide bonding for the placenta.

Cell differentiation of the embryo continues during and after implantation, with formation of three germinal layers. The outer layer, the ectoderm, will form the basis for the skin, the cells lining the glands that open into it, parts of the eye, most of the nervous system, the adrenal medulla, the pituitary, epithelium of the nose and mouth, salivary glands, and tooth enamel. The endoderm will ultimately develop into the epithelial lining of most of the alimentary canal, most glands that open into it, as well as epithelium of ears, thyroid, parathyroids, thymus, respiratory tract, urinary tract, and prostate. The mesoderm will give rise to the remaining organs and tissues, including bone, cartilage, connective and sclerous tissue, teeth (except enamel), musculature, vascular and lymphatic systems, most of the genitourinary system, adrenal cortex, and the mesothelial lining of the pericardial, pleural, and peritoneal cavities. By the fourth week the main organs begin to form, and differentiation continues until the eighth to twelfth weeks, when the foundation of all organs will have been laid down. Thereafter, until the end of gestation, principal changes are those of further elaboration, development, and growth.

Development of the fetus occurs in a cephalocaudal progression. Changes in structure and function begin in the head and upper body and proceed downward toward the legs. The embryo seems topheavy, and even at birth the neonate has a larger head in proportion to the rest of the body than does the adult. The early rapid growth of the nervous system, including the spinal cord, makes it particularly vulnerable to alterations in environment during this early phase of gestation. At 8 weeks the embryo is perhaps 2 to 3 cm long and weighs 1 to 4 g; the central nervous system constitutes 25 percent of body weight.

Development is also proximodistal, beginning near the central axis and progressing toward the extremities. The head and trunk are fairly well developed when the limb buds appear, and the arms and legs are formed before fingers and toes.

The survival and proper development of the embryo depend on an interplay of hereditary, physiological, and environmental factors in the mother, the developing placenta, and the embryo itself. During this period mortality is probably higher than at any other time of life.[14] Growth of the embryo during the first trimester is primarily by hyperplasia, with rapid increase in DNA and protein synthesis indicative of the proliferation of cells. Nutrient requirements are quantitatively small but qualitatively critical. The embryo is extremely vulnerable to alterations in oxygen or nutrient supply, to radiation, drugs, or infection, and to variations in hormonal, nervous, and vascular functions. Many physical defects have their origin in abnormal genes or chromosomes or in any disturbance in cell differentiation or growth during the embryonic period. During the first few weeks, the embryo is dependent on its own supply of nutrients and on those obtained from uterine fluids, but with the establishment of the placenta and the first embryonic heart beat early in the fourth week, the placenta becomes the vital source of nutrition for the fetus.

THE PLACENTA

The placenta[11-24] is a specialized organ that is formed primarily from embryonic tissue for the purpose of supplying the embryo/fetus with oxygen, nutrients, hormones, and other vital substances, and of removing waste products to prevent their accumulation in the fetus. After the trophoblast has penetrated into the uterine mucosa, changes occur in both embryonic and maternal tissue to provide a link between the two.

The chorion, which surrounds the cluster of embryonic cells, begins to develop capillary-containing villi. The layers of decidua and the blood vessels of the uterus undergo alteration, forming pools of blood into which the villi project. The placenta, then, is bounded on the fetal side by the chorion and on the maternal side by the decidual plate, as shown in Figure 3.1. As the embryo grows, the villi become longer and more branched, providing greater surface area exposed to maternal blood. Maternal blood flow to the uterus increases to provide a greater supply of nutrients. Maternal and fetal blood do not mingle but are separated by the membranes of the villi, across which nutrients and other materials must be transported.

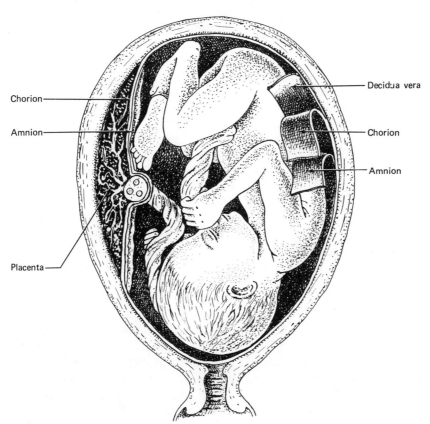

Figure 3.1 Diagrammatic representation of fetus, placenta, and uterine tissues.

The placenta becomes functional early in the fourth week, when the heart of the embryo begins to beat and its circulation becomes established. By the eighth week a distinct umbilical cord is in place between the chorion and the fetus. The cord contains a vein that carries materials to the fetus and two arteries which carry waste products, such as carbon dioxide, urea, creatinine, and uric acid, from the fetus back into the maternal circulation for disposal.

Placental growth and function are obviously difficult to measure in situ, but a combination of animal experiments, analyses of placentas from terminated pregnancies, and studies of maternal, fetal, and cord blood has provided data directly or by inference. The placenta is formed, grows, serves its purposes, ages, and is expelled at delivery. The weight, protein, and RNA content of the placenta continue linearly to term. However, cell multiplication ceases at 35 to 36 weeks, as estimated by DNA content. At that age the placenta weighs approximately 300 g and the fetus approximately 2300 g.[21] The reduction in nucleic acid synthesis after the 35th week is consistent with in vitro studies that indicate a shift in the glucose metabolic pathway in the placenta away from the hexose monophosphate shunt.[24] Therefore, the steep increase in fetal weight during the last weeks of gestation is sustained by a placenta with a constant number of cells; however the size of cells continues to increase. There are signs that the placenta may not be able to provide the fetus with enough nutrients to maintain its previous rate of growth, which begins to fall off after about the 36th week.[22]

Interpretation of available data on the transport of nutrients across the placenta and availability of maternal nutrients for the fetus must take into account the high rate of growth and metabolism of the placenta itself, particularly in early pregnancy. The placenta may alter organic substances during their passage and needs a supply of nutrients for its own synthesis of proteins, enzymes, nucleic acids, high-energy phosphates, and hormones.[16] It has been estimated that 10 to 30 percent of the oxygen delivered by maternal blood is utilized by the placenta. The placenta has a high concentration of both essential and nonessential amino acids[18] and during most of pregnancy maintains a storage of some nutrients. By the 12th week the placenta produces its own hormones.

Until approximately the 16th week, the placenta grows faster and weighs more than the embryo. Thereafter the fetus gains at a faster rate, and by term the ratio of fetal to placental weight is approximately 7:1.[22] When expelled at delivery, the placenta is a discoid mass that resembles a flattened cake (the Latin word placenta means cake). Its diameter averages 16 to 20 cm, with a thickness at its center of 3 to 4 cm.[12] The average weight is 500 g, but there is wide individual variation in placental weight and size. Placental weight at term has been variously reported between 325 and 1000 g. Since placental weight has been shown to correlate better with fetal weight than

120

with gestational age, it was suggested that placental size is a factor in determining fetal size, and that a small placenta could limit fetal growth. However, it is now believed that, since the fetus and placenta are both parts of the conceptus, they are subject to a common mechanism of growth regulation or that the fetus regulates growth of the placenta just as it controls the growth of its own internal organs.[17,18,22]

NUTRIENT TRANSFER

The transfer of nutrients from mother to fetus follows a pathway from the maternal blood into the intervillous spaces in the placenta, across the membranes of the villi, through placental capillaries to the umbilical vein, and finally into the fetal circulation. Therefore, several factors are involved in the transfer. The quantity, quality, and composition of the maternal blood determine the availability of oxygen, nutrients, and other materials. The degree of perfusion of blood in the intervillous spaces and the integrity and capability of the placenta to concentrate, synthesize, and transport nutrients, as well as the hydrostatic pressure in the intervillous spaces influence transfer. The surface area of the villi affects the amounts of nutrients that may cross the membrane, and finally the amount of umbilical blood flow influences the ease of transport into the fetal circulation.

Pathology may alter placental transfer. Circulatory changes in the mother, as in hypertension, or hormonal disturbances, as in diabetes, may alter the concentrations and availability of nutrients. Deficits in oxygen supply, as observed in pregnancy at high altitudes or in anemia, may limit fetal growth. The effects of pathology in the placenta itself, such as hemangiomata or infarcts, may alter the efficiency of the organ. Since the mechanisms of transfer under normal conditions are not well understood, it is even more difficult to evaluate the effects of aberrations in function.

The fetus is totally dependent on the supply of nutrients from the maternal organism. The fetus can synthesize its own carbohydrate, fat, and protein, but it must have a supply of glucose, amino acids, other short-chain metabolites, minerals, and vitamins. Placental transfer of each nutrient depends in part on its chemical properties. Water, gases, ions, or compounds with molecular weight under 1000 tend to cross the placenta by simple diffusion. Some nutrients, like glucose, require a specific carrier to facilitate diffusion. When passage of a nutrient is against an electrochemical gradient, energy (adenosine triphosphate) is needed to accomplish active transport. Pinocytosis may assist the transfer of some compounds and is believed to accomplish the transport of some amino acids or polypeptides.

Methods and rates of transfer of specific nutrients have been largely inferred from comparison of the concentrations in maternal and fetal blood.

For example, equilibrium between maternal and fetal blood suggests that the transfer is by simple or facilitated diffusion from the more concentrated maternal blood to the less concentrated fetal blood until the concentrations are equal. When fetal blood has a higher concentration than maternal blood, passage of the nutrient must be accomplished against an electrochemical gradient, requiring energy (adenosine triphosphate) for pumping, as in active transport. However, several mechanisms control the concentrations of some nutrients and limit the return of nutrients from the fetus to the maternal circulation. Some examples of these controls have been observed in animal experimentation and speculated upon in human physiology.

Glucose is the principal metabolic fuel for the fetus, and a continuous supply crosses the placenta with the aid of a highly specific carrier. Although some fructose also may cross the placenta, it is at a rate of only 10 percent of that of glucose, and galactose is not believed to be transferred to the fetus. The rate of transfer of glucose increases during gestation and may rise to more than 20 mg/min near term. Normally the level of glucose in fetal blood is lower than in maternal blood, but Widdowson has suggested that this may be a result of differences in the rate of removal of glucose from the blood on the fetal and maternal sides of the placenta.[17] Plasma glucose may be elevated in both the fetus and mother if she is diabetic.

The concentration of free amino acids is higher in fetal than in maternal blood, especially in early gestation, with the exception of cyst(e)ine, which is higher in maternal blood.[18] The differences in concentration suggest that a specific transport system requiring energy is involved in amino acid transport. Transfer of amino acids becomes more efficient later in pregnancy. It is possible that some polypeptides or maternal albumin may cross the placenta, perhaps by pinocytosis. No other intact maternal proteins are known to be transferred to the fetus with the exception of the immunoglobulin IgG, which may depend on specific receptors on the surface of the villi. The placenta synthesizes its own proteins, but there is no evidence that they are transferred to the fetus. It has been observed, however, that the ratio of essential to nonessential amino acids is significantly greater in the placenta than in other components of the feto-maternal system, although the significance is not clear.[18]

Urea, creatinine, and uric acid readily cross the placenta from the fetal to the maternal circulation, either by diffusion or by active transport. There is also evidence that some amino acids may be returned from the fetal to the maternal circulation.[18]

The placenta appears relatively impervious to lipids, and there is general agreement that phospholipids, triglycerides, and cholesterol esters do not cross the placenta intact. It is possible that free cholesterol may cross the

122

placenta, however, and that the placenta may break down phospholipids and resynthesize them for passage to the fetus. The fetus can synthesize fatty acids. In most other species there is evidence of placental transfer of fatty acids, and "it is tacitly assumed that essential fatty acids must reach the fetus from the mother and that the fetus cannot synthesize them."[23] However, the data on the maternal-placental-fetal relationship in regard to lipids are very limited.

The concentrations of calcium and phosphorus are higher in fetal plasma than in maternal plasma, suggesting that active transport mechanisms for these minerals exist. The interplay of hormonal control and placental passage has been suggested as a factor in increasing the amount of calcium retained by the fetus. With removal of calcium from maternal plasma, the secretion of parathyroid hormone, which does not cross the placenta, stimulates withdrawal of calcium from the mother's bones to increase her level of plasma calcium. In the fetus, secretion of calcitonin increases calcium deposition in bone. Magnesium, potassium, sodium, and chlorine pass freely through the placenta.

Iron is released from transferrin in the maternal blood at the placenta, and is rapidly transferred to the fetus. The transfer is against a gradient, since the fetal level is higher than the maternal level. There is no reverse transfer from fetal to maternal blood. The fetus requires a reserve of iron, especially in the third trimester. The level of hemoglobin in the fetus and newborn seems to be independent of the maternal level. The neonatal hemoglobin level is usually in the normal range even if the mother is anemic.

Oxygen transfer is easily accomplished. Fetal hemoglobin has greater oxygen-combining power than adult hemoglobin, so the higher affinity for oxygen is in the direction from maternal blood to fetal blood. The passage of oxygen to the fetus is also facilitated by the transfer of carbon dioxide from fetal to maternal hemoglobin, so that in essence the fetus exchanges carbon dioxide for oxygen.

The placental transfer of vitamins varies with their characteristics of solubility. Water-soluble vitamins are readily transferred, although at different rates, dependent in part on the levels in maternal blood. Concentration of water-soluble vitamins is higher in fetal than in maternal blood; for example, free riboflavin concentration has been reported to be as much as four times higher in fetal blood although flavin adenine dinucleotide is lower. Therefore, passage is probably by active transport requiring energy. In addition, there is some evidence that fetal retention may be protected after passage by modification of the molecular structure. The placenta seems to be more permeable to the oxidized form of ascorbic acid, dehydroascorbic acid, which may then be reduced by the fetal liver to prevent its return to the maternal circulation.

The mechanisms and rates of transfer of the fat-soluble vitamins are not well understood, but evidence suggests that vitamin A, at least, has a poor transfer rate. Fat-soluble vitamins are usually higher in concentration in maternal than in fetal blood. Their transfer is believed to be accomplished by binding to protein. There are indications that carotene may be more readily transported than retinol, and that the fetus itself then converts carotene to retinol. It is not known whether the fetal kidney can synthesize 1,25-dihydrocholecalciferol or whether it is transported across the placenta.[18]

As pregnancy progresses, fetal requirements increase. During the third trimester the fetus nearly doubles its length and has a fivefold increase in weight. Most of the calcium and iron deposition occurs during the last three months. Alterations in the maternal-placental-fetal blood flow favor greater availability of nutrients to the fetus. Blood flow to the uterus increases. The vascular bed of the placenta expands; at term its surface area is estimated to be approximately 3 to 4 square meters per kilogram of fetal weight, or a total area of 10 to 13 square meters. The rate of blood flow through the intervillous spaces near term is 400 to 500 ml/minute. Blood flow through the umbilical cord is also increased. In addition, the placental membrane becomes progressively more permeable. These adaptations lead to greater nutrient supply to the fetus when its need is greater.

AMNIOTIC FLUID

The fetus also has an interchange of nutrients, hormones, enzymes, and other compounds with the amniotic fluid.[15,25] In the first half of pregnancy the composition of amniotic fluid is similar to that of extracellular fetal fluid, and there is free exchange. Following the keratinization of fetal skin in the middle of pregnancy, there is no longer equilibrium, but amniotic fluid is ingested by the fetus, and some studies have shown that amniotic proteins may be absorbed by the fetus. The concentration of urea, uric acid, and creatinine in amniotic fluid as a result of urinary excretion by the fetus has sometimes been used as an index of fetal maturity. It is believed that the contents of amniotic fluid come from both fetal and maternal sources.

PLACENTAL HORMONES

In addition to its functions of transfer between maternal and fetal blood, the placenta both synthesizes and metabolizes hormones. The largest proportion of hormones is found in the fetal (chorionic) rather than the maternal (decidual) part. Steroid hormone production begins early in gestation, and by the third month the placenta is the main source of estrogens (primarily estriol) and progesterone for the conceptus. The concentration of both increases during pregnancy and reaches a maximum a few days before parturition. They are believed to aid in implantation and in enhancing the capacity of the uterus to expand, as well as contributing to development of the mammary glands in preparation for lactation. The placenta also synthesizes protein hormones, primarily human chorionic gonadotropin (HCG), human chorionic somatomammotropin (HCS), and human chorionic thyrotopin (HCT), and possibly other hormones as well.

FETAL GROWTH IN THE LAST TWO TRIMESTERS

Size, body composition, and degree of maturity of the fetus are difficult to evaluate. The inaccessibility of the fetus in utero has led to use of a number of sources of data. Direct evidence of body composition has been obtained from chemical analysis of the bodies of aborted and stillborn fetuses.[26-33] Studies of the DNA and protein content of cells to estimate the number and size have thus far been done primarily on the brain,[31] although some data are available on cellular growth of heart, liver, kidneys, muscle, and adrenal glands.[32,33] Measurements of weight and length of abortuses and prematurely born infants have been used to generate growth curves when gestational age was known.[22] The data from these sources must be evaluated in view of possible pathology related to the suboptimal outcome of the pregnancies.

Since size is an index to the sum of somatic processes and is related to cell proliferation, cell constituents, and the physiological action of enzymes and hormones, it has often been used to evaluate maturity of the fetus. However, maturity of function and structure are not necessarily directly proportional to size, and some caution must be used in this application of physical measurements. Prematurely born infants of the same weight and gestational age may vary widely in maturity. There are marked differences in body composition and maturity between premature infants and those who are small for gestational age, even though the criterion of weight under 2500 g at birth is used for both groups of infants. Indeed, individual variation in maturity as well as in physical size occurs during fetal life just as in any other period.

The traditional method of estimating fetal size has been by abdominal palpation of the mother. However, variations in the amount of amniotic fluid, the presentation and position of the fetus, the length of the maternal abdomen, the tone of the uterus, and the thickness of maternal soft tissues may result in errors of estimation.[34] Radiology has sometimes been used, but potential genetic and somatic damage now limit its application. Ultrasound techniques are a recent advance in the measurement of fetal size. Fetal biparietal diameter, crown-rump measurement, and the ratio of head circumference to abdominal circumference, especially when taken serially, can provide an estimate of fetal growth.[34]

Biochemical assays of maternal urine and plasma are an index to fetal maturity. These include levels of estrogens, placental lactogen, and enzymatic activity of leukocytes.[35] Amniocentesis allows evaluation of cellular and biochemical components of amniotic fluid, in which creatinine content may be used as an index of fetal renal function.

After the differentiation of body tissues has been accomplished in the first 8 to 12 weeks, the rest of the period in utero is characterized by continued growth of the fetus, with expansion of structure and function of organs. Increase in body size and maturation are critical to the survival of the infant, whether born prematurely or at full term. Table 3.1 summarizes the average size and some aspects of physical and physiological development of the fetus.[12] More detailed descriptions of fetal development are available from other sources.[11,14]

Growth in length is essentially linear from the third week to term, but increase in weight is relatively slow during the first half of gestation, as was shown in Figure 1.5. By 20 weeks the fetus has attained approximately 50 percent of its probable birth length but only 10 percent of its probable birth weight. The major acceleration in weight occurs in the second half of pregnancy. Fetal weight doubles in the last 10 weeks of gestation.

Although all parts of the body contribute to the sharp increase in fetal weight during the last half of pregnancy, the progressively greater deposition of fat than of other components makes a major difference in weight, as shown in Table 3.2. Fat provides less than 1 percent of body weight at 20 weeks, but 16 percent at term. When fetal weight has reached 1 kg, at approximately 26 weeks, only 10 g is due to body fat, most of which occurs as essential lipids in cell membranes and in the nervous system. When the fetus has reached 2 kg of body weight, around 33 weeks, fat content of the body is close to 100 g. At a fetal weight of 3 kg, body fat has increased to 360 g, and thereafter exceeds the body content of protein. The newborn with a weight of 3.5 kg has an average body content of 560 g, two-thirds of which has been deposited in the last 5 weeks of gestation.[29] The rapid fat deposition toward the end of pregnancy becomes important in evaluating the problems of the prematurely born infant, who has a fat deficit in addition to an immature body structure and functioning; it is also important in evaluating some term infants who are small for gestational age with inadequate body fat.

With such rapid deposition late in pregnancy, there must be some adjustment in the availability of fat for the fetus. It is presumed that transplacental passage of fatty acids increases, and it is possible that as much as 40 percent of fetal lipid is derived from maternal blood.[18] The ability of the fetus

126

Table 3.1 Summary of Main Events of Embryonic and Fetal Growth and Development in Man

Ferti-lization Age (Weeks)	Crown–Rump Length (Approx.)	Crown–Heel Length (Approx.)	Weight (Approx.)	Gross Appearance	Internal Development
Embryonic Stage					
1	0.5 mm	0.5 mm	?		Early morula; no organ differentiation
2	2 mm	2 mm	?	Ovoid vesicle superficially buried in endometrium	External trophoblast; first embryonic disc forming 2 inner vesicles (amnioectomesodermal and entodermal)
3	3 mm	3 mm	?	Early dorsal concavity changes to convexity; head, tail folds form; neural groove closes partially	Optic vesicles appear; double-chambered heart recognized; 14 mesodermal somites present
4	4 mm	4 mm	0.4 gm	Head at right angles to body; limb rudiments obvious; tail prominent; all somites present	Vitelline duct only communication between umbilical vesicle and intestines; organ development in initial stages; heartbeat begins
8	3 cm	3.5 cm	2 gm	Eyes, ears, nose and mouth recognizable; digits formed; tail almost gone	Sensory organ development progressing; ossification beginning in occiput, mandible, and humerus; small intestines coil within umbilical cord; pleural, pericardial cavities forming; testes and ovaries distinguishable

Continued

127

Fetal Stage

Fertilization Age (Weeks)	Crown–Rump Length (Approx.)	Crown–Heel Length (Approx.)	Weight (Approx.)	Gross Appearance	Internal Development
12	8 cm	11.5 cm	19 gm	Skin pink, delicate, resembles a human being, but head is disproportionately large; sex readily recognizable upon external inspection	Brain configuration roughly complete; internal and external sex organs now specific; blood forming in marrow; upper cervical to lower sacral arches and bodies ossify
16	13.5 cm	19 cm	100 gm	Face looks "human," scalp hair appears; motor activity; arm–leg ratio now proportionate; body outgrowing head	Heart muscle well developed; lobulated kidney attains final situation; meconium first appears in bowel; vagina and anus open; eye, ear, nose grossly approach typical appearance; general sense organs differentiated
20	18.5 cm	22 cm	300 gm	Legs lengthened appreciably; distance from umbilicus to pubis increased; lanugo hair present	Sternum ossifies; gross brain architecture completed; myelination of cord begins

Continued

	cm	cm	gm		
24	23 cm	32 cm	600 gm	Skin reddish and wrinkled; slight newly deposited subcuticular fat; vernix appears; primitive respiratory-like movements begin	Cerebral cortex layered typically; blood formation increasing in bone marrow and decreasing in liver (gradual process continuing until birth)
28	27 cm	36 cm	1100 gm	Skin less wrinkled; more fat present; nails first appear; if delivered, breathes, cries, moves poorly; rare possibility of survival with optimal care	Testes at internal inguinal ring or below in their descent toward the scrotum; astragalus ossifies; cerebral fissures and convolutions appearing rapidly; retinal layers completed and light receptive
32	31 cm	41 cm	1800 gm	Fetal weight increases proportionately more than length	Middle fourth phalanges ossify; permanent teeth primordia indicated; taste sense present
36	35 cm	46 cm	2200 gm	Skin pale, body rounded; general lanugo disappearing; umbilicus now in center of ventral portion of body	Distal femoral ossification centers present
40	40 cm	52 cm	3200 + gm	Skin smooth and pink; copious vernix often present; moderate to profuse hair on head; lanugo hair on shoulders and upper back only; nasal and alar cartilages apparent; nails extended over tip of digits; testes in scrotum, or labia major well developed	Proximal tibial ossification centers present; cuboid, tibia (proximal epiphysis) ossify; some fetal blood passages discontinued; myelination of brain begins; pulmonary branching only 2/3 completed; ear deaf at birth

Source: Timiras, P. S. *Developmental Physiology and Aging,* Macmillan, New York, 1972.

Table 3.2   Total Amounts of Water, Fat, Nitrogen, and Minerals in the Body of the Developing Fetus

Body Weight (gm)	Approximate Fetal Age (Weeks)	Water (gm)	Fat (gm)	N (gm)	Ca (gm)	P (gm)	Mg (gm)	Na (meq)	K (meq)	Cl (meq)	Fe (mg)	Cu (mg)	Zn (mg)
30	13	27	0.2	0.4	0.09	0.09	0.003	3.6	1.4	2.4	—	—	—
100	15	89	0.5	1.0	0.3	0.2	0.01	9	2.6	7	5.1	—	—
200	17	177	1.0	2.8	0.7	0.6	0.03	20	7.9	14	10	0.7	2.6
500	23	440	3.0	7.0	2.2	1.5	0.10	49	22	33	28	2.4	9.4
1000	26	860	10	14	6.0	3.4	0.22	90	41	66	64	3.5	16
1500	31	1270	35	25	10	5.6	0.35	125	60	96	100	5.6	25
2000	33	1620	100	37	15	8.2	0.46	160	84	120	160	8.0	35
2500	35	1940	185	49	20	11	0.58	200	110	130	220	10	43
3000	38	2180	360	55	25	14	0.70	240	130	150	260	12	50
3500	40	2400	560	62	30	17	0.78	280	150	160	280	14	53

Source: Widdowson, E. M. Growth and composition of the fetus and newborn. In: Assali, N. S. (Ed.) Biology of Gestation, Vol. II. Academic Press, New York, 1968

to synthesize fats must also become more efficient. The fetus itself can synthesize fats from glucose, pyruvate, acetate, or citrate.[23]

Protein deposition in the fetus is basic to growth, and continues throughout gestation. In the first half of pregnancy, body composition is primarily fluids and lean tissue, and in the last half of pregnancy the proportions of water and protein decrease as the proportion of fat increases. The amount of protein in the body has been estimated to be 385 to 435 g in the full-term infant at birth,[10,29] although lower values have been reported for infants born to undernourished mothers in India.[30]

Calcium and phosphorus content of the fetus increases with mineralization of bones. Calcification of the fetal cartilage begins about the eighth week, but by midgestation the fetus contains only approximately 1 g of calcium, which increases to 30 g by 40 weeks. The fetal need for calcium in the last trimester is 13 mg/hour.[29] The calcium-to-phosphorus ratio remains close to 1.8 throughout the last half of fetal development. Similar increases in body content, especially in the last trimester, have been reported for other minerals, including magnesium and potassium.

The full-term newborn has a body content averaging 280 to 300 mg of iron,[10,29] of which 40 to 50 mg are stored in the liver. Hemoglobin concentration of the newborn is 16 to 22 g/100 ml blood, a level higher than at any time during later life. The marked increase in iron content of the fetus occurs primarily in the last trimester, with some evidence that maternal absorption of dietary iron intake may increase up to fourfold toward the end of pregnancy to meet the greater demand. Iron levels in the fetus seem to have little relationship to maternal hemoglobin levels.

At term the newborn has a body content of 50 to 60 mg of zinc. Since plasma zinc is usually bound to albumin, which does not cross the placenta to any appreciable extent, the mechanism of transfer of maternal zinc to the fetus is not known.[18] The newborn body contains approximately 14 mg of copper, about half of which is in the liver, apparently bound in a complex with protein in the mitochondria. The concentration of copper in the newborn liver is 10 times higher than found in the adult.[18]

MATERNAL PHYSIOLOGICAL ADJUSTMENTS

Preparation of the uterus for potential pregnancy occurs during the menstrual cycle under normal estrogen and progesterone control, with increase in blood supply as the major change. Once the ovum has been fertilized and implanted in the uterus, progressive alterations in physiology affect many systems of the maternal body as it adapts to the needs of the growing embryo. The woman may not be aware of change until after the first missed period or even later if she has some bleeding at the time when a menstrual period might have been expected. Changes in maternal physiology are at first largely under hormonal control but as the fetus becomes larger and has increasing needs, and as placental growth and function play a greater role, the interplay of mother-placenta-fetus leads to further physiological adjustments.

NAUSEA AND VOMITING

Nausea is often the first symptom of pregnancy. The cause is not well understood. Hormonal effects and adaptation to the presence of foreign material, because half the genes in the conceptus are of paternal origin, have been suggested as possible causes. Nausea does not occur in all women, and the timing and degree of nausea, with or without vomiting, vary from one woman to another. The most common pattern is one of onset after the first missed period and cessation in the third month. Many women experience nausea on rising in the morning, before eating, which suggests that hunger contractions may play a part. However, some women have nausea at any time of the day or night without relation to food ingestion, and sometimes in response to odors or taste. Therapy varies from physician to physician, and none has proved totally satisfactory. Vitamins of the B complex, either orally or by intramuscular injection, have been sometimes successful. A number of drugs, including tranquilizers, have been administered, but the hazards of fetal damage currently rule against the use of drugs except under careful medical supervision. Many women find that eating before rising from bed is a simple solution, and dry food such as crackers may dispel the nausea.

Although nausea is an uncomfortable sensation, its only hazard to health lies in its effects on food consumption. Gastric discomfort may result in lower food intake, usually only intermittently. However, vomiting may have a more drastic effect on intake, especially if it is severe and persistent, resulting in weight loss or ketonuria. The woman who enters pregnancy in good nutritional status has greater reserves to buffer the adverse effects of vomiting. The woman in poor or marginal nutritional state at conception who then has severe vomiting may experience weight loss during the first trimester or longer. Since this is a critical period of embryonic development, weight loss during the first trimester may cause an inadequate supply of essential nutrients to the placenta and embryo and may compromise both growth and organ formation. Special attention is needed for the woman with severe vomiting. Unfortunately many women do not seek medical care at this early stage of pregnancy.

132

BLOOD VOLUME AND BLOOD COMPONENTS

Maternal blood volume begins to increase shortly after conception to supply the added nutrients, oxygen, hormones, and enzymes needed by the conceptus.[36] However, the increase in plasma volume and the increase in red cell volume are of different orders of magnitude, as can be seen in Table 3.3. Plasma volume rises to a peak of 39 to 50 percent above the nonpregnant level early in the third trimester, after which there is little or no increase,[37] or even a decrease.[10] In contrast, red cell volume increases in essentially a linear pattern throughout pregnancy, and by term is 17 to 40 percent above the initial level.[38] As a result, the percentage increase in plasma volume may be four times as great as that of red cell volume, but toward the end of pregnancy the ratio of increments is closer to 2:1.[10]

With the differential in rates of increase of these two blood components, the concentration of many substances in the blood decreases. For example, even though there is an absolute increase in red cell volume and in total hemoglobin, the dilution of cells in more plasma causes a drop in hemoglobin concentration since it is expressed as g/100 ml blood. Hemoglobin concentration rises toward term when the increase in red cell volume continues while there is no increase in plasma volume.

Other factors affect the concentration of nutrients in maternal blood. The demand for nutrients by the conceptus, both the fetus and the placenta, increases with growth, so that the drain on maternal blood is higher as pregnancy progresses. In addition, maternal renal function is altered; excretion of some nutrients falls, and excretion of other nutrients or their metabolites rises. Therefore, the evaluation of levels of various components of maternal blood must take into account a variety of influences that are peculiar to

Table 3.3   Plasma Volume, Red Cell Volume, Total Blood Volume, and Hematocrit in Pregnancy

		Weeks of Pregnancy		
	Nonpregnancy	**20**	**30**	**40**
Volume (ml)				
Plasma	2600	3150	3750	3600
Red Cell	1400	1450	1550	1650
Total blood	4000	4600	5300	5250
Hematocrit (%)	35.0	31.5	29.5	31.5

Source: Committee on Maternal Nutrition, Food and Nutrition Board. *Maternal Nutrition and the Course of Pregnancy*. National Academy of Sciences, Washington, D.C., 1970.

pregnancy. This has led to controversy about the interpretation of prenatal blood levels and recommendations for mineral–vitamin supplementation of the diet.[36,39]

There is no clear dividing line between normal prenatal levels and values that could be diagnostic of deficiency. Many of the physiological changes that characterize pregnancy simulate pathology (deviation from normal) in the nonpregnant state.[36] If the decrease is an expected and natural accompaniment of pregnancy, should an effort be made to maintain nonpregnant levels of those nutrients that can be elevated by supplementation? Alternatively, should different standards be used for the pregnant woman than for the nonpregnant woman? Should each nutrient be considered separately in the light of current knowledge of its clinical significance? There is no consensus, and practice varies from time to time. For example, early reports of increased pregnancy wastage attributed to folacin deficiency led to recommendation of routine folacin supplementation.[10] However, when further study failed to confirm fetal risk, the rationale for special attention to folacin has been questioned.[39]

Iron supplementation during pregnancy has been widely recommended as routine practice. Mean hemoglobin concentrations of nonpregnant women in most of the studies reviewed by Bowering et al.[38] were between 12.8 and 14.5 g/100 ml. In 16 studies during all stages of pregnancy, mean levels did not fall below 11 g, and several group averages did not fall below 12 g, except in two studies that reported means of 10.4 and 10.9 in late pregnancy. In normal pregnancy, the hemoglobin concentration, red cell count, serum iron, and packed cell volume decrease during the first 7 to 8 months, then rise again. Total iron-binding capacity increases during pregnancy. The decrease in hemoglobin, serum iron, and hematocrit can be lessened but not prevented by supplementation of the diet with iron.[37] In discussing the enthusiasm for routine iron supplementation, especially in the United States, Hytten and Leitch stated in 1971 that "in general, there is no convincing published evidence that the normal pregnant woman is at an advantage if she takes extra iron."[36] However, the controversy about routine iron supplementation continues.

Fasting levels of blood glucose decrease during pregnancy, and on the average are 10 to 15 percent lower by the third trimester than in the nonpregnant state. In contrast, pregnancy represents a hyperlipemic state, and elevated levels of total lipids, triglycerides, phospholipids, and cholesterol are typical. Total serum protein decreases gradually in the first two trimesters, primarily because of a decrease in albumin, and remains essentially constant during the third trimester. Plasma amino acids also tend to be lower in pregnancy, except arginine, which rises, and histidine, which remains unchanged.[37]

134

The pattern of decrease in the first two trimesters followed by an increase in concentration in the third trimester has been observed for serum levels of calcium, magnesium, phosphorus, and potassium. Serum chloride drops in early pregnancy, then rises to a level above the nonpregnant concentration by the middle of gestation, possibly because of a decrease in serum bicarbonate concentration, which shifts the chloride ion from intracellular to extracellular fluids and plasma. The sodium level decreases early but then remains fairly constant. Plasma zinc seems to show a steady decline from the tenth week, although data on zinc are still limited. In contrast to other elements, serum copper rises during pregnancy from the second month to term, although wide individual variations have been observed.[37,40]

Serum levels of ascorbic acid, folacin, vitamin B_{12}, and pyridoxine tend to decrease during pregnancy. Serum vitamin A concentration remains relatively unchanged. However, serum tocopherol increases an average of 40 to 50 percent during the second trimester, evidently unrelated to changes in dietary intake.[37]

TOTAL BODY WATER AND RENAL FUNCTION

The increase in blood volume is one component of the increase in total body water. Approximately 7 liters of water are added to the total body fluids during pregnancy. This accounts for 60 percent of the weight gain. The increase in fluids to approximately 30 weeks can be accounted for by the conceptus, maternal blood volume increase, and the increase in the reproductive organs. However, at term 1 to 2 liters of surplus water cannot be so accounted for. It is possible that much of the fluid acquisition is due to sodium retention in response to increased aldosterone secretion. Women with edema retain more water, especially when the edema is generalized. It has been estimated that 40 percent of normotensive women have some degree of recorded edema.[36] The excess fluid is lost in the first few weeks after delivery.

Restriction of sodium intake and administration of diuretics to promote water loss have been common in the treatment of edema for many years. However, sodium requirement increases during pregnancy with the increase in body fluids, and this treatment stresses normal renin–angiotensin–aldosterone adjustments, leading to exhaustion of aldosterone-producing cells. Therefore, routine salt restriction and diuretic therapy are no longer recommended.[41,42]

Both anatomical and functional changes that affect excretion are observed in the maternal body.[36] The whole renal tract from the kidney to the bladder becomes dilated as pregnancy progresses, so that it is capable of handling the increased urinary load. Renal blood flow is approximately one-third higher by the end of gestation. Glomerular filtration rate rises to a level about 50 percent higher than in the nonpregnant state. The activity of the renin–angiotensin system is greatly enhanced. The net result is an increased ability to handle the excretion of urea, uric acid, and creatinine from the conceptus and the maternal body itself. However, there is also increased excretion of nutrients, which seems inconsistent with the higher requirement of these substances. The urinary content of glucose, several amino acids, inorganic iodine, ascorbic acid, riboflavin, niacin metabolites, and folate rises during pregnancy.

The increased urine volume, at least during early pregnancy, may be a factor in the unusual thirst that many women experience. However, the relaxation and dilatation of the urinary tract with its higher nutrient concentration may create greater susceptibility to urinary tract infections.

CARDIAC FUNCTION

With a greater volume of blood to circulate and a larger body mass to service, adjustments in cardiac function are also characteristic of pregnancy. Cardiac output rises from a nonpregnant mean of 4.5 to 5.0 liters per minute to a level of 6.0 to 7.0 liters per minute. Heart rate increases from 70 to 85 beats per minute and stroke volume from 64 to 71 ml.[36] There may be some enlargement of heart size during pregnancy.

RESPIRATORY FUNCTION AND OXYGEN NEEDS

Growth of tissue, especially lean body mass, places greater demands on oxygen supply. The combined metabolic requirements of the mother with her increase in body tissues, the placenta, and the fetus result in an increase in the basal or resting metabolic rate and in the function of the lungs. There have been conflicting reports of the degree of elevation of the basal metabolic rate, but the general consensus is that the increase by the end of pregnancy is approximately 15 percent, or 30 ml of oxygen per minute above the nonpregnant oxygen consumption.[10] However, the ventilation rate rises progressively throughout pregnancy from about 7 liters per minute to about 10 liters per minute, an increase of more than 40 percent. Vital capacity of the lungs is not increased, but tidal volume is greater, mainly at the expense of expiratory reserve volume, so that the lung is more collapsed than usual at the end of normal expiration as a result of "overbreathing." Carbon dioxide is washed out from the alveolae and alveolar pCO_2 falls from approximately 38 mm Hg to about 30 mm Hg by midpregnancy[10] with a parallel decrease in blood bicarbonate. The pregnant woman may experience dyspnea, with a conscious need to breathe.

The increase in basal metabolic rate may be offset by a gradual decrease in physical motion, especially toward the end of pregnancy.

GASTROINTESTINAL FUNCTION

Several changes occur in the gastrointestinal tract. Increased appetite may be observed beginning early in pregnancy, sometimes despite the concomitant presence of nausea. Thirst also becomes more pronounced. Unless there is interference by pathology or by deliberate limitation of food and/or fluids, the normal appetite of the pregnant woman leads to higher intake of foods and liquids to meet the increased nutrient requirements.

The relaxation of smooth muscles, probably as a result of progesterone secretion, has both positive and negative effects. Hypomotility and the relaxation of the cardiac sphincter may contribute to nausea and vomiting as well as to the reversal of stomach contents to the esophagus, resulting in "heartburn." The slower passage of food through the gastrointestinal tract may also result in constipation.

On the other hand, the slower emptying time provides greater opportunity for digestive enzymes to break down the complex molecules of food. The intestinal contents are in contact with the epithelial cells of the intestinal lining for an extended time period and absorption of nutrients is increased. Some studies have shown increased absorption, particularly of nitrogen and minerals, during pregnancy. This greater efficiency in the utilization of food components is especially important when dietary intake is marginal.

MATERNAL WEIGHT GAIN

The increase in maternal body weight during pregnancy is due to a large number of components, many of which can only be estimated and some of which have not been identified. It is, therefore, difficult to establish either a single value or a range of values that might be considered "optimal" weight gain. Wide individual variations are consistent with health of both the mother and her fetus, and a single goal or weight increment should not be applied to all women. Among the factors that must be considered in evaluating the weight gain of an individual woman are height, preconceptional weight and nutritional status, age, parity, previous reproductive record, race, and physiological status (including adolescent growth, multiple fetuses, diabetes, edema, and toxemia). Monitoring gain during pregnancy is an important part of medical care, but rigidity in standardizing weight gain should be avoided.

Studies of weight gain in pregnancy have been done in several population groups, both in developed and in developing countries. Weight gain is one of the major determinants of infant weight, but the relationship is modified by many of the factors listed above, as well as by other physiological adjustments peculiar to pregnancy. The aim of medical care and nutritional support during pregnancy is twofold: to ensure the health of the mother during pregnancy and after parturition, including lactation, and to produce a healthy term infant whose weight does not compromise his survival and development. The common practice in the 1950s and 1960s to limit maternal weight gain to 12 to 18 lb (5 to 8 kg) by dietary restriction is now viewed as of little value in the control of toxemia[42] or edema and as potentially hazardous to cell growth of the fetus and placenta. A review of studies in the literature has shown that weight gains that average 10 to 12.5 kg are consistent with good reproductive performance.[10,42]

The pattern and components of "average" maternal gain of 11 kg are shown in Figure 3.2. When birth weight is 3.0 to 3.5 kg, the fetus itself may account for less than one-third of maternal gain. Adding placenta and amniotic fluid to fetal weight, the total of the products of conception contribute less than 50 percent of gain to term; maternal increases in uterine and breast tissue and body fluids contribute most of the remainder. In this type of factorial calculation, 1 to 3 kg of weight gain cannot be accounted for. Early balance studies[43] showed higher nitrogen retention during pregnancy

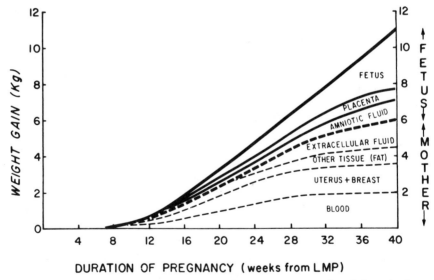

Figure 3.2   Pattern and components of average maternal weight gain during pregnancy. (Reprinted from Pitkin, R. M. Nutritional support in obstetrics and gynecology. Clin. Obstet. Gynecol. 19:489–513, 1976.)

138

than expected, and the additional weight gain was attributed to storage of protein, probably in preparation for lactation. The theory that the extra weight was due to protein increment in the maternal body was challenged, and it was theorized that fat deposition was more likely to account for the 1 to 3 kg additional gain.[44] However, recent nitrogen balance studies of King, Calloway, and associates[45,46] confirm that the maternal body retains nitrogen in excess of that required for synthesis of new tissue, and that protein storage does occur in pregnancy. It is logical that, under the influence of progesterone, somatomammotropin, insulin, and/or growth hormone, amino acids may be transferred from extracellular to intracellular pools and that uptake of amino acids by the liver is increased. The compartment in Figure 3.2 designated "other tissue" is now thought to be a combination of fat and protein.[18]

The timing of weight gain is related to growth of maternal, placental, and fetal tissues and to increments in maternal fluids. During the first trimester a gain of 1 to 2 kg is common. Loss of weight during the first trimester, because of vomiting or some other cause, implies a limitation of caloric intake and a consequent diversion of protein to energy, as well as inadequate supplies of other nutrients. This may contribute to loss or defective development of the embryo. If the mother has adequate reserves in her body prior to conception, they may provide a buffer during this early period, but weight loss is not desirable either at this or at any later stage of pregnancy. In a study of women in the last five months of pregnancy, Oldham and Sheft[47] found that nitrogen balance was precarious when caloric intake fell below 36 to 40 kcal/kg (0.15 to 0.17 MJ/kg), and that on intakes of 30 kcal/kg (0.13 MJ/kg) or less there was no appreciable retention of nitrogen.

Weight gain during the second and third trimesters, according to the calculated averages in Figure 3.2, is essentially linear, with a 5 kg increment in each trimester, or 350 to 400 g/wk. The maternal component is responsible for much of the gain in the second trimester and the conceptus for close to 90 percent of the gain in the third trimester. However, there is wide individual variation, both in the amount of gain and in the timing of increments. The tendency of a woman to repeat her pattern of weight gain in successive pregnancies was shown by a correlation coefficient of 0.64 in a study of women during 2 to 4 pregnancies each.[48]

Monitoring weight gain during the last half of pregnancy is recommended to provide an index of edema. A sudden large gain (3 kg or more/month) may indicate excessive retention of extracellular fluids. Dependent or gravitational edema of the ankles and pretibial areas is often seen in late pregnancy, in part due to pressure of the uterus on pelvic veins and the inferior vena cava; it usually lessens or disappears with a recumbent position. However, generalized edema may be an early sign of developing toxemia.[42] When edema is accompanied by elevation of blood pressure and albuminuria, which are the other symptoms of toxemia, or preeclampsia, it is of greater concern because of its relationship to premature delivery and risks to the health of both mother and fetus. Unfortunately, in most studies of maternal weights, no estimation of edema is included in the published results. If the increase in weight of an individual woman is evaluated, however, the contribution of edema to weight must be taken into account.

Maternal age, height, and preconceptional weight influence gain during pregnancy. The adolescent who has not yet completed growth continues to add to her own body mass during pregnancy, and her gain in weight is not totally the result of reproduction, so additional leeway in gain should be allowed for increment in her own tissues. The underweight woman constitutes an obstetric hazard since she has a greater chance of premature delivery.[49] If preconceptional weight is 10 percent or more below ideal weight for age and height, additional gain during pregnancy should be allowed, since the woman is likely to retain some of the gain if her nutritional intake is improved during pregnancy. Perinatal mortality is higher among infants of young adolescents, especially under 15 years of age, and underweight women than among infants of mature women of average weight. For both groups, efforts should be made to encourage extra weight gain during pregnancy.[50]

BIRTH WEIGHT

The weight of the infant at birth is critical to survival. Mortality rates are especially high for infants under 2.5 kg, lowest for weights between 2.5 and 4 kg, and rise somewhat again for infants with birth weights above 4 kg. Although the average birth weight in a population is often used as a standard, the lowest mortality is observed when birth weight is close to the 75th percentile.[34] Newborn infants vary not only in weight and length, but also in degree of maturity. Maturity is a better index of survival than weight, but weight is easily measured and is a valuable indicator of fetal experience.[22] An analysis of infant mortality data by the National Center for Health Statistics[51] showed that 7.8 percent of infants born in one year weighed less than 2.5 kg at birth, but this small group accounted for 59 percent of all deaths in the first year of life. Limiting analysis to infants of at least 36 weeks gestation, the British Perinatal Mortality Survey[52] found a mortality rate for infants more than two standard deviations below the mean birth weight six times higher than for infants in the average range; the rate for infants more than two standard deviations above the mean was twice the rate for infants in the average range.

LOW BIRTH WEIGHT

Of all live births in the United States, 8 to 10 percent have weights under 2.5 kg. These infants have a sharply higher death rate than infants of normal weight, especially in the first 24 hours, and mortality rates are higher as birth weight is lower. They have a higher incidence of congenital defects, neurological and cognitive problems, mental retardation, and susceptibility to infection and neonatal hypoglycemia. However, all deficits of birth weight do not have the same significance. Since the 1960s distinction has been made between low birth weight (LBW) infants who are delivered before the 37th week of gestation (preterm or premature infants) and LBW infants born at term, or after the 37th week.

The first group, premature infants, have not completed fetal growth because of limitation of time in utero. Since the fetus acquires two-thirds of its weight but only one-third of its length in the last 12 weeks of gestation, early delivery results in greater deficit in weight than in length, with low body fat content. The size, physical characteristics, biochemical status, and organ capabilities of the preterm infant are usually consistent with gestational age. The structure and function of organs are immature, and there is limited body content of calcium, iron, and other minerals that are normally deposited in large amounts during the last trimester of gestation. Developmental defects and impairment of motor and intellectual function may persist to varying degrees. Mortality is closely related to gestational age and to body weight.

The second group of LBW infants are more difficult to categorize. There has thus far been no consensus on terminology. LBW infants have in various reports been called small for gestational age (SGA), small for dates (SFD), fetal growth retardation (FGR), or intrauterine growth retardation (IUGR or IGR). With a longer gestational period, LBW infants tend to be more mature and have a better survival rate than those born prematurely. With more mature metabolic rate and central nervous system development, metabolic needs of the LBW infants are higher and they are more susceptible to neonatal hypoglycemia. However, in contrast to term infants of greater weight, they have a deficit in fetal growth, which is an index of total somatic growth. Body organs are smaller, enzyme and hormone production may be limited, and bone age retarded. Since the factors that caused a distortion of normal growth vary from one infant to another, and the pattern of retardation of one fetus may be different from that of another, each SGA infant must be evaluated individually. There is no description that is characteristic of all SGA babies.

However, some anthropometric relationships of the SGA baby give clues to possible etiology. When length, head circumference, and weight are in normal proportion to each other, fetal growth may have been at a consistent, though reduced, rate throughout gestation. This infant probably has a general reduction in cell numbers in all organs and uniformly limited biochemical function. However, when length is proportionately higher than weight and head circumference, it implies that fetal growth was normal or close to normal during the first two trimesters and that the interruption in growth occurred in the third trimester when weight and head growth would normally have accelerated. If the only deficit is in weight and the skin appears loose, it suggests an actual loss of weight late in pregnancy after it had been acquired. Present rapid advances in methodology for monitoring fetal growth can be expected to provide more precise knowledge of the patterns and timing of aberrations in fetal growth as well as normal growth.

FACTORS AFFECTING BIRTH WEIGHT

Sex of Infant
Males, on the average, weigh 100 to 200 g more than females at birth, although there is wide overlap in weight distributions. Sex differences in fetal size are negligible until about 33 weeks, after which the weight increase of males exceeds that of females, presumably under the influence of sex hormones.

Ethnic Differences
The data on ethnic differences in birth weight are somewhat difficult to evaluate because of concomitant differences in socioeconomic status and consequent environmental influences. In the Collaborative Perinatal Study of nearly 56,000 women and their infants,[53] the mean birth weight of black infants was 3.04 kg and of white infants 3.27 kg; however, gestation was 8 days shorter for blacks. Further analysis revealed that fetal weights of blacks exceeded those of whites to 35 weeks of gestation, after which relative positions were reversed.

In a summary of the mean weights of infants from various areas of the world, Hytten and Leitch[36] reported highest values in American Indians, at nearly 3600 g. Infants with Down's syndrome had a mean birth weight of approximately 3100 g, Africans 3000 g, and Asian Indians 2900 g.

Multiple Fetuses
When two or more fetuses share a uterus at the same time, the stress on maternal capacity and blood supply is greatly increased. Multiple fetuses are almost invariably smaller than single infants, and gestation is usually shorter in duration. Twins have a combined weight greater than single in-

fants, but usually not twice as much. The pregnancy is associated with a considerable increase in perinatal deaths and in such complications as pre-eclampsia and anemia.[36] Few studies have been done on pregnancies with more than two fetuses.

Length of Gestation

The length of gestation is the largest determinant of birth weight. The infant who is prematurely delivered has a weight deficit closely proportional to the degree of prematurity.

Compiling data from a variety of sources on birth weight in relation to gestational age, Gruenwald[22] developed the thesis that toward the end of pregnancy the placenta becomes insufficient as a supply line to the fetus. As a result, fetal growth, which had been progressing on a straight line, has a slower rate toward term and, in the postmature infant, after 40 weeks. As shown in his illustration of this phenomenon (Figure 3.3), deviation of the adjusted mean birth weight from the extrapolated straight line (E) varies in timing in different populations. Swedish infants (S) maintain linear increase almost to 40 weeks. Infants in Portland, Oregon (P) begin to slow growth about one week earlier. A group in Baltimore (B), which presumably included a large number of black infants, deviated at the 38th week. In Denver (D) the effect of altitude on oxygen tension is believed to be the cause of earlier deviation and lower birth weight. Two curves of data from Japan in 1945 (J45) and in 1963 (J63) reflect the increase in birth weight observed during the time interval, similar to reported increases in heights of older children. The lowest curve (T) is from Gruenwald's data on twins, indicating the lower birth weights usually seen in multiple fetuses.

Maternal Weight Gain

The second largest factor in birth weight, as determined in several epidemiological studies, is the weight gain of the mother during pregnancy. In the Collaborative Perinatal Study of nearly 56,000 women and their infants,[53-55] when maternal weight gain was 15 lb (7 kg) or less, 16 percent of the infants weighed less than 2.5 kg. The incidence dropped to 8 percent when the maternal gain was 16 to 25 lb (7 to 11 kg), to 4 percent with a maternal gain of 26 to 35 lb (11 to 16 kg), and to 3 percent when the maternal gain during pregnancy was 36 lb (16 kg) or higher. A positive linear relationship between maternal weight gain and infant birth weight has been confirmed in many studies, leading to the conclusion that emphasis on weight restriction in an effort to reduce preeclampsia has instead increased the prevalence of low birth weight. The Collaborative Perinatal Study also showed that low prenatal weight gain was associated with higher perinatal mortality.

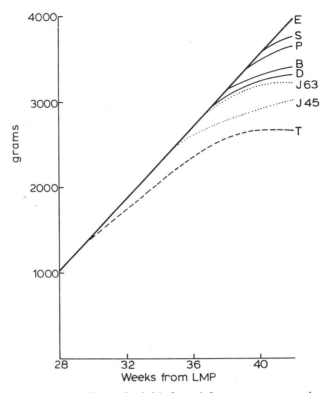

Figure 3.3 Smoothed birth weight curves suggesting that in each population departure from the straight line occurs when the supply line becomes insufficient to support the growth potential. Data: E = extrapolated curve; S = Sweden; P = Portland, Oregon; B = Baltimore, Md.; D = Denver, Colo.; J63 = Japan, 1963; J45 = Japan, 1945; T = Twins. (Reprinted from Gruenwald, P. Pathology of the deprived fetus and its supply line. In: Size at Birth. Ciba Foundation Symposium 27. Elsevier, Associated Scientific Publishers, Amsterdam, 1974.)

Preconceptional Weight

The preconceptional weight of the mother modifies the effect of gain during pregnancy. The woman who was underweight at the start of pregnancy and has a small prenatal gain has the greatest risk of delivering an infant with low birth weight. If the thin woman has a larger gain during pregnancy, the risk of low birth weight is lessened. However, in women with average pre-

144   PREGNANCY

conceptional weights, the impact of prenatal gain on birth weight is not so great. Women who were overweight before conceiving tend to have large babies, and prenatal weight gain has even less effect. In other words, the lower the preconceptional weight, the greater the importance of weight gain during pregnancy. When we translate these findings into nutritional terms, it is clear that a woman who is undernourished both before and during pregnancy cannot supply adequate nutrients for satisfactory growth of the fetus and has few reserves from which to draw; this limitation of somatic growth in the fetus is reflected in a small baby. However, if the undernourished woman is well fed during pregnancy, fetal growth increases; supplementation of the diets of undernourished women in both developing[3,56] and developed[50,57] countries has lowered the incidence of low birth weights. On the other hand, the woman who was well-nourished prior to conception has reserves large enough to buffer the effects of low intake during pregnancy. The higher mortality rates for infants of obese women may be related to the greater frequency of associated medical complications, including chronic hypertension and diabetes mellitus.

From their study of more than 1000 fetal autopsies, Naeye et al.[33] suggested that there is no discernible relationship of fetal size to maternal weight or weight gain prior to 33 weeks, but that after 33 weeks the size of the fetus and many of its organs as well as the size and weight of the placenta are directly related to maternal weight, weight gain, and dietary restrictions. This is consistent with the timing of the greatest increment in fetal weight and nutrient demand.

Analysis of successive full-term pregnancies in the same women in the Collaborative Perinatal Study[58] showed that the impact of weight gain during pregnancy on birth weight was 1.4 times greater than the impact of preconceptional weight. When weight gain during pregnancy was 5 lb (2.3 kg) higher, birth weight was increased by 80 g. When prepregnant weight was 5 lb higher, the increase in birth weight was 57 g, on the average. When both prepregnant weight and weight gain increased by 5 lb, the average increase in birth weight was 137 g, indicating an additive effect.

Maternal Height

The genetic component of fetal size may be determined by the height of the mother. In addition, maternal height has been used in some studies as an indicator of the level of nutritional intake during childhood. However, analysis of data from the Collaborative Perinatal Study[53] showed that the contribution of maternal height to birth weight was less than the effect of either maternal weight or weight gain. It appeared that the effect of height might be mediated through weight. Paternal size has been shown both in animal experimentation and in human epidemiological studies to have relatively little effect on fetal growth.

Maternal Age

Fetal development, birth weight, and infant mortality rates are influenced by maternal age. Mothers past the age of 35 years suffer more fetal loss and infant mortality and are more likely to give birth to infants with congenital malformations, birth injuries, and chromosomal abnormalities, such as Down's syndrome.

Mothers under 15 years of age have increased rates of preeclampsia and premature delivery, are more likely to deliver infants of low birth weight, and have higher rates of fetal loss and infant mortality. The risks are higher when there is a short time interval between menarche and conception.[59] Peak height velocity in the adolescent precedes menarche, so the young adolescent has recently passed through a period of accelerated anabolism and nutrient demands, and may still be in a decelerating phase of growth with nutrient requirements above those of the adult woman. Physical and gynecological immaturity, compounded by psychological immaturity and the stress of pregnancy, makes the young adolescent subject to risk. Nearly 20 percent of all liveborn infants in the United States with birth weights under 2.5 kg are born to mothers under 15 years of age. A high proportion of these mothers are nonwhite and from low economic status, factors that contribute to the risk. When growth ceases and maturity of physical and gynecological status has been attained, at 17 years or later, on the average, the risk of low birth weight drops markedly. Epidemiological data on adolescents suggest that maturational age is more critical than chronological age although it is rarely determined.

Insofar as birth weight is concerned, the best reproductive records have been reported for women between 18 and 35 years, or more narrowly between 20 and 29 years.

Parity

The greater reproductive risk among older women is associated with a larger number of pregnancies, especially if they have been closely spaced. The reasons for higher perinatal mortality and morbidity are not clear, but may arise from a combination of advanced age, hormonal insufficiency, chromosomal damage, and nutritional depletion.

Prior Obstetric Record

A woman often repeats her past reproductive history. If she has previously experienced fetal loss, premature delivery, or delivery of an infant with low birth weight, there is a greater chance of a similar occurrence in subsequent pregnancies. Therefore, prior obstetric performance is a clue to a "high risk" pregnancy.

Maternal Pathology

Severe chronic hypertension and severe renal disease in the mother interfere with the supply of nutrients and their clearance from the fetus and placenta, and tend to limit fetal growth.

Diabetic mothers tend to have large babies, with cells that are both hyperplastic and hypertrophic. The alteration of carbohydrate metabolism in pregnancy is associated with a decrease in the fasting level of blood glucose and alteration of the glucose tolerance test in the direction of a higher peak in blood glucose and a longer elevation of the rise. A rise in circulating insulin and increased insulin response to glucose form part of the pattern of physiological alterations in early pregnancy, and an increased need for insulin in late pregnancy places greater demands on the pancreas. The incidence of diabetes is higher among women who have had a large number of pregnancies. There is some controversy about whether pregnancy itself is diabetogenic or whether the stress of pregnancy reveals latent diabetes.[36]

Toxemia, or preeclampsia, is a pathological state specific to pregnancy in humans. It is diagnosed by a triad of symptoms: generalized edema that may cause a sudden rise in weight gain, albuminuria, and blood pressure elevated above 140/90. Toxemia is more common among primiparas, adolescents (especially those under 15 years), underweight women, and in pregnancies with multiple fetuses. It is one of the major factors in premature delivery and is associated with higher frequency of perinatal mortality. Progression of the condition to eclampsia presents great risk to both mother and fetus.

Cigarettes

It is now well established that the smoking of cigarettes tends to limit fetal development and lower birth weight in direct relation to the number of cigarettes smoked. The mechanism of action is not clear, although several hypotheses have been proposed.

Alcohol

Alcohol consumption during pregnancy has been associated with deficiencies in both fetal and postnatal growth of the offspring, as well as with mental retardation, microcephaly, and other physical anomalies. At the present time it is unclear whether the fetal alcohol syndrome (FAS) is due to the direct effect of the placental transfer of ethanol, to other teratogenic components of alcoholic beverages, or to associated factors, such as hypoglycemia, malnutrition, or cigarette smoking. Studies are now under way to investigate possible mechanisms, the amount of alcohol that may produce characteristics of the syndrome, and the time elements of greatest vulnerability.

Dietary Intake

Good nutritional status, both before and during pregnancy, is essential to provide an adequate supply of nutrients for the growth and function of the maternal body, for the maintenance of maternal stores, and for the growth of the fetus and placenta. Severe starvation is likely to result in cessation of the menstrual cycle, anovulation, and infertility. A marginal level of intake permits conception but may not allow continuation of the pregnancy. However, reproductive efficiency in the face of malnutrition has been demonstrated by the high birth rates even among poorly nourished populations. The remarkable adaptation of the body to chronically low dietary intakes and the ability of the maternal organism to buffer the effects of inadequate intake in order to supply nutrients to the fetus have made it difficult to delineate with any degree of clarity the relationship between nutritional intake and fetal growth. However, the high rates of maternal and infant mortality in populations with inadequate food supply attest to the importance of nutrition. The maternal organism may draw upon reserves to meet the stress of pregnancy and produce a live infant, but the long-term effects of inadequate intake on the health of both the mother and her child are undesirable.

As indicated earlier, the three major determinants of fetal growth and infant birth weight are length of gestation, maternal weight gain, and preconceptional weight. Nutrition is a major influence on each of these factors. Epidemiological and physiological studies have shown that the effects of diet during pregnancy[2] and the supplementation of the diet[3,7,50,57] are greatest when prenatal stress is superimposed on poor preconceptional nutritional status; the effects of prenatal diet are less obvious when preconceptional nutritional status was good.[1] The clear implication is that the nutrition of the female throughout her early life is important in her reproductive success, but that improvement in diet during pregnancy can moderate effects of earlier malnutrition.

Poor nutrition is found most often when socioeconomic status is low, and the multiple negative aspects of poverty make it difficult to sort out the effects of each.

Socioeconomic Status

Gordon[60] has used the term matroenvironment to encompass the diverse influences of the mother upon her developing fetus and on the infant after she has given birth. The physiological and biochemical environments have

148

long been recognized and evaluated by the maternal anthropometric, psychological, pathological, and obstetric complications. "Recognition grows, however, that the third classical component of environment, the sociocultural, also provided by the mother, has equal significance if not an overriding importance in development of the fetus. Poverty governs food supply, education determines the direction of health maintenance and the management of illnesses, and the extent of child training and experiences derived from preceding pregnancies affect the care afforded the as yet unborn. Social and economic influences acting on the mother are thus reflected directly or indirectly on the fetus."

Low economic status is related to poor diet, higher parity at younger ages, shorter intervals between pregnancies, increased morbidity and infectious diseases, and less medical care during pregnancy, all of which contribute to the risk of inhibition of fetal development and low birth weight.

NUTRIENT REQUIREMENTS AND DIETARY ALLOWANCES

During pregnancy the basic requirements of the woman to maintain her own body continue. In addition, she must supply nutrients for the growth of new tissue of the placenta and fetus as well as the reproductive tissues to support pregnancy and prepare for lactation. The increases in blood volume and total body water constitute approximately one-third of total weight gain and have a high requirement of protein, minerals, and electrolytes. Metabolic demands for the formation and maintenance of new tissue and more energy for the increased work load of movement add to dietary needs during gestation. Storage of additional fat and protein in her own body, whether as a physiological concomitant of pregnancy or for the purpose of supporting lactation, must also be supplied. The percentage increment to nonpregnant needs is not equal for all nutrients, but is specific to each nutrient in relation to its functions and to the timing of each of the growth aspects for which it is essential.

SOURCES OF DATA

Inadequate information is available for defining requirements of the pregnant woman, resulting in calculations based largely on the interpretation and judgment of individuals or committees. As discussed in Chapter 2, variations in recommendations from one country or agency to another, and within a country from time to time, testify to the paucity of firm data. Differentiation between mean levels and optimal levels is ultimately essential, but at the present time difficult.

Balance studies have usually been limited to a few nutrients, primarily nitrogen, calcium, and phosphorus. Potential errors have led some authorities to question results, but they have provided more detailed values than are otherwise available. Much of the knowledge of nutrient requirements during pregnancy was derived from the studies of Macy and associates[61] at the Children's Fund of Michigan in the 1930s and 1940s. Among the few balance studies in recent years have been the nitrogen studies of Calloway, King, and associates.[45,46]

Biochemical studies of the effects of diet or supplementation on blood levels and urinary excretion have contributed much valuable data, especially in regard to iron and vitamins. These have enlarged knowledge about the metabolism of nutrients and indirectly about requirements.

Dietary surveys have been conducted on various population groups throughout the world. These have most often been limited to intakes during relatively few days, usually late in the gestation period. In a few studies dietary intake data have been obtained at repeated intervals during pregnancy. This epidemiological approach is most valuable when the outcome of pregnancy is also evaluated, which allows some distinction between usual intake and that which might be considered optimal. When the clinical course of pregnancy and delivery, birth size, condition of the infant, and biochemical evaluations can be compared to levels of dietary intake, the value of dietary studies is greatly enhanced. Since dietary intake studies are relatively easily accomplished, reports of nutrient intakes and their distribution in various population groups have provided the bulk of the literature on nutrition during pregnancy.

Factorial calculation of nutrient requirements has been attempted by a number of individuals and committees in the absence of more precise data. These calculations are based on a summation of the known or estimated content of tissues and on the timing of their increments. It is obvious from the gaps in knowledge about physiological changes in the mother, actual tissue content, and variations in growth that such calculations contain a very large margin of error and can be accepted only as tentative estimates while more accurate information is unavailable.

Requirements have been estimated for some nutrients, based only on evidence of increased need during pregnancy, with information derived from alterations in blood level or clinical reports of increased risk with low intakes. This method of establishing tentative recommendations has been used primarily for trace elements and vitamins which have only recently been considered of importance in human nutrition and for which little data are available. Such estimations are usually conservative and with further studies can be expected to change.

150

So many factors affect nutrient requirements of the individual woman during pregnancy that a single figure in a table can be used only as a rough approximation of need. Changes in tissue content are a major basis for estimating prenatal needs, but the few tissue analyses that have been done give inadequate knowledge of individual variation or of optimal content. Therefore the actual nutrient needs of each added component of the pregnant woman's body are not known. Body storage and nutritional status prior to conception affect the requirements of a woman and interpretation of findings in prenatal studies. This is demonstrated both in balance studies and in studies of the efficiency of absorption as measured by blood levels. Renal conservation of some nutrients and wastefulness of others vary as pregnancy progresses, altering requirements in various stages of pregnancy.

Most studies of pregnant women have been done during the last half of gestation, and the preconceptional baseline is unknown, so individual changes in dietary intake or in measurements of physiological, biochemical, or metabolic adjustments cannot be evaluated. Some studies of postpartum status have been used as a substitute for preconceptional baselines,[37] but there is little knowledge about alterations in physiology or metabolism that result from having been pregnant. Postpartum body functions may differ from preconceptional functions.

The establishment of allowances for the pregnant woman involves some considerations that are not applicable to other members of the population. Since there are decreases in blood levels of nutrients, some as the result of normal hemodilution and some at present unexplainable, the allowances may be set high enough to attempt to maintain blood levels close to those of the nonpregnant woman, or alternatively they may be set at a level that accepts the lower levels as normal but aims to prevent deficiency. The latter method implies using separate blood standards for pregnant and nonpregnant women. An additional consideration is that the maternal body may draw on its storage of some nutrients, probably with replenishment after pregnancy is completed. This raises the question of whether the allowances should be set high enough to protect maternal storage reserves. These unanswered questions have contributed to the differences in allowances established by different groups.

ENERGY

The Recommended Dietary Allowance (RDA) for pregnancy provides 300 kcal (1.26 MJ) above the age-specific nonpregnant recommendation (Table 3.4). Since the first edition of the RDAs in 1943, when the extra allowance for pregnancy was 400 kcal, the allowance was decreased in 1958 to 300

Table 3.4   Recommended Dietary Allowances during Pregnancy

	Increment during Pregnancy	11–14 years	15–18 years	19–22 years	23 years +
Energy, kcal	300	2500	2400	2400	2300
MJ	1.26	10.50	10.04	10.04	9.62
Protein, g	30	76	76	74	74
Vitamin A, I.U.	1000	5000	5000	5000	5000
Retinol equiv., μg	200	1000	1000	1000	1000
Vitamin D, I.U.	200	600	600	500	400
Vitamin E, mg α T.E.	2	10	10	10	10
Ascorbic acid, mg	20	70	80	80	80
Folacin, μg	400	800	800	800	800
Niacin, mg N.E.	2	17	16	16	15
Riboflavin, mg	0.3	1.6	1.6	1.6	1.5
Thiamin, mg	0.4	1.5	1.5	1.5	1.0
Vitamin B_6, mg	0.6	2.6	2.6	2.6	2.6
Vitamin B_{12}, μg	1.0	4.0	4.0	4.0	4.0
Calcium, g	0.4	1.6	1.6	1.2	1.2
Phosphorus, g	0.4	1.6	1.6	1.2	1.2
Iodine, g	25	175	175	175	175
Iron, mg	Suppl.	18 + Suppl.	18 + Suppl.	18 + Suppl.	18 + Suppl.
Magnesium, mg	150	450	450	450	450
Zinc, mg	5	20	20	20	20

Source: Recommended Dietary Allowances. National Academy of Sciences, Washington, D.C. Ninth Edition, in press, 1979.

kcal, and then further decreased to 200 kcal in 1963 and 1968, rising again to 300 kcal in 1974 and 1979. The timing of increase has varied from the latter half to the last two trimesters, and in the 1974 edition[63] was recommended for the entire pregnancy, adjusted for a weight gain of 11 kg.

The energy allowance is an example of factorial calculation, based on known or estimated increments of body tissue and oxygen consumption,[36] as shown in Tables 3.5 and 3.6. These values were based on a "standard" primigravida, 24 years of age, with a height of 163 cm, prepregnant weight of 56 kg, and prepregnant basal metabolic need of 1400 kcal/day. The estimated increment of protein in the mother and conceptus was 935 g and of fat 3825 g (Table 3.5). This was based on the assumption that the 1 to 3 kg of weight gain that could not be accounted for is entirely fat; adjustment should probably be made to divide the compartment labeled "Maternal stores" between protein and fat, thus elevating the amount of added protein and lowering the amount of fat. Calculating the energy cost of these tissues, using 5.6 kcal/g protein and 9.5 kcal/g fat, and adding the energy value of oxygen consumed, the total net cost of the pregnancy itself is 67,761 kcal (288 MJ). With a further adjustment for a respiratory quotient of 90, thereby adding 10 percent, the total metabolizable energy cost of pregnancy is calculated as 74,537 kcal (311.6 MJ). This figure has often been rounded to 80,000 kcal (335 MJ) as the gross energy cost of a nine-month pregnancy. If protein were factored in maternal stores, the caloric cost would be lowered.

The Food and Nutrition Board committee, in using this as a basis for calculation of the RDA, pointed out that this did not take into consideration

Table 3.5 Addition of Body Tissue During Pregnancy

	Added Protein in Pregnancy, g. Weeks of Pregnancy				Fat Storage in Pregnancy, g. Weeks of Pregnancy			
	10	20	30	40	10	20	30	40
Fetus	0.3	27	160	440	negl.	2	80	440
Placenta	2	16	60	100	negl.	1	3	4
Amniotic fluid	0	0.5	2	3				
Uterus	24	55	102	166	0.5	1.3	2.4	3.9
Breasts	9	36	72	81	1.4	5.4	10.8	12.2
Blood	0	30	102	135	0.4	3.9	17.4	19.6
Maternal stores[a]					326	2050	3480	3345
Total	36	165	498	925	328	2064	3594	3825

[a]Based on assumption that maternal tissue storage is entirely fat.

Source: Hytten, F. E., and I. Leitch. *The Physiology of Human Pregnancy.* Blackwell Scientific Publishing Company, Oxford, Second Edition, 1971.

Table 3.6   Calculation of the Energy Cost of Pregnancy

	Mean Daily Increments (g) and Energy Cost				Cumulative Total, g	Cumulative Total, kcal
	Weeks of pregnancy					
	0–10	10–20	20–30	30–40		
Mean daily increments						
Protein, g	0.64	1.84	4.76	6.1	925	
Fat, g[a]	5.85	24.80	21.85	3.3	3825	
Energy cost[b]						
Protein, kcal	3.6	10.3	26.7	34.2		5,180
Fat, kcal	55.6	235.6	207.6	31.3		36,337
Oxygen consumption	19.9	62.0	110.9	186.1		26,244
Total net energy	79.1	307.9	345.2	251.6		67,761
Metabolizable energy[c]	87	339	380	277		74,537

[a]Based on assumption that maternal tissue storage is entirely fat.
[b]Values of 5.6 kcal/g protein and 9.5 kcal/g fat were used.
[c]Total net energy + 10 percent, assuming RQ of 0.90.

Source: Hytten, F. E., and I. Leitch. *The Physiology of Human Pregnancy.* Blackwell Scientific Publishing Company, Oxford, Second Edition, 1971.

any decrease in the physical activity of some women, and further considered a weight gain of 11 kg a desired average. They concluded that an increment of 300 kcal/day is sufficient for most women, to be taken throughout pregnancy.

In contrast, in citing the same data, the committee that set the 1976 Dietary Standard for Canada[63] pointed out that approximately half of the total energy cost of pregnancy as calculated in Table 3.6 is attributed to fat deposition. "In countries where food supply is abundant and where few women breast-feed their child, there is a tendency to consider this storage of energy as non-essential, and perhaps undesirable." They estimated from these data of Hytten and Leitch that a supplementary allowance of 40,000 kcal (167 MJ) would cover the extra energy needs of pregnancy. However, in view of the risk of diversion of protein to energy when caloric intake is low, and the dangers of undernutrition to the fetus, they suggested a total additional intake of 65,000 kcal (272 MJ) throughout pregnancy. The division allowed for 100 kcal (0.42 MJ) daily in the first trimester, and 300 kcal (1.3 MJ)/day in the second and third trimesters.

When the RDA is adjusted for age (Table 3.4), greater allowance is provided for the adolescent than for the mature woman. The woman who is thin at the start of pregnancy should also be given greater leeway, since some of her weight gain during pregnancy is likely to be incorporated into her own body tissues. Physical activity also demands individual adjustment of the allowance. A primigravida who is not working outside the home may have more time for resting; the multigravida who has young children may find limitation of physical activity difficult. As pregnancy progresses, the additional energy cost of motion may be offset by a slower pace or lowered activity. The woman who has outside employment may not be able to reduce physical activity.

Weight reduction during pregnancy is not recommended. The incidence of infants with low birth weight is higher among women whose weight gain is low. Oldham and Sheft[47] showed that adequate utilization of nitrogen was imperiled when caloric intake fell below 36 kcal/kg of pregnant weight.

PROTEIN

Whereas the energy allowance during pregnancy is increased only 14 to 15 percent above the nonpregnant level, for protein the increment is approximately 65 to 68 percent. The RDA provides for an addition of 30 g of protein per day from the second month to term. This allowance is based on 1.3 g/kg body weight for mature women, 1.5 g/kg for adolescents between 15 and 18 years, and 1.7 g/kg for those under 15 years of age. The higher allowance for adolescents takes into account their own continued growth in addition to pregnancy needs. Roche and Davila[64] reported that adult stature was attained in girls in the Fels Research Institute study at a median age of 17.3 years, with a range from the 10th to the 90th percentiles of 15.8 to 21.1 years. Although peak height velocity preceded menarche by more than one year, slower growth continued for a median of 6 years following menarche. Therefore, to support both maternal and fetal growth, extra provision of protein should be recommended for the adolescent. The allowance for protein for both adolescents and mature women assumes adequacy of caloric intake.

Protein requirements have been established by both factorial and nitrogen balance study methods, and interpretation of available data has resulted in changes in the concept of the amount of additional protein needed. From 1943 to 1958, the allowance for the mature woman was 60 g/day in the non-pregnant state and 85 g/day during pregnancy, a difference of 25 g. In 1964 and 1968 the allowances for the nonpregnant woman were lowered to 58 and then to 55 g/day and the added allowance for pregnancy was lowered to 20 g and then to 10 g. However, in 1974, when the nonpregnant allowance was lowered still further to 46 g, the extra recommendation for pregnancy was raised to 30 g, giving a total of 76 g daily for the mature woman. In the 1979 revision, the allowance for the nonpregnant mature woman was decreased to 44 g, but the 30 g differential for pregnancy was retained.

The factorial calculation of the protein increments attributed to pregnancy is shown in Table 3.6, with estimate of a total accumulation of 925 g in nine months to the maternal body, the placenta, and the fetus.[36] This makes no concession to protein deposition in maternal stores. With adjustment for a margin of safety in regard to protein quality and individual variation, this calculation was considered justification in 1968 for the extra allowance of only 10 g protein daily in the RDA. However, further balance studies[45,46] have shown that, at the caloric allowance recommended, 10 g was not sufficient in view of increased retention during pregnancy on higher protein intakes. In young primiparas maximum nitrogen retention was not attained on intakes as high as 125 g/day. Assuming that the estimation of 925 g of protein in fetal and maternal reproductive tissues and blood during pregnancy is correct, it now seems evident that additional allowance must be made for maternal stores. In addition, limitation of either calories or protein during pregnancy has repeatedly been shown to interfere with fetal growth. On the basis of this evidence, the protein increment was raised to 30 g/day in 1974.

CALCIUM AND PHOSPHORUS

The recommended increase in dietary calcium and phosphorus during pregnancy is 400 mg/day for each, representing an increase of 50 percent. The increment for calcium, however, has undergone change. Between 1943 and 1958 the nonpregnant level was 0.8 g, except for one edition, and the pregnancy intake recommended was 1.5 g, an increase of nearly 90 percent. The allowance during pregnancy was lowered to 1.3 g in 1964 and has been 1.2 g since 1968. Phosphorus was not included in the RDA table until 1968.

Like protein, both factorial calculations and balance studies have been used to estimate requirements during pregnancy, and balance studies have usually shown greater retention than can be accounted for in fetal and placental increments. The calcium content of the infant body at term was determined by Widdowson[29] as 30 g (Table 3.2). In a review of the literature, Irwin and Kienholz[65] reported that analysis of more than 100 full-term fetuses showed variation of 13 to 33 g calcium, but that most were between 21 and 28 g. Placental content was 0.65 g. Most of the calcium deposition in the fetus occurs during the last 1 to 2 months of gestation, when deposition has been estimated to occur at rates of 200 to 300 mg/day.[36,65,66] However, calcium balance studies of women during the last half of pregnancy have shown retention of 34 to 53 g total during that period. Macy and Hunscher[43] found that maternal retention exceeded the estimated fetal requirements except in the last 4 weeks of pregnancy, when fetal deposition was estimated to be 200 mg/day above maternal retention. These studies suggest that maternal retention begins early in pregnancy for later use by the fetus. It is also possible that the maternal body may be storing calcium in bones for lactation.[66]

Estimating calcium requirements during pregnancy is also complicated by several other factors. Urinary excretion of calcium may be more pronounced early in gestation than later when fetal requirements are high. Large individual differences in percentage absorption of dietary calcium have been reported, influenced by the food source, the level of calcium in the diet, previous diet and adaptation to low or high levels, and other components of the diet, including vitamin D, protein, fat, phosphorus, phytin, and magnesium. In addition, the removal of calcium from maternal bone to supply fetal needs is possible. The amount of calcium needed by the fetus represents only 2 to 3 percent of the total maternal body calcium[36] and would not be a large drain on maternal storage for a single pregnancy, although the effect of repeated pregnancies might be appreciable.

Despite lower calcium allowances and intakes without evidence of deficiency in many areas of the world, the RDA in the United States for calcium during pregnancy has been maintained at a level to ensure maternal storage as well as fetal growth.

Less concern has been expressed about phosphorus requirements, partially because of its widespread availability in foods, so that deficiency of intake is unknown.[66] The RDA is set to provide a calcium:phosphorus ratio of 1.

IRON

Greater uncertainty exists about the metabolism of iron than of most other nutrients. The complexities of the bioavailability of iron in single foods or in mixed diets, changes in rate of absorption under differing physiological conditions, identification of anemia, and the clinical significance of levels of iron-related blood components have led to differences of opinion and repeated revisions of recommendations in the past two decades.

Data on which recommendations have been based have included balance studies, epidemiological evidence of blood levels in relation to dietary intake and of the hematopoietic response to administration of iron supplements, and factorial calculations. In a survey of the literature, Bowering et al.[67] proposed three generalizations: (1) the rate of absorption is inversely proportional to the size of the dose; (2) absorption tends to increase as pregnancy progresses; and (3) the increase in absorption is greater in iron-deficient and anemic women than in nonanemic.

The fetus triples its iron deposition in the last 10 weeks of gestation (Table 3.2). Since hematocrit and other blood indices at birth tend to be within the normal range regardless of the mother's iron intake, it is assumed that the fetus takes priority in demands for available iron. Therefore the maternal reserves must be drawn upon if intake is not adequate. The need for iron during the first two trimesters is primarily for increase in maternal and placental erythrocyte mass, and in the last trimester mainly for fetal deposition. In the last 3 months, 2 to 4 mg/day may be transferred to the fetus.

Estimations of increase in efficiency of absorption have varied widely, usually rising from an assumed absorption of 10 percent average in the nonpregnant state to 20–40 percent in the third trimester. Since absorption rate is influenced by maternal iron storage, type of foods or supplement, the presence of a variety of substances in the gastrointestinal tract, and the degree of need, there is wide individual variation in absorption and it is difficult to estimate mean absorption rates. The RDA[62] is presumably based on "an average availability of 10 percent of the food iron" even during pregnancy, while the Canadian standard[63] has assumed absorption during pregnancy to be 20 percent.

Wide ranges of estimates for the components of a factorial calculation of the need for iron during pregnancy are evident in Table 3.7, in which there is a threefold difference in the sums of the lowest and highest estimated needs. The average total need for absorption during a full-term pregnancy is approximately 1 g of elemental iron, including maternal maintenance.[67,68] The need directly associated with pregnancy is close to 800 mg. However, some factorial calculations take into account the finding that most of the iron accumulated in the increased maternal red blood cell volume is returned to maternal stores after delivery. Therefore, some figures in the literature refer to the "cost" of pregnancy itself as including only the placenta, the fetus, and the blood lost at delivery. From a physiological standpoint, then, the iron that will leave the mother's body when she delivers may range between 300 and 800 mg. From the viewpoint of dietary recommendations, the total amount of iron needed during the nine-month period is close to 1 g, including maternal maintenance.

From 1943 through 1958 the RDA for iron was 12 mg for the nonpregnant woman and 15 mg for the pregnant woman. In 1963 the nonpregnancy allowance was raised to 15 mg and the pregnancy allowance to 20 mg for the last two trimesters. In 1968 the allowance for both categories of women was 18 mg, and the text stated that "it is impractical to supply these needs with ordinary food, and iron supplementation is required." In 1974 and 1979 the allowance for the nonpregnant woman was 18 mg, and for the pregnant woman 18 + mg with the statement that "this increased requirement cannot be met by ordinary diets; therefore the use of supplemental iron is recommended" and the amount of supplement was specified as 30 to 60 mg daily.

The WHO recommendation[69] for supplementary iron is based on the characteristics of the population and their diets. "Variations in the dietary intake of iron, and in iron stores, in different population groups make it necessary to recommend iron supplementation at different dosage levels. In women more than 25% of whose caloric intake comes from animal sources and who have iron stores at the beginning of pregnancy, a daily supplement of 30 mg of iron is sufficient to maintain optimal haemoglobin concentrations. However, there is evidence that these conditions seldom exist, even in developed countries, and it is probable that a daily supplement of 60 mg of

Table 3.7   Iron Requirements for Pregnancy

	Average mg	Range mg
External iron loss (maintenance)	170	150–200
Expansion of red blood cell mass	450	200–600
Fetal iron	270	200–370
Iron in placenta and cord	90	30–170
Blood loss at delivery	150	90–310
Total requirement[a]	980	580–1340
Cost of pregnancy[b]	680	440–1050

[a]Blood loss at delivery not included.
[b]Expansion of red cell mass not included.

Source: Committee on Iron Deficiency, Council on Foods and Nutrition. Iron deficiency in the United States. JAMA *203*:407–412, 1968.

iron is desirable." For populations where less than 10 percent of calories is derived from animal foods and iron deficiency is prevalent, the recommended dosage is 120 to 240 mg per day.

In contrast, the Canadian dietary recommendation[63] is 14 mg for the nonpregnant woman and 15 mg in the second half of pregnancy for the woman whose iron stores are adequate and 15 + mg with less than adequate stores, and no specific recommendation for supplementation is made. Hytten and Leitch[36] stated that "in general there is no convincing published evidence that the normal pregnant woman is at an advantage if she takes extra iron." There is, then, no universal agreement on the need for routine supplementation with iron during pregnancy in developed countries. Women with diagnosed anemia or high risk of anemia should undoubtedly receive iron supplementation.

FLUORINE

The efficacy of fluorine in preventing dental caries has led to the suggestion that it be administered to pregnant women. However, since the amount of calcification in the fetal tooth buds is relatively small, it seems unlikely that prenatal fluoride would have any beneficial effects.[42] Studies have failed to show any effect of prenatal intake of fluorine on later incidence of caries in children.

IODINE

With alteration in the metabolic rate during pregnancy, there are major changes in iodine metabolism. Blood levels of thyroid-stimulating hormone (TSH), thyroxine (T4), and triiodothyronine (T3) are elevated.[37] The Food and Nutrition Board has recommended that only iodized salt should be used. Slightly more than half of the table salt consumed in the United States is iodized, and salt added to processed foods usually does not contain iodine.[62] The RDA for pregnancy is 25 μg above the allowance of 150ug for the nonpregnant woman.

SODIUM

The total added sodium requirement in pregnancy, based on a weight gain of 11 kg, of which 70 percent is water, has been estimated at slightly more than 1000 mEq, or an additional 25 g Na or 60 g NaCl. Sodium restriction stresses the renin-angiotensin-aldosterone mechanism in an effort to maintain homeostasis. Therefore, restriction of sodium intake is not recommended as a routine procedure. Specific contraindications include diagnosis of pathology, such as hypertensive cardiovascular and renal disease.

160

OTHER MINERAL ELEMENTS

It is currently believed that a diet meeting the requirements for major nutrients will supply adequate amounts of other electrolytes and trace elements.

FOLACIN

Folacin is the only nutrient for which the RDA during pregnancy is twice the nonpregnancy allowance. The functions of folate in DNA synthesis and in erythrocyte maturation are particularly important during pregnancy. Early studies associated the fall in serum folate with abruptio placentae, late pregnancy bleeding, fetal malformation, and abortion, although more recent research has failed to confirm a relationship betweeen folate deficiency and any of these complications of reproduction.[39] However, megaloblastic anemia as a result of folacin deficiency is not uncommon in undernourished women, especially in developing countries, and is a hazard in pregnancies with multiple fetuses. Although megaloblastic anemia due to folate deficiency is relatively uncommon in the United States, it does occur and must be considered in the differential diagnosis of any anemia encountered during pregnancy.[10] Infants born to women with megaloblastic anemia of pregnancy tend to have normal hemoglobin values.[39]

The level of serum folate usually decreases during pregnancy, particularly in the third trimester. However, since serum folate is extremely labile and sensitive to fluctuations in dietary intake, it is probably a poor indicator of folate deficiency or folate reserves.[37] Low serum folate levels are not necessarily associated with megaloblastic anemia or any biochemical changes. Serum folate levels of less than 3 ng/ml have been observed in 20 to 25 percent of otherwise normal pregnancies.[39]

Erythrocyte folate, on the other hand, is relatively stable, and decreases with the formation of new red cells.[37] It is therefore regarded as a more accurate and less variable quantitative index to the severity of folacin deficiency. Megaloblastic changes in bone marrow appear only after 4 months or more of deficiency, and a level of 20 ng/ml or less is indicative of folacin deficiency.

Evaluations of dietary adequacy of folacin are tentative with present data, because of the multiple chemical forms of the vitamin, differences in absorption and utilization, and losses of folacin in processing of foods. The RDA of 800 μg during pregnancy is based on total folate, including both the free and polyglutamate forms.

Supplementation with 500 μg folic acid daily is recommended by WHO, starting not later than the second trimester of pregnancy.[69] However, Pritchard[10] has suggested that the goal of supplementation should be clearly delineated before a decision is made on routine folic acid supplementation. If the goal is to raise blood folate levels to normal nonpregnant levels where megaloblastic anemia is rare, 100 μg/day is adequate. In populations where megaloblastic anemia is common, 350 μg may be recommended. In women with severe megaloblastic anemia, including those with twins, daily administration of 1 mg orally can be expected to produce hematologic remission. A Committee on Nutrition of the American College of Obstetricians and Gynecologists[42] has suggested that folic acid supplementation is "probably a reasonable prophylactic measure, particularly in high risk patients, such as those with low socioeconomic class and those with multiple pregnancy and chronic hemolytic anemia." Supplements in the recommended dose of 200 to 400 μg/day would diminish the incidence of megaloblastic anemia of pregnancy but whether it would have additional beneficial effects is problematic.

VITAMIN B$_{12}$

Megaloblastic anemia in pregnancy is most often due to a deficiency of folacin, but vitamin B$_{12}$ must be considered in making the diagnosis. The serum level of vitamin B$_{12}$ falls during pregnancy, seemingly without relation to dietary intake levels, and supplementation does not affect the level in normal women.[37] Although data on requirements are limited, the recommendation of 3 μg/day for the nonpregnant woman is increased to 4 μg/day during pregnancy.[62]

Concern about meeting the recommendations is probably unnecessary in women whose diets contain animal products. The sole source of vitamin B$_{12}$ in nature is synthesis by microorganisms. Except for incorporation of microorganisms in the root nodules of some legumes, uncontaminated fruits, vegetables, and grains are devoid of the vitamin.[70] Therefore, strict vegans who consume no animal products will be unable to meet the recommended allowance. The length of time a vegan diet has been followed may play a role, since vitamin B$_{12}$ can be stored in the body, and presumably the reserves may be drawn upon.

VITAMIN B$_6$

The RDA for vitamin B$_6$ has been increased from the nonpregnant level of 2.0 mg to 2.5 mg in pregnancy. Several aspects of the metabolism of this vitamin are of particular importance during pregnancy, and concern has been expressed that dietary intake may not meet the added needs.

The placenta concentrates vitamin B$_6$, and levels of the vitamin in cord blood are at least twice as high as in maternal blood, ensuring a supply to the fetus. Plasma levels of pyridoxal phosphate are lower in the third trimester than nonpregnant levels, and urinary excretion of tryptophan metabolites is increased.[37] These alterations may be moderated by supplements, although such effect has not been reported in all studies.

The need for vitamin B_6 increases with high protein intakes, and therefore the requirement during pregnancy is elevated. Some studies have shown beneficial effects on nausea and preeclampsia of pregnancy with administration of vitamin B_6. An additional factor of concern is that many biochemical parameters associated with vitamin B_6 metabolism are altered with the use of anovulatory steroids,[62] so that special attention may need to be given to the woman who has taken these contraceptives for an extended period of time and has not allowed sufficient time for normalization of B_6 metabolism before conceiving.

OTHER VITAMINS

Table 3.8 summarizes the percentage increment recommended during pregnancy for each of the nutrients. Except for folacin, the increased need for vitamins is estimated to range from 15 to 33 percent above the nonpregnant allowances. In general, the need for protein and minerals is increased to a greater extent than the need for vitamins.

Vitamin D is not included in this listing. The 1979 RDA provides an addition of 5 μg during pregnancy. Thus the allowance is 600 I.U. (15 μg) to 18 years, 500 I.U. (12.5 μg) between 19 and 22 years, and 400 I.U. (10 μg) after 22 years. Excessive prenatal intakes of vitamin D have been related to hypercalcemia in infants, although confirmation of this finding remains controversial.[65]

MEETING NUTRIENT NEEDS

The diet during pregnancy should be carefully selected to provide all nutrients for optimal growth of the fetus, placenta, and new maternal tissues as well as for maintenance of the mother's reserves. If the woman enters preg-

Table 3.8   Percentage Increase in RDA during Pregnancy (Adult)

Percent Increment	Nutrients[a]
100	Folacin
68	Protein
50	Calcium, phosphorus, magnesium
40	Thiamin
30–33	Zinc, ascorbic acid, vitamin B_6, vitamin B_{12}
20–25	Vitamin A, vitamin E, riboflavin
15–17	Energy, niacin, iodine

[a]For iron and vitamin D, see text.

nancy in poor nutritional status, special attention should be given to provision of foods with high nutrient density to compensate for her limited reserves. The adolescent requires a higher intake of energy and nutrients to allow for her own continued somatic growth in addition to the special needs associated with pregnancy. The obese woman needs guidance in the selection of a diet that provides enough energy not to compromise the growth functions of protein, and all of the protein, minerals, and vitamins essential for pregnancy; the only limitation is of foods high in simple carbohydrates and fat that may have contributed to her obesity.

Most women are very receptive to nutrition teaching during pregnancy, if they are given an understanding of the importance of nutrition to the growth and health of the fetus. The health worker who merely distributes a printed list of foods to be consumed is missing one of the best opportunities for education. A simple explanation of fetal growth and its mechanisms, along with the application of the functions of nutrients, may provide a real stimulus toward dietary improvement. When the woman improves her own diet, she is likely to improve the diets of other family members as well. This type of teaching takes more time, but the benefits to be accrued are probably greater than at any other stage of the life span.

Caloric needs increase only 14 to 15 percent, but the allowance for protein is 65 to 68 percent higher during pregnancy. This necessitates careful attention to satisfying the higher appetite primarily with foods high in protein. Protein foods are also high in minerals and the vitamins of the B complex, so primary emphasis on these foods provides for the intake of those nutrients as well. The pregnant woman should be encouraged to include milk, eggs, and meat, fish, or poultry in her daily diet. It is more difficult, although not impossible, to meet protein allowances with a totally vegetarian diet, and emphasis must be given to the complementary values of plant proteins. However, the provision of calcium and vitamin B_{12} and the absorption of iron may be compromised on a vegan diet. Although a carefully selected vegan diet has been shown to be adequate for adults, the amino acid, mineral, and vitamin requirements of growth are difficult to meet without inclusion of milk at least.

The inclusion of milk in the diet is also the most effective means of meeting the allowance of calcium. One quart of whole milk supplies 1.15 g of calcium; slightly higher values are found in low-fat milk. Without milk or milk products, the calcium content of the usual diet in the United States rarely exceeds 0.3 g. The woman who dislikes milk will often accept 3 or 4 ounces at a time and rebels only with larger amounts; additional milk may be consumed in creamed foods or puddings or as cheese. Lactase deficiency rarely involves total avoidance of milk. Since the deficiency is usually a comparative one, women with lactase deficiency can often consume small amounts at a time without discomfort, and most will tolerate yogurt or buttermilk.

Dependence on calcium supplements is not recommended. Many supplements contain relatively small amounts of calcium in relation to need; it is essential to check the calcium content so that an adequate intake is assured. In addition, women are often erratic about taking supplements, and they do not supply the protein, vitamins, and other minerals found in milk.

Four additional nutrients require special consideration because of the limited food categories that are major sources. Irradiated milk supplies vitamin D. If milk is not included in the diet, vitamin D assumes greater importance in the absorption and utilization of a reduced intake of calcium, and should be taken as a supplement. Vitamin A is supplied primarily as retinol in the lipid of milk and eggs and in organ meats such as liver; plant sources contain the provitamin, carotene, especially in green leafy and yellow varieties. Fortified margarines usually contain both carotene and preformed vitamin A. Ascorbic acid is high in citrus fruits, but may also be obtained in appreciable amounts from tomato, potato, and a variety of other fruits and vegetables. Vitamin B_{12}, as previously indicated, is obtained almost exclusively from animal products.

Other minerals and vitamins are present in varying amounts in many foods. A diet adequate in energy and protein will provide reasonable assurance of meeting the needs for these nutrients, with the possible exception of iron, as discussed earlier.

There is no single list of foods that must be taken to meet nutrient requirements. Selection of foods by the individual is often based on cultural, social, and economic factors. Dietary advice during pregnancy should be based on evaluation of customary intake of the woman, with as little distortion of usual food patterns as possible. Evaluation will indicate which specific foods need to be increased or decreased and whether additional foods should be introduced into the pattern. Attempts to make major changes in the diet are unlikely to be acceptable. It is wiser to build on the strengths of a diet that is familiar and has psychological meaning for the woman and to explain the rationale for alterations.

As a guide to the foods that will meet the nutrient needs during pregnancy, based on the most common pattern of food consumption in the United States, the following listing is suggested:

Milk: One quart daily, whole, low-fat, or skim, or buttermilk. Equivalent values of cheese or yogurt may be used. Milk may be used on foods or in cooking.
Meat (including organ meat), fish, or poultry: At least four ounces daily. Nuts or legumes may be substituted.

Egg: One daily.

Fruits: At least one citrus and one other fruit daily.

Vegetables: One potato and two to four servings of others daily. A green leafy or yellow vegetable should be included at least three to four times a week.

Butter or fortified margarine: One to two tablespoons daily.

Bread and cereal: Two to four servings daily, preferably whole grain or enriched. Enriched pasta may be a substitute.

Additional foods to meet energy needs.

The total amount of food consumed is usually determined by appetite, and extra allowances should be made for the adolescent and for the underweight woman. Individual attention will be needed by the woman whose usual diet is markedly different or limited to a small variety of foods. Idiosyncrasies, allergies, and food intolerance will also require special counseling.

The goal of dietary advice during pregnancy is to correct preexisting deficiencies, to provide nutrients for optimal growth of the fetus, and to maintain or improve the health of the mother. Although we have incomplete knowledge of the specific functions of nutrients in the reproductive process, maternal nutrition is a major determinant in the successful outcome and should be a component of all prenatal care.

REFERENCES

1. Smith, C. A. The effect of wartime starvation in Holland upon pregnancy and its product. *Am. J. Obstet. Gynecol. 53*:599–608, 1947.
2. Antonov, A. N. Children born during the siege of Leningrad in 1942. *J. Pediat. 30*:250–259, 1947.
3. Habicht, J.-P., A. Lechtig, C. Yarbrough, and R. E. Klein. Maternal nutrition, birth weight and infant mortality. In: *Size at Birth. Ciba Foundation Symposium 27.* Associated Scientific Publishers, Amsterdam, 1974.
4. Burke, B. S., V. A. Beal, S. B. Kirkwood, and H. C. Stuart. The influence of nutrition during pregnancy upon the condition of the infant at birth. *J. Nutr. 26*:569–583, 1943.
5. Tompkins, W. T. The significance of nutritional deficiency of pregnancy. *J. Internat. Coll. Surg. 4*:147–154, 1941.
6. Balfour, M. I. Supplementary feeding in pregnancy. *Lancet 1*:208–211, 1944.
7. Ebbs, J. H., F. F. Tisdall, and W. A. Scott. The influence of prenatal diet on the mother and child. *J. Nutr. 22*:515–526, 1941.

8. Interim Report of the People's League of Health. Nutrition of expectant and nursing mothers. *Lancet 2*:10–12, 1942.

9. Warkany, J., B. B. Monroe, and B. S. Sutherland. Intrauterine growth retardation. *Am. J. Dis. Child. 102*:248–279, 1961.

10. Committee on Maternal Nutrition, Food and Nutrition Board. *Maternal Nutrition and the Course of Pregnancy*. National Academy of Sciences, Washington, D.C., 1970.

11. Giroud, A. *Nutrition of the Embryo*. Charles C Thomas, Springfield, Ill., 1970.

12. Timiras, P. S. *Developmental Physiology and Aging*. Macmillan, New York, 1972.

13. Hunt, E. E., Jr. The developmental genetics of man. In: Falkner, F. (Ed.) *Human Development*. W. B. Saunders, Philadelphia, 1966.

14. Vaughn, V. C., III. Developmental pediatrics. In: Vaughn, V. C., III, R. J. McKay and W. E. Nelson (Eds.) *Nelson Textbook of Pediatrics*. W. B. Saunders, Philadelphia, 1975.

15. Gruenwald, P. (Ed.) *The Placenta and Its Maternal Supply Line. Effects of Insufficiency on the Fetus*. Univ. Park Press, Baltimore, 1975.

16. Behrman, R. E. Placental function and malnutrition. *Am. J. Dis. Child. 129*:425–426, 1975.

17. Widdowson, E. M. Prenatal nutrition. *Ann. N. Y. Acad. Sci. 300*: 188–196, 1977.

18. Metcoff, J. Maternal nutrition and fetal growth. In: McLaren, D. S., and D. Burman (Eds.) *Textbook of Paediatric Nutrition*. Churchill Livingstone, Edinburgh, 1976.

19. Rosso, P. Maternal nutrition, nutrient exchange, and fetal growth. In: Winick, M. (Ed.) *Nutritional Disorders of American Women*. John Wiley and Sons, New York, 1977.

20. Winick, M. (Ed.) *Nutrition and Development*. John Wiley and Sons, New York, 1972.

21. Winick, M., A. Coscia, and A. Noble. Cellular growth in the human placenta. 1. Normal placental growth. *Pediat. 39*:248–251, 1967.

22. Gruenwald, P. Pathology of the deprived fetus and its supply line. In: *Size at Birth. Ciba Foundation Symposium 27*. Associated Scientific Publishers. Amsterdam, 1974.

23. Hahn, P. Lipid metabolism and nutrition in the prenatal and postnatal period. In: Winick, M. (Ed.) *Nutrition and Development*. John Wiley and Sons, New York, 1972.

24. Beaconsfield, P., J. Ginsburg, and N. Jeacock. Glucose metabolism in the pentose phosphate pathway relative to nucleic acid and protein synthesis in the human placenta. *Devel. Med. Child Neurol. 6*:469–474, 1964.

25. Pitkin, R. M., and Reynolds, W. A. Fetal ingestion and metabolism of amniotic fluid protein. *Am. J. Obstet. Gynecol. 123*:356–363, 1975.

26. Givens, M. H., and I. G. Macy. The chemical composition of the human fetus. *J. Biol. Chem. 102*:7–17, 1933.

27. Swanson, W. W., and L. V. Iob. The growth of the fetus and infant as related to mineral intake during pregnancy. *Am. J. Obstet. Gynecol. 38*:382–391, 1939.

28. Kelly, H. J., R. E. Sloan, W. Hoffman, and C. Saunders. Accumulation of nitrogen and six minerals in the human fetus during gestation. *Human Biol. 23*:61–74, 1951.

29. Widdowson, E. M. Growth and composition of the fetus and newborn. In: Assali, N. S. (Ed.) *Biology of Gestation.* Vol. II, Academic Press, New York, 1968.

30. Apte, S. V., and L. Iyengar. Composition of the human fetus. *Brit. J. Nutr. 27*:305–312, 1972.

31. Winick, M., J. A. Brasel, and P. Rosso. Nutrition and cell growth. In: Winick, M. (Ed.) *Nutrition and Development.* John Wiley and Sons, New York, 1972.

32. Widdowson, E. M., D. E. Crabb, and R. D. Milner. Cellular development of some human organs before birth. *Arch. Dis. Child. 47*:652–655, 1972.

33. Naeye, R. L., W. Blanc, and C. Paul. Effects of maternal nutrition on the human fetus. *Pediat. 52*:494–501, 1973.

34. Campbell, S. Physical methods of assessing size at birth. In: *Size at Birth. Ciba Foundation Symposium 27.* Associated Scientific Publishers, Amsterdam, 1974.

35. Metcoff, J. Maternal leukocyte metabolism in fetal malnutrition: Nutrition and malnutrition, identification and measurement. *Adv. Exp. Med. Biol. 49*:73–118, 1974.

36. Hytten, F. E., and I. Leitch. *The Physiology of Human Pregnancy.* Blackwell Scientific Publishers, Oxford, Second Edition, 1971.

37. Committee on Nutrition of the Mother and Preschool Child, Food and Nutrition Board. *Laboratory Indices of Nutritional Status in Pregnancy.* National Academy of Sciences, Washington, D.C., 1978.

38. Bowering, J., A. M. Sanchez, and M. I. Irwin. A conspectus of research on iron requirements of man. *J. Nutr. 106*:985–1074, 1976.

39. Pitkin, R. M. Nutritional support in obstetrics and gynecology. *Clin. Obstet. Gynecol. 19*:489–513, 1976.

40. Kaminetzky, H. A., and H. Baker. Micronutrients in pregnancy. *Clin. Obstet. Gynecol. 20*:363–380, 1977.

41. Pike, R. L., and H. A. Smiciklas. A reappraisal of sodium restriction during pregnancy. *Internat. J. Gynaec. Obstet. 10:*1–7, 1972.

42. Pitkin, R. M., H. A. Kaminetzky, M. Newton, and J. A. Pritchard.

Maternal nutrition. A selective review of clinical topics. *Obstet. Gynecol. 40*:773–785, 1972.

43. Macy, I. G., and H. A. Hunscher. An evaluation of maternal nitrogen and mineral needs during embryonic and fetal development. *Am. J. Obstet. Gynecol. 27*:878–892, 1934.

44. Thomson, A. M., and F. E. Hytten. Caloric requirements in human pregnancy. *Proc. Nutr. Soc. 20*:76–83, 1961.

45. King, J. C. Protein metabolism during pregnancy. *Clin. Perinatol. 2*:243–254, 1975.

46. Calloway, D. H. Nitrogen balance during pregnancy. In: Winick, M. (Ed.) *Nutrition and Fetal Development.* John Wiley and Sons, New York, 1974.

47. Oldham, H., and B. B. Sheft. Effect of caloric intake on nitrogen utilization during pregnancy. *J. Am. Dietet. Assoc. 27*:847–854, 1951.

48. Beal, V. A. Nutritional studies during pregnancy. II. Dietary intake, maternal weight gain, and size of infant. *J. Am. Dietet. Assoc. 58*:321–326, 1971.

49. Hunscher, H. A., and W. T. Tompkins. The influence of maternal nutrition on the immediate and long-term outcome of pregnancy. *Clin. Obstet. Gynecol. 13*:130–144, 1970.

50. Primrose, T., and A. Higgins. A study in human antepartum nutrition. *J. Reprod. Med. 7*:257–264, 1971.

51. Armstrong, R. J. A Study of Infant Mortality from Linked Records by Birth Weight, Period of Gestation, and Other Variables, United States. Vital and Health Statistics Series 20, Number 12. DHEW Publ. No. (HSM) 72-1055. Supt. of Documents, U.S. Government Printing Office, Washington, D.C., 1972.

52. Butler, N. R., and E. D. Alberman. *Perinatal Problems. The Second Report of the 1958 British Perinatal Mortality Survey.* Churchill Livingstone, Edinburgh, 1969.

53. Niswander, K. R., and M. Gordon. *The Women and Their Pregnancies. The Collaborative Perinatal Study of the National Institute of Neurological Diseases and Stroke.* W. B. Saunders, Philadelphia, 1972.

54. Singer, J. E., M. Westphal, and K. Niswander. Relationship of weight gain during pregnancy to birth weight and infant growth and development in the first year of life. *Obstet. Gynecol. 31*:417–423, 1968.

55. Niswander, K., and E. C. Jackson. Physical characteristics of the gravida and their association with birth weight and perinatal death. *Am. J. Obstet. Gynecol. 119*:306–313, 1974.

56. Lechtig, A., C. Yarbrough, H. Delgado, J.-P. Habicht, R. Martorell, and R. E. Klein. Influence of maternal nutrition on birth weight. *Am. J. Clin. Nutr. 28*:1223–1233, 1975.

57. Higgins, A. C. Montreal Diet Dispensary Study. In: *Nutritional Sup-*

plementation and the Outcome of Pregnancy, Proceedings of a Workshop. National Academy of Sciences, Washington, D. C., 1973.

58. Weiss, W., E. C. Jackson, K. Niswander, and N. J. Eastman. The influence on birthweight of change in maternal weight gain in successive pregnancies in the same women. *Int. J. Gynaecol. Obstet. 7*:210–223, 1969.

59. Grant, J. A., and F. P. Heald. Complications of adolescent pregnancy. Survey of the literature on fetal outcome in adolescence. *Clin. Pediat. 11*:567–570, 1972.

60. Gordon, J. E. Nutritional individuality. *Am. J. Dis. Child. 129*:422–424, 1975.

61. Macy, I. G., and H. C. Mack. Implications of nutrition in the life cycle of women. *Am. J. Obstet. Gynecol. 68*:131–150, 1954.

62. *Recommended Dietary Allowances,* Eighth Edition, National Academy of Sciences, Washington, D.C., 1974.

63. *Dietary Standard for Canada.* Minister of Supply and Services Canada, Ottawa, 1976.

64. Roche, A. F., and G. Davila. Prepubertal and postpubertal growth. In: Cheek, D. (Ed.) *Fetal and Postnatal Cellular Growth.* John Wiley and Sons, New York, 1975.

65. Irwin, M. I., and E. W. Kienholz. A conspectus of research on calcium requirements of man. *J. Nutr. 103*:1019–1095, 1973.

66. Pitkin, R. M. Calcium metabolism in pregnancy: A review. *Am. J. Obstet. Gynecol. 121*:724–737, 1975.

67. Bowering, J., A. M. Sanchez, and M. I. Irwin. A conspectus of research on iron requirements of man. *J. Nutr. 106*:985–1074, 1976.

68. A.M.A. Council on Foods and Nutrition. Iron deficiency in the United States. *JAMA 203*:407–412, 1968.

69. World Health Organization. *Nutritional Anemias. WHO Technical Report Series No. 503.* World Health Organization, Geneva, 1972.

70. Herbert, V. Folic acid and vitamin B_{12}. In: Goodhart, R. S., and M. E. Shils (Eds.) *Modern Nutrition in Health and Disease.* Lea and Febiger, Philadelphia, Fifth Edition, 1973.

4

LACTATION

From earliest history breast milk has been ess ntial to the continuation of the human race. Until the past century the mortality rate was very high among infants who were for any reason deprived of mother's milk; a high rate persists in areas of the world where nutritionally adequate substitutes for human milk are unavailable or unsafe. The incidence of protein-energy malnutrition and enteric diseases of young children are closely related to the lack of breast milk, due to early weaning and the growing practice of bottle feeding in developing countries.

The nutritional needs of the infant are better met by human milk than by any substitute, and breast milk has not been improved on as a reference standard.[1] Throughout the world milks of many mammals have been used for feeding infants when the mother could not or wished not to nurse her infant. However, the milk of each species is biologically designed to meet the needs of the young of that species.[2] Size and degree of metabolic maturity at birth, length of the lactation period, early postnatal growth rate, and susceptibility to specific diseases vary from one species to another. For example, the calf is heavier at birth and doubles birth weight twice as fast as the human infant; cow's milk contains approximately three times as much protein and ash as human milk. Therefore, when cow's milk is fed to the human infant, it must be adapted to the physiological capabilities and requirements of the infant.

Efforts to duplicate human milk by alteration of the components of cow's milk have not yet been successful. Adaptation of cow's milk involves changes in nutrient content and concentration and in the balance of nutrients. The formulation of commercial substitutes for breast milk has continually changed with the expansion of nutrition knowledge, and further changes can be expected. More than 100 constituents of human milk have been identified, not only nutrients but also nonnutritive components. The enzymes, hormones, and immunological factors in breast milk affect digestion, absorption and utilization of nutrients as well as resistance to enteric and respiratory diseases and to allergy, and have an effect on the nutritional status and health of the infant. Therefore, although attempts have been made, it is impossible to "humanize" cow's milk. However, the availability of safe formulas has provided mothers with a choice of whether to feed their infants by breast or bottle. In the United States and other technologically advanced countries this choice became practical in the 1920s with the marketing of evaporated cow's milk, providing a safe and standardized base for adaptation, followed later by commercially premodified formulas. As a result, major changes have occurred in infant feeding practices, and the prevalence of breast feeding has declined.

BREAST FEEDING IN THE UNITED STATES

PREVALENCE

At least 90 percent of infants in the United States were breast fed in the early twentieth century.[3] Unfortunately, studies on the prevalence of breast feeding have seldom used comparable timing or methodology, but a composite picture can be drawn from a variety of sources to show trends. Figure 4.1 summarizes a number of reports on the percent of mothers breast-feeding in the neonatal period. Major national surveys and smaller surveys with at least 90 subjects were included in the graph. Sources of data in the surveys were questionnaires to hospitals or to mothers, clinic or home interviews, and records of pediatricians. Hospital survey data were based on the method of feeding at discharge, which ranged from eight days or more in the 1946 survey to two or three days in recent surveys. The data from smaller studies were based on initiation of breast feeding in the neonatal period. When the economic level of a group was specified, it is indicated on the graph. Despite the limitations of the data, trends can be identified.

The longest time span in a single survey, indicated by the dotted line, is from the 1965 National Fertility Survey.[4] Nearly 5,000 women born between 1910 and 1950 and still living with their husbands in 1965 provided retrospective information on whether they had breast-fed their first-born; only single births were included. The data show a decrease from 81 percent of mothers initiating breast feeding in 1926–1930 to only 32 percent in 1961–1965.

172

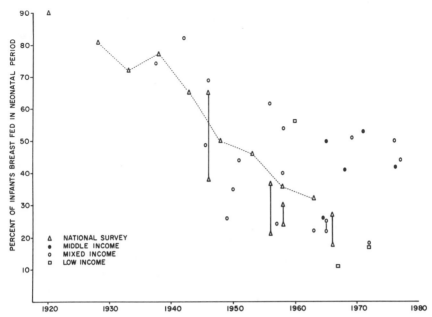

Figure 4.1   Breast feeding on hospital discharge in the United States. Vertical lines for surveys indicate percentage of infants totally breast fed (lower point) and percentage fed a combination of breast milk and formula (higher point). Each study includes at least 90 subjects.

National surveys[5-8] between 1946 and 1966 are indicated by vertical lines connecting two triangles. The lower triangle represents mothers who breast-fed totally and the higher connected triangle includes mothers who breast-fed with supplementary bottle feedings. A study with comparable data from the North Central region[9] is indicated by a vertical line connecting two circles. In more recent years fewer mothers combined both methods of feeding, tending instead to discontinue breast feeding if the milk supply was inadequate. In the national surveys regional analysis consistently showed the lowest incidence of breast feeding in New England and the highest in the southern and western areas of the United States.

The trend toward the decreasing practice of breast feeding in this country was clear. By 1965 only one-fourth of mothers initiated lactation. Similar trends have been reported from other countries when commercial infant formulas became available.[10-16] The few published studies in the past 15 to 20 years, representing small and sometimes selected groups of subjects, suggest a reversal of the downward trend in the United States. Increased interest in breast feeding was first reported among women of middle and upper income and educational levels,[17-19] but more recently women in lower economic levels are also tending to choose breast feeding over bottle feeding.[10] In some studies as many as 50 percent of the women have elected to breast feed. Further data are needed to confirm the reversal of the downward trend.

DURATION OF BREAST FEEDING

There are few published reports on the duration of breast feeding in the United States. Figure 4.2 summarizes available literature on the percentage of mothers still nursing after hospital discharge.

In 1920 it was estimated that more than 75 percent of infants were still breast-fed at 6 months of age and 10 percent at 12 months. In the period between 1940 and 1960 an average of approximately one-third of mothers surveyed discontinued breast feeding in the first month and an additional third in the second month. Few were still breast feeding at 6 months. Therefore, not only did fewer mothers initiate breast feeding, but those who did weaned their infants at earlier ages.

In the past decade, as the prevalence of breast feeding seems to be increasing, so too is the duration of breast feeding. The few published reports in the 1970s suggest that approximately 80 percent of infants started on breast milk were still nursed at one month and 60 percent at two months. Published data on older infants are too meager to discern trends, but informal reports suggest that breast feeding to at least six months is no longer unusual.

FACTORS INFLUENCING CHANGE

Reasons for the decrease in the prevalence of breast feeding in technologically advanced countries between 1920 and 1960 have been reported extensively. The availability of evaporated milk and later premodified formulas, refrigeration, safe water supplies, and techniques for bacteriological protection markedly decreased the mortality and morbidity of bottle-fed infants, and for the first time gave mothers an alternative to breast feeding that did not threaten the lives of their children.

Changes in life-style and women's views of their own roles accentuated the trend toward bottle feeding. More women were working outside the home and returned to work soon after delivery. By 1978, nearly 50 percent of women in the United States were gainfully employed. The bottle became the symbol of woman's emancipation.

174

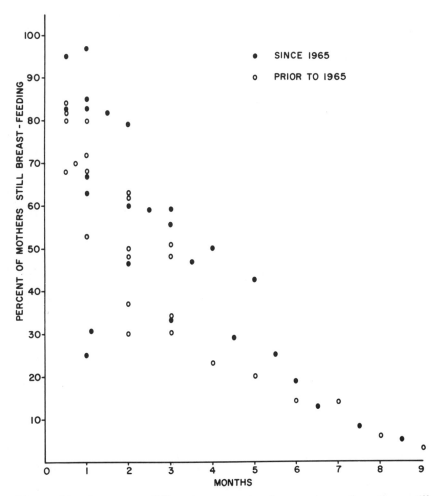

Figure 4.2   Summary of literature reports of percentage of mothers still breast-feeding when surveyed during first 9 months after delivery.

The trend toward the nuclear family decreased contacts with grand-mothers and other relatives who had themselves experienced lactation and could give support and advice to the nursing mother. An increasing number of young women had never even observed breast feeding. No longer was breast feeding considered the expected sequel to reproduction.

Specialization in medicine often meant that the family physician was replaced by an obstetrician whose primary concern was the woman during pregnancy and delivery, and a pediatrician whose role began after the birth of the infant. As a result the prenatal-postnatal transition necessary for successful lactation was often missing.

Delivery in hospitals replaced delivery at home. The separation of mother and infant into different rooms and routine adherence to a time schedule of feeding were common practices. Babies were brought to their mothers at four-hour intervals during the day but usually not at night. The few hospitals that permitted mother and infant to share a room tended to have a higher proportion of mothers successfully nursing.[21] The length of the hospital stay after delivery became shorter. In the 1940s mother and infant remained in the hospital 8 to 13 days, which allowed time for lactation to become well established. By 1970 the hospital stay was sometimes as short as one or two days. The mother then resumed home activities with the added responsibility of a newborn infant when milk production was still very tentative and the relationship of mother and infant in lactation not yet established. Stress was increased at a critical period when relaxation would be more beneficial.

As breast feeding became less common, women had less exposure to the practice and problems of lactation and became more dependent on the advice and counsel of physicians. At the same time, physicians themselves had progressively less experience and training with which to guide mothers, and pediatric textbooks devoted little space to breast feeding. The attitudes of women and their husbands also changed. Bottle feeding became the norm, and lactation was viewed as an unusual practice. The breast became a sexual rather than a functional organ. Breast feeding, however discreet, was rarely practiced in public places and even within the family it sometimes became a source of embarrassment.

The reasons for the decrease in breast feeding, then, were social, cultural, emotional, and psychological, not physiological. There was no evidence that fewer women were capable of breast feeding; fewer women chose to breast feed.

The increased interest in breast feeding in the past two decades originated with mothers themselves, especially young mothers. Widespread resistance to a "plastic" society led to enthusiasm for a "natural" way of life. As part of this cultural change, more women have preferred to experience labor and delivery without anesthesia and to breast feed their infants. This was first evident among women with higher educational attainment, but recent reports indicate that the trend has spread to a wider socioeconomic range. Initial lack of support from some physicians led to the formation of organizations such as La Leche League,[22] in which women banded together to share ideas and provide mutual support. Childbirth Education Association chapters were organized in many communities. Within the past few years larger numbers of physicians, nurses, and other health personnel are recommending and supporting the practice of breast feeding. The values of breast milk for the infant are receiving greater emphasis.

DEVELOPMENT AND FUNCTION OF THE BREASTS

The adult breast is composed of glandular and fatty tissue interspersed with fibrous tissue. In each breast the gland has 15 to 20 lobes, each made up of a number of lobules. Scattered in the lobules are groups of alveoli, which secrete milk. Small ducts lead from these collections of alveoli to form lactiferous ducts, one from each lobe. Each duct leading toward the nipple widens under the pigmented areola to form a lactiferous sinus which then opens directly into the surface of the nipple (Figure 4.3).

Milk is provided by the cytoplasm of the alveolar cells. Surrounding the alveoli are myoepithelial cells which contract, forcing milk from the alveoli into the ducts. The milk travels through the ducts and collects in the sinuses, where it becomes available to the suckling infant.

The development of the breast is under the control of a variety of hormones, and its function is determined by hormonal, reflex, and psychological influences. Although the breast endocrinology of the human is not

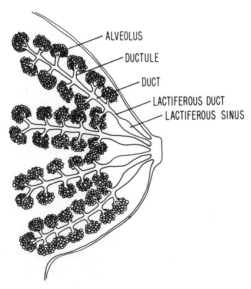

Figure 4.3   Diagram of breast structures essential to lactation process.

known precisely, a combination of human and animal studies provide a description of thc processes involved in the eventual production and ejection of milk.[23-26]

During fetal development the mammary glands originate from the skin as specialized ectodermal structures beginning about the fourth week. Under a complex of hormonal stimulating influences, by the end of the fetal period lactiferous ducts, the ducts and acini of the gland, the areola, and the nipple have been differentiated. After delivery, for perhaps 15 to 20 days, there is an episode of proliferation, growth and dilatation of the ducts and lobules in the infant, with secretion of so-called witch's milk, composed mainly of water, fat and cellular debris. The gland then involutes to a quiescent state with almost no mammary growth until puberty.

At puberty the hormonal changes that result in the establishment of ovarian cycles and the initiation of reproductive function are also responsible for mammary growth and the appearance of other secondary sex characteristics. During this period there is extension and branching of the duct system, proliferation of lobules, deposition of adipose tissue around the glands, enlargement and change in contour of the breast, and pigmentation of the areola and nipple. The increase in fatty and connective tissues is greater than the increase in glandular elements.

The sensitivity of the breast to estrogen and progesterone becomes evident during the menstrual cycle. The pre-ovulatory phase is characterized by a moderate degree of proliferation of ducts and lobules, which then regresses. In the premenstrual phase increased blood flow and edema of the fibrous tissue sometimes give rise to sensations of fullness or tightness.

During pregnancy further maturation of the breast occurs under the influence of a delicate equilibrium of ovarian, adrenal, hypophyseal, and placental hormones. Changes start very soon after conception and continue until delivery, when the fully developed organ is now capable of synthesizing and transporting milk. The secretory and transport potential of the alveolar-ductal system are enhanced by hyperplasia of the distal epithelial elements of the ductal tree, enlargement of the lumina of the ducts, mitotic formation of new alveoli, enlargement of the cytoplasm of epithelial cells, and increase in the number of ducts in each lobule. The gland becomes a compact mass of lobules of alveoli separated from each other by connective tissue. The vascular bed around the alveoli increases, with proliferation and engorgement of capillaries and venules. As the epithelial cells mature they have more mitochondria and ribonuclear protein particles. The apical surface of the cell forms cytoplasmic projections extending into the lumen with numerous microvilli and large aggregates of ribosomes. Lipid inclusions increase, associated with elements of rough endoplasmic reticulum. Toward the end of gestation alveolar cells enlarge further; their cytoplasm becomes very rich and dense due to development of most of the organelles. The Golgi system is enlarged. Myoepithelial cells have an increased content of ribosomes, related to the synthesis of contractile protein. By the end of the gestation period, the mammary gland is mature, prolactin concentration has increased, and the breasts are ready for activation by neurohormonal influences.

It has been estimated that 90 to 95 percent of mothers are capable of breast feeding. Contraindications to breast feeding include: unwillingness of the mother; severe chronic disorders in the mother, such as active tuberculosis, septicemia, nephritis, convulsive disorder, or severe neurosis or psychosis; some medications given to the mother; or a defect in the infant, such as severe cleft palate or a metabolic disease requiring specially formulated food. Mastitis was formerly considered a reason for weaning, but the belief now is that continued nursing prevents engorgement during treatment for the infection. Although another pregnancy does not necessitate weaning, the physiological and nutritional stress of concomitant pregnancy and lactation suggest that lactation should not be continued beyond the first half of pregnancy. Unconjugated hyperbilirubinemia has been reported in less than one percent of breast-fed infants, attributed to an unusual steroid metabolite of progesterone, which *in vitro* inhibits glucuronyl transferase activity. However, after two or three days of substitute feedings, breast feeding may be safely continued.[27,28]

THE PROCESS OF LACTATION

Lactation involves the synthesis of milk components in the alveoli, the release of milk from the alveoli to the ducts, passage of milk through the ducts to the lactiferous sinuses, removal of milk from the sinuses, and the continued production and release of milk during the nursing period. Although some of the specific mechanisms in lactation have not been fully defined, much of the process is known.[25,26,29] A complex series of activities in lactation involve hormones, enzymes, nerves, muscles, and reflexes. The breast must be capable of initiating lactation in the immediate postpartum period, supplying milk continually during each nursing period, altering composition of the milk over time, and maintaining lactation for a extended time period.

HORMONAL CONTROL

Prolactin is the major hormone for lactogenesis, although a number of other hormones are involved also. Growth hormone and chorionic somatomammotrophin are essential for the initiation of lactation. Mineralocorticoids and glucocorticoids from the adrenals, thyroid hormone, thyroid-stimulating hormone, and insulin are essential to the continuation of lactation. Oxytocin is the major hormone responsible for milk ejection.

Prolactin production begins during pregnancy, both by the anterior pituitary and by the placenta, and the plasma level increases progressively during pregnancy. Its effect on mammary function, however, is inhibited until delivery. The interaction of hormones during pregnancy may be inferred from animal studies and from human postpartum studies. Estrogen is essential for the production of prolactin, but the high level of circulating estrogen during pregnancy inhibits release of prolactin. Estrogen and progestogen in oral contraceptives have been shown to decrease milk volume in lactating women. Estrogen is commonly administered to suppress lactation in women who choose not to breast feed their infants. Therefore the high levels of circulating estrogen and progesterone during pregnancy inhibit the effects of the rising concentration of prolactin. The ovarian and placental steroids may act by limiting the release of lactogenic hormones from the pituitary, by inhibiting the response of mammary epithelial cells to prolactin, or by inhibiting the formation of a-lactalbumin.[24,30,31]

A fall in the concentration of estrogen and progesterone in the maternal blood at delivery permits the response of mammary epithelial cells to lactogenic factors. There is a prompt rise in prolactin release from the anterior pituitary, enhanced by hypothalamic stimulation as a result of the infant's suckling. Therefore, milk production is stimulated and lactation is initiated.

Oxytocin is produced by the posterior pituitary. This hormone is concerned primarily with the transfer of milk from the epithelial cells of the alveoli into the ducts and then to the sinuses, where it becomes available to the infant. This is a complex psycho-neuro-hormonal process with a series of phases of milk release. At the start of the nursing period the infant's sucking elicits the let-down reflex in the breast, and milk that is in the sinuses and large ducts may be withdrawn easily. However, milk in the smaller ducts and alveoli is retained until the second phase, sometimes called the draught.

The mammary gland is of cutaneous origin and has nerve receptors. The nipple, areola, and peripheral skin of the nursing mother are believed to be among the most highly innervated tissues of the body. The tactile stimulus of sucking triggers nerve impulses from the breast receptors to the hypothalamus. The hypothalamus stimulates the pituitary to release oxytocin. Oxytocin is carried by the blood both to the uterus, where it stimulates involution, and to the mammary gland, where it causes contraction of the myoepithelial cells surrounding the alveoli and small ducts, forcibly expelling milk down the ducts. During nursing increased blood supply in the breast, evidenced by increases in pressure and temperature, provides greater access of the circulating oxytocin to the myoepithelium. Changes in blood level of oxytocin during a nursing period have been observed,[32] suggesting that it may be released in spurts, providing repeated refilling of the sinuses.

The infant draws the nipple into the back of the mouth, circling the areola with the lips. When the lower jaw is elevated, breast tissue is compressed between the tongue and upper jaw, pressure is exerted from the front of the mouth to the back, and milk is drawn from the nipple. Suction is believed to be secondary to the motions. When the mandible is lowered, pressure on the nipple and areola is decreased, allowing the sinuses to fill again. Repetition of the sucking process causes waves of stimuli to the hypothalamus which in turn stimulates the posterior pituitary to release more oxytocin.

REFLEX ACTION

In the early postpartum period the let-down reflex depends primarily on the tactile stimulation of the infant's sucking. When lactation becomes well established the reflex becomes conditioned and may be elicited by a variety of other factors associated with the nursing process. Milk may be ejected at the sound of the baby's cry, at the thought of the baby, at the usual time of feeding even if the baby is not present, or with any occurrence usually associated with nursing.

The let-down reflex may be inhibited by a variety of factors; this is often the reason for failure in lactation. Anesthetics or sedatives may weaken the reflex and cause difficulty in the initiation of nursing in the immediate postpartum period. Ethanol (1–2 g/kg) has been shown to inhibit the reflex.[33] Emotional disturbances and stress are major impediments; many women have reported difficulty in let-down under situations of embarrassment or family disagreements. An increase in adrenaline may cause vasoconstriction, thus making oxytocin less available to myoepithelial cells. The weakness or inhibition of the reflex may be a cause of the inability to produce an adequate amount of breast milk in a mother who is not really interested in nursing. The sensitivity of the let-down reflex to multiple personal and environmental factors is a critical element in the success or failure of lactation.

THE NURSING INFANT

During the period when total anesthesia was commonly used for delivery, the first mother-infant contact was delayed and the baby was not put to the breast for 12 to 24 hours or longer. Total anesthesia is now less commonly used, and the initial nursing contact of infant with mother is often within a few hours after delivery. It has been postulated that early contact, preferably within six hours, is important in mother-infant bonding and increases the likelihood of successful lactation.[34]

Lactation depends on glandular and ductal tissue and therefore has little relation to the size of the breasts, which is determined largely by adipose and connective tissue. Eversion of the nipple must be sufficient for the infant to grasp and retain it, and inversion may be aided by prenatal attention.[35] During pregnancy and especially after delivery the nipple becomes more prominent as a result of the fibromuscular tissue surrounding the lactiferous ducts. Although prenatal preparation of the breasts by rubbing, application of creams, or expression of colostrum is sometimes recommended, it has not been demonstrated to have a measurable effect on nipple sensitivity during nursing.[36]

Success in nursing depends on the combination of the baby's sucking characteristics, the mother's personality and her response to her baby's individuality, and the interactions of mother and baby with others, whether hospital personnel or family. The variations in infants' approach to nursing has been well described by Barnes et al.,[37] who categorized babies under five main headings:

1. "Barracudas": When put to the breast, these babies vigorously and promptly grasp the nipple and suck energetically for from 10 to 20 minutes. There is no dallying. Occasionally this type of baby puts too much vigor into his nursing and hurts the nipple.

2. "Excited Ineffectives": These babies become so excited and active at the breast that they alternately grasp and lose the breast. They then start screaming. It is often necessary for the nurse or mother to pick up the baby and quiet him first, and then put him back to the breast. After a few days the mother and baby usually become adjusted.

3. "Procrastinators": These babies often seem to put off until the fourth or fifth postpartum day what they could just as well have done from the start. They wait until the milk comes in. They show no particular interest or ability in sucking in the first few days. It is important not to prod or force these babies when they seem disinclined. They do well once they start.

4. "Gourmets or Mouthers": These babies insist on mouthing the nipple, tasting a little milk and then smacking their lips, before starting to nurse. If the infant is hurried or prodded, he will become furious and start to scream. Otherwise, after a few minutes of mouthing he settles down and nurses very well.

5. "Resters": These babies prefer to nurse a few minutes and then rest a few minutes. If left alone, they often nurse well, although the entire procedure will take much longer. They cannot be hurried.

The strength of some reflexes in the infant is also important to the initiation and maintenance of lactation. The rooting reflex causes the infant to turn his head in the direction of a touch on the cheek. If the cheek is touched by the breast or a hand, his head will rotate in that direction as he seeks the nipple. A person unaware of the rooting reflex may try to push the infant's face toward the breast by pressure on the outside cheek; by reflex action the infant turns toward the touch and away from the breast.

The sucking reflex affects both the infant's acquisition of milk and the maternal stimulus to the hypothalamus. An infant with a strong sucking reflex is more likely to stimulate greater milk production, although the mother may find vigorous nursing somewhat painful until the nipples become accustomed to it. On the other hand, an infant with a weak sucking reflex or one affected by anesthetics or sedatives given to the mother during labor and delivery may not get enough milk to satisfy him, may not empty the breast, and may not adequately stimulate further milk production. Some infants suck well the first time they are put to the breast; others may not display true sucking ability or interest until the second or third day or even later. The timing of breast engorgement also varies. Some women may not experience engorgement or secretion until the fourth to the sixth day. If the breasts become engorged before the infant sucks well, it may be advisable to relieve the breasts by manual expression.

FREQUENCY OF NURSING

The timing of feedings in the neonatal period should be individualized for each mother-infant combination. The stomach capacity of the newborn is only 10 to 20 ml, but increases rapidly to 80 ml by two weeks and to 100 ml average by the end of the first month.[38] The infant may want to be nursed every two or three hours in the first few weeks. Unrestricted or self-demand feedings are the practice in most preliterate cultures. However, in westernized countries, it became common to restrict breast feeding to a four-hour schedule, which Newton calls "token breast feeding."[39] Rigid scheduling may have been a factor in the decreased incidence of breast feeding.[40-42] Milk production is higher and infant weight gain is more rapid, after the initial weight loss, when true self-demand is practiced. Since sucking is a stimulus to both milk production and ejection, limitation in frequency of feedings may lead to the "not enough milk" syndrome. The interdependence of mother and baby is a guide to the frequency of feedings. The baby becomes hungry and needs milk; the mother's breasts fill and she needs the baby to nurse. As the stomach capacity of the infant increases, the time interval between feedings is lengthened, and by the end of the first month many babies on self-demand schedules are satisfied with feeding every four hours. The primiparous mother who is anxious may need some guidance in interpreting signs of hunger.

SUPPLY AND DEMAND

Most women who wish to nurse are capable of breast feeding if they are given understanding of the physiological mechanisms, adequate support from hospital personnel and family, and relative freedom from anxiety and stress. Secretion is usually well established by the end of the first week.

The next problem of many mothers occurs usually between the second and sixth week postpartum. The mother and infant in the first few weeks develop a synchronization of supply and demand. Toward the end of the first month or early in the second month the infant may have a sudden increase in demand, perhaps related to increased stomach capacity or a spurt in growth. Even if the mother offers both breasts at a feeding, the infant is not satisfied. The mother becomes anxious, which may inhibit let-down. Breast feeding is too often discontinued at this point because the mother or her physician decides that she cannot produce an adequate amount of milk. In many cases weaning is not necessary. Time is needed for the neurohormonal system to respond to the increased sucking by producing more prolactin and oxytocin. This will usually be accomplished within 24 hours and a greater yield of milk results. In the meantime, either of two procedures may be followed. Putting the baby to the breast at shorter time intervals will sometimes be adequate stimulation. On the other hand, offering a bottle after a breast feeding (not in place of nursing) allows the baby to be satisfied; the mother becomes more relaxed, and the lowered stress helps to increase the milk supply. With either method it is important to continue the stimulus of sucking. Bottles should not replace breast feedings, and care should be taken to avoid giving fluids or solids between nursing periods so that the infant is hungry when put to the breast. Within a day or two milk yield is likely to increase. It is possible, of course, that a woman may not increase her milk supply, but a hasty decision to wean the infant is too often made at the first sign of difficulty.

Women vary widely in their capacity to produce milk. Some can successfully nurse twins, while others must use formula to supplement an inadequate supply for a singleton. For some infants a single breast supplies enough for a total feeding so that breasts can be alternated for successive feedings. If both breasts are needed at each feeding, the first breast offered should be alternated. That is, if the mother started one feeding with the left breast and finished with the right, at the next feeding she should offer the right breast first. This would ensure complete emptying of one breast at each feeding. Although there was formerly controversy about the value of complete emptying of the breast, it is now generally accepted that retention of milk in the breast may inhibit further milk production.

Once lactation is well established the mother may have more freedom for social activities or even for working outside the home without discontinuing breast feeding. Extra breast milk may be manually expressed and frozen for later feeding by bottle when the mother is away, or a bottle of formula may be substituted for a breast feeding. Convenient day care facilities for the working mother are rare, but many working mothers breast feed morning and night and provide frozen breast milk or a formula substitute during the day. This schedule is more successful with older infants; an extended span of time between feedings may inhibit milk production in the early months. The working mother may need to express milk during the day to relieve engorgement until she adapts to the schedule.

The amount of milk actually consumed by an infant is very difficult to determine. Collection of milk samples interferes with the usual pattern of infant feeding and alters the psychological state of the mother. Maternal physiological response to a mechanical pump or manual expression is different than to the sucking of the infant, and the volume of samples collected by these methods may not reflect the amount that the infant would have obtained. Different collection techniques and environments may affect the volume because of the sensitivity of the neurohormonal control of milk production. Diurnal variation is so great that the sample from a single feeding may not be proportionately representative of total volume, and 24-hour collection is usually impractical. Most available data on milk volume are indirect, calculated from weights of the infant before and after feedings.

Volume of milk increases rapidly in the first month as lactation becomes established. Using data of Fomon, Widdowson[43] calculated that median daily intakes of fully breast-fed infants were: 600 ml in the first month, 840 ml in the second, 930 ml in the third, 960 ml in the fourth, 1010 ml in the fifth, and 1100 ml in the sixth month. These values represent increases of 40 percent in the second month, 11 percent in the third, 3 percent in the fourth, and less than 1 percent in the fifth and sixth months. The increase in total volume is consistent with the increasing weight of the infant, and the progressive drop in percentage increase is consistent with the slowing rate of growth.

Somewhat lower volumes were reported in Swedish women, estimated from infant weights. Lönnerdal et al.[44] estimated means of 558 ± 83 ml in the first two weeks, 724 ± 117 ml between 2 and 6 weeks, 752 ± 177 ml between $1\frac{1}{2}$ and $3\frac{1}{2}$ months, and 756 ± 140 ml between $3\frac{1}{2}$ and $6\frac{1}{2}$ months.

Lower volumes of breast milk have been reported from developing countries, reflecting the poorer milk production of chronically malnourished women.

Milk volume may be somewhat lessened by menstruation, but nutrient content of the milk is probably unaffected. Resumption of both menstruation and ovulation occur later in lactating than in nonlactating women, so breast feeding provides some protection against conception. The period of infertility has ranged from 2 to 14 months in various populations that have been surveyed and is related to the duration and intensity of breast feeding. Longer periods of total breast feeding without food supplements to the infant are associated with later renewal of the estral cycle. However, the nutritional status of the woman may be a factor in the timing. In tropical countries the first menses after delivery were found to be earlier in women who were given extra food during pregnancy and lactation than in controls,[45] suggesting greater delay in resumption of menstruation and ovulation in chronically malnourished women than in well-nourished women. Because of wide individual variation, lactation is not a dependable contraceptive means, especially for women in good nutritional state. It is, however, an important factor in limiting the birth rate in developing countries.

The effects of oral contraceptives on the volume and nutrient content of breast milk have not been clearly defined. Inconsistencies in the results of published studies may be due to differences in the type of compound used, dosage, stage of lactation, duration of study, nutritional status of the women, and cultural practices that affect either lactation or early conception after a delivery.[46] However, it appears that during the establishment of lactation the impact of the sucking stimulus overrides the inhibitory effects of gestogens. On the other hand, the maintenance of lactation may be imperilled by estrogen or by progestational agents which have an estrogenic effect when metabolized.[46,47] Most studies have shown shorter duration of lactation, inhibition of milk production, and lower infant weight gain, particularly with the extended use of the estrogenic compounds.

NONNUTRITIVE COMPONENTS

Immune Factors

Breast milk not only supplies the infant with nourishment, but also gives immunologic protection against respiratory and gastrointestinal infections.[10,48,49] The higher incidence of infections in bottle-fed infants has long been recognized, but bacterial contamination was considered a major factor, as it still is in developing countries. However, in the past two or three decades a number of anti-infective agents have been identified in human milk, although the precise actions of some have not yet been determined.

186

Immunoglobulins, especially secretory IgA, in colostrum and mature milk confer passive mucosal immunity against pathogens in the intestine and protect the infant until his own immunity is developed. Secretory IgA may also prevent absorption of dietary antigens, lowering the risk of allergy. Lactoferrin is an iron-binding glycoprotein which appears to be bacteriostatic. Human milk contains a mucopolysaccharide growth factor for Lactobacillus bifidus, which reduces the pH of the intestinal contents by production of acetic and lactic acids and inhibits growth of potential pathogens. Human milk also contains living leukocytes, primarily macrophages but also some lymphocytes; they contain many lysozymes that inhibit bacterial growth, especially E. coli and salmonella. Lactoperoxidase has been shown to inhibit growth of streptococci *in vitro*. Complement components and antibodies to poliomyelitis virus have also been found in human milk. These anti-infective factors are of critical importance in countries with poor standards for bacteriological safety, but their value to all infants is increasingly being recognized.

Contaminants

Concern has been aroused by the transmission of environmental contaminants in breast milk. Pesticide residues have received the most attention because they become more concentrated in the higher levels of the animal kingdom. Recently there has been evidence of other commercial chemical residues in breast milk. However, no harmful effects have been demonstrated to date. Concern about environmental contaminants in human milk is also being extended to the investigation of placental transfer of chemical substances as well as their presence in cow's milk and other infant foods. Most of the publicity has focused on breast milk, but the infant is exposed to other sources of contaminants as well.

Some drugs taken by the mother may be transported via blood to breast milk, so care should be taken in the prescribing of medications to the lactating woman.[50-52]

NUTRIENT COMPOSITION OF COLOSTRUM AND MATURE MILK

COLOSTRUM

In the first few days after delivery the mammary gland changes from a quiescent state to one of active secretion. The first secretions include cellular constituents and debris from the alveoli and ducts and become progressively diluted with newly secreted milk. This early secretion, colostrum, is different from later milk. It is a thick, alkaline fluid with a deep lemon yellow color and a higher specific gravity than mature milk. Colostrum is effective in clearing meconium from the infant's gastrointestinal tract and is designed to meet the immediate specific needs of the neonate. It is high in IgA and other protective factors and is suited to the relative immaturity of the digestive enzyme system of the newborn.

Colostrum is higher than mature milk in total protein, nonprotein nitrogen, and globulin. Energy value is lower, due to its low fat content, but the fat has a higher percentage of phospholipids. Colostrum is higher than later milk in ash, especially sodium and potassium, and in vitamins A and E, and carotene, but lower in ascorbic acid and some B vitamins. The changing nature of colostrum makes it impossible to assign specific nutrient values. Table 4.1 shows the ranges of mean values which were summarized by Macy et al.[53] from the literature; in different studies there is nearly a threefold difference in observed mean values for some nutrients. These values must be considered tentative, not only because of the change in nutrient content of colostrum in the first five days, but also because the number of determinations on which the means are based varies from fewer than 10 for cholesterol, NPN, and some minerals, to more than 400 for total protein.

The amount of colostrum produced varies widely among women. Macy[54] reported secretions varying from negligible to more than 80 ml on the first postpartum day and from 56 to 385 ml on the second day.

Because of the gradual change from colostrum to transitional milk and then to mature milk, definition of time periods has been arbitrary. Macy[54] defined colostrum as the secretion in the first five days, and transitional milk as the secretion from the sixth to the tenth days. Mature milk values in most tables were obtained after 30 days; relatively few studies have been reported on the content of mature milk before that age.

MATURE MILK

The most extensive studies of the nutrient content of milk were done by the Children's Fund of Michigan. Macy published the first compilation in 1949;[54] Macy and Kelly published a second compilation in 1961.[55] All data available in the literature were reviewed by a committee of the National Academy of Sciences and published in The Composition of Milks in 1950 and revised in 1953.[53] These values are the basis of most of the tables in current use. Much of the research on breast milk in the past two decades has been done in the developing countries because of the critical value of breast milk to infant health and survival. Until the effect of chronic malnutrition on the composition of breast milk has been defined more clearly, it is advisable to continue to use data from healthy well-nourished women. Table 4.2 was selected for presentation here because the standard deviations and ranges are included as well as the mean values.[56]

Table 4.1   Composition of Human Colostrum, 1–5 days

	Reported Means per 100 ml		Reported Means per 100 ml
Energy, kcal	49–67	Vitamin A, μg	51–161
Lactose, g	4.4–6.4	Carotenoids, μg	85–137
Fat, g	2.2–4.1	Vitamin E, mg	1.1–1.5
Total choles-		Ascorbic acid	
terol, g	13–36	mg	1.4–7.2
Total protein, g	2.0–5.5	Thiamin, μg	2–35
Non-protein		Riboflavin, μg	26.7–32.0
nitrogen, mg	91	Nicotinic	
Ash, g	0.30–0.36	acid, μg	75
Calcium, mg	23–48	Biotin, μg	0.1
Phosphorus, mg	13–16	Folic acid, μg	0.05
Magnesium, mg	3–4	Pantothenic	
Potassium, mg	74	acid, μg	183
Iron, mg	0.04–0.13	Vitamin B_{12}, μg	0.045
Copper, mg	0.04–0.06		
Zinc, mg	0.56–0.74		
Iodine, mg	12.2		
Chlorine, mg	59–159		
Sodium, mg	47–50		
Sulfur, mg	20–23		

Source: Macy, I. G., H. J. Kelley, and R. E. Sloan. *The Composition of Milks.* Publ. 254. National Academy of Sciences, Washington, D.C., 1953.

The transition from colostrum to mature milk is only one aspect of variation in its nutrient content. Even mature milk changes in composition, as the needs of the infant change with age. In addition, there is variation between women unrelated to diet, presumably genetically determined similar to the variations in fat content of cows of different breeds. Maternal factors that have been related to milk composition include age, parity, number of prior lactations, nutritional status, dietary intake, and stage of lactation. Seasonal variations may be related to dietary intake. Diurnal variation was shown by Hytten,[57] who reported a rise in fat content between 6 A.M. and 10 A.M., followed by a decline during the rest of the day.

The change in composition of milk during a single feeding was well demonstrated by Hall,[58] who pumped milk from the right breast at the same pace as the mother's five-week-old infant nursed from the left breast in a 16-minute nursing period. In the first five minutes 60 percent of the total milk volume was secreted, containing 60 percent of the total protein and carbohydrate, more than 40 percent of the total lipid, and more than half of

Table 4.2 Composition of Mature Human Milk and Cow's Milk

Constituent (g/l Except Where Stated)	Mature Human Milk			Cow's Milk		
	Mean	Range	s.d.	Mean	Range	s.d.
Energy (kcal/l)	747	446–1192	93	701	587–876	
(MJ/l)	3.127	1.867–4.989	0.389	2.934	2.457–3.666	
Protein						
Total	10.6	7.3–20	4.6	32.46	28.16–36.76	
Casein	3.7	1.6–6.8	0.8	24.9	21.90–28.0	
Lactalbumin	3.6	1.4–6.0	1.0	2.4	1.40–3.3	
Lactoglobulin	2.0[a]			1.70	0.7–3.7	
Amino acids						
Total	12.8	9.0–16.0		33.0	27.0–41.0	
Essential total	5.39[b]			19.59[b]		
Histidine	0.24	0.12–0.30	0.041	1.2	1.1–1.3	
Isoleucine	0.61	0.41–0.92	0.121	2.5	2.1–2.9	
Leucine	0.97	0.65–1.47	0.174	3.6	3.2–3.9	
Lysine	0.70	0.36–0.93	0.127	2.6	2.3–3.1	
Methionine	0.12	0.07–0.16	0.023	0.8	0.6–0.9	
Cystine	0.29[a]	0.23–0.25		0.29[a]		
Phenylalanine	0.40	0.24–0.58	0.069	1.8	1.5–2.2	
Tyrosine	0.62[a]	0.46–0.52		1.9[a]		
Threonine	0.52	0.30–0.66	0.085	1.7	1.3–2.2	
Tryptophan	0.19	0.14–0.26	0.030	0.6	0.4–0.8	
Valine	0.73	0.45–1.14	0.155	2.6	2.4–2.8	

Continued

Fats					
Total (g)	45.4	13.4–82.9	10.0	38.0	34.0–61.0
Essential total (% weight of total fatty acids)	12.02[b]			4.2[b]	
Linoleic (18:2)	10.6		2.9	2.1	0.7
Linolenic (18:3)	0.85			1.7	0.7
Arachidonic (20:4)	0.57			0.4	
Saturated total	50.3[b]			70.9[b]	
C4:0–C10:0	1.4			9.1	1.1
Lauric (12:0)	4.7		2.2	3.6	1.5
Myristic (14:0)	7.9		1.5	11.8	4.7
Palmitic (16:0)	26.7		2.7	36.6	3.2
Stearic (18:0)	8.3		1.7	8.1	
Arachidic (20:0)	1.3			1.7	
Unsaturated					
C10:1–C16:1	3.8			5.2	
Oleic (18:1)	37.4		3.7	17.7	4.2
Eicosenoic (20:1)	0.9			1.0	
Cholesterol	0.139	0.088–0.202	0.025	0.110	0.070–0.170
Carbohydrates					
Lactose	71	49–95		47	45–50
Citric acid		0.35–1.25		2.45	2.15–2.90

Continued

191

Constituent	Mature Human Milk			Cow's Milk		
(g/l Except Where Stated)	Mean	Range	s.d.	Mean	Range	s.d.
Minerals						
Electropositive (mEq/l)	41			149		
Sodium (g/l)	0.189	0.080–0.350	0.006	0.768	0.392–1.390	
Potassium (g/l)	0.553	0.425–0.735	0.070	1.430	0.380–2.870	
Calcium (g/l)	0.271	0.207–0.372	0.030	1.370	0.560–3.810	
Magnesium (g/l)	0.035	0.018–0.057	0.007	0.130	0.070–0.220	
Electronegative (mEq/l)	28			108		
Phosphorus (g/l)	0.141	0.068–0.268	0.025	0.910	0.560–1.120	
Sulphur (g/l)	0.140	0.050–0.300	0.030	0.300	0.240–0.360	
Chlorine (g/l)	0.375	0.088–0.734	0.090	1.080	0.930–1.410	
Excess electropositive						
Elements (mEq/l)	13			41		
pH	7.01	6.4–7.6		6.6		
Trace elements						
Cobalt (μg/l)	trace			0.6		
Iron (mg/l)	0.50	0.20–0.80		0.45	0.25–0.75	
Copper (mg/l)	0.51		0.046	0.102		
Manganese (mg/l)	trace			0.02	0.005–0.067	
Zinc (mg/l)	1.18	0.17–3.02		3.9	1.7–6.6	
Fluorine (mg/l)	0.107	0.0–0.24			0.10–0.28	
Iodine (mg/l)	0.061	0.044–0.093		0.116	0.036–1.05	
Selenium (mg/l)	0.021			0.04	0.005–0.067	

Continued

Vitamins

Vitamin A (mg/l)	0.610	0.150–2.260	0.230	0.270	0.170–0.380
Carotenes (mg/l)	0.250	0.020–0.770	0.110	0.370	0.120–0.790
Vitamin D (μg/l)		0.1–2.5			0.1–1.0
Tocopherol (mg/l)	2.4	1.0–4.8		0.6	0.2–1.0
Thiamine (mg/l)	0.142	0.081–0.227	0.024	0.430	0.280–0.900
Riboflavine (mg/l)	0.373	0.198–0.790	0.087	1.560	1.160–2.020
Vitamin B_6 (mg/l)	0.180	0.100–0.220		0.510	0.400–0.630
Nicotinic acid (mg/l)	1.83	0.66–3.30	0.48	0.74	0.50–0.86
Vitamin B_{12} (μg/l)	trace			6.6	3.2–12.4
Folic acid (μg/l)	24.0	7.4–61.0		37.7	16.8–63.2
Biotin (μg/l)	2	1–3		22	14–29
Pantothenic acid (mg/l)	2.46	0.86–5.84	0.63	3.4	2.2–5.5
Ascorbic acid (mg/l)	52	0–112	19	11	3–23

[a]Macy and Kelly (1961).
[b]Calculated by author.

Source: Documenta Geigy Scientific Tables, Seventh Edition. Ciba-Geigy Ltd., Basle, Switzerland, 1970.

the total energy. The next six minutes provided 26 percent of the volume, more than 33 percent of the lipid, and about one-fourth of the protein, carbohydrate, and calories. In the final five minutes, 13 percent of the total volume, 16 percent of the protein and calories, and 25 percent of the total lipids were secreted. Hytten[59] had previously shown a rise in lipid concentration between early and late milk in a single feeding. These changes are consistent with observations that milk early in the feeding has a thin watery appearance and late in the feeding is thicker and whiter. Despite the increase in lipid concentration, fatty acid composition of the lipid does not change during a nursing period.[60] Hall postulated that the change in chemical composition, taste, and texture may be a cue for the infant to stop feeding, implying an appetite control mechanism. Formulas, being constant in compositon, would not have this effect and might result in a different development of hunger-satiety control.

Changes in the composition of milk over time (Table 4.3) were shown by analysis of samples taken serially from 17 women between 14 and 84 days of lactation and 12 women at 112 days.[11] The relatively low fat content may reflect sampling only at the beginning of a nursing period, but the high standard deviations indicate wide variability between women. The decrease in concentration of protein and some minerals is evident from these data.

It is obvious, then, that nutrient values of breast milk vary with many factors inherent in the lactation process. Nutrient analyses reported in the literature depend on the subjects selected and the time of sample collection. In addition, analyses are altered by the procedures of collection, handling, and preservation of samples, as well as by the methods of analysis for specific nutrients. As with all food value tables, precision is impossible, and the user must be aware of factors that affect variation.

Despite the limitations of available data, some comparisons of the content of human and cow's milk can be made. Caloric values are similar; both supply approximately 20 kcal (84 kJ)/ounce or 67 kcal (280 kJ)/100 ml. However, a larger proportion of energy in human milk is derived from lactose and lipids than from protein. Human milk is lower in all minerals with the exception of copper and perhaps iron. Human milk is higher in vitamin A (but not carotene), tocopherol, niacin, and ascorbic acid but lower in other vitamins than cow's milk.

Protein

Human milk has approximately one-third as much protein as cow's milk (1.1 percent in contrast to 3.3 percent). Milk-specific proteins, such as lactoferrin, a-lactalbumin, and casein are synthesized by the mammary gland, but some proteins, such as serum albumin, are derived from maternal blood.[44] The component proteins change as lactation progresses. Total ni-

Table 4.3   Composition of Human Milk at Various Stages of Lactation

	Day of Lactation											
	14		28		42		56		84		112	
Content per Liter	m.	S.D.	m.	S.D.	m.	S.D.	m.	S.D.	m.	S.D.	m.	S.D.
Protein (N x 6.25), g	15.4	1.8	13.8	1.8	12.6	1.4	10.9	1.8	10.2	2.6	8.7	2.6
NPN, g	0.49	0.13	0.40	0.13	0.41	0.12	0.46	0.16	0.38	0.11	0.32	0.09
Fat, g	26.3	9.1	29.4	12.3	26.8	15.9	22.3	11.9	21.0	13.3	28.4	12.5
Carbohydrate, g	83.2	9.0	82.3	11.1	81.3	12.0	80.7	12.5	88.4	14.5	88.6	18.5
Ash, g	2.32	0.28	2.18	0.47	1.81	0.52	2.15	0.60	2.22	0.54	1.84	0.83
Calcium, mg	278	45	261	64	255	78	266	56	247	56	236	38
Phosphorus, mg	188	33	169	45	151	30	150	28	130	33	132	26
Magnesium, mg	30	3	28	5	28	4	31	6	30	6	32	5
Sodium, mg	204	58	161	62	151	64	135	79	125	52	120	48
Potassium, mg	421	90	347	121	367	129	374	66	343	90	296	129
Chloride, mg	410	119	441	193	427	137	378	98	406	165	399	147
Zinc, mg	3.7	1.2	2.6	1.1	2.2	0.9	2.0	0.7	2.0	1.2	1.1	0.5

Source: Fomon, S. J. Infant Nutrition, second edition. W. B. Saunders, Philadelphia, 1974.

trogen and total protein are highest in concentration in colostrum and decrease rapidly in the first month and then more slowly. However, milk volume increases, so the infant takes a larger volume of milk with less protein per unit of volume. A similar rate of decrease has been observed for immunoglobulins and lactoferrin, and a relatively steady decrease in a-lactalbumin, but little change in the concentration of serum albumin and non-protein nitrogen. Non-protein nitrogen (NPN) comprises 15 to 25 percent of the total nitrogen in breast milk, as compared to 6 percent in cow's milk. Its significance to the infant is unclear, but NPN is also higher in colostrum than in mature milk. The calculation for total protein in milk is overestimated by the Kjeldahl method (N x 6.25). If NPN has been determined, and deducted from total nitrogen, the remaining nitrogen is converted to protein by the factor 6.37, which is specific for milk protein.

The relative proportions of whey proteins (lactalbumin and lactoglobulin) and casein in human and cow's milk have been given considerable attention. In human milk the ratio is 60:40 and in cow's milk 18:82. The higher level of whey proteins in human milk results in smaller and more flocculent curds in the infant's intestinal tract, resulting in easier digestion, greater absorption, and softer stools. Nitrogen absorption from human milk reaches 90 percent by the end of the second week.[55] When cow's milk is fed to young infants, some procedures may be used to alter the larger and harder curds due to its higher casein content. There are also differences in the proportions of amino acids as well as in their concentrations in the two milks (Table 4.2), but nitrogen balance can be maintained on both. "Humanized" formulas in which the ratio of casein to whey protein is adjusted to simulate human milk still have profoundly different protein composition.[44] The high nucleotide content of human colostrum and milk may enhance protein synthesis by the infant.[61]

Carbohydrate

The carbohydrate in milk is primarily lactose and the concentration in human milk is higher (6.5 to 7 percent) than in cow's milk (4.5 to 5 percent). The rate of lactose synthesis may be related to the rate of protein synthesis and may also be one of the controlling factors determining the amount of milk produced. Lactose synthesis is the last step in the transfer of galactose to glucose by means of the enzyme lactose synthetase, which is composed of two protein subunits, one of which is a-lactalbumin.[24] The concentration of lactose is lower in colostrum than in mature milk. Early studies had indicated that lactose remains relatively constant in mature milk as lactation progresses, but Lönnerdal et al.[44] found that lactose increased from 7.0 to 7.6 percent in the milk of a group of Swedish women. Lactose lowers intestinal pH, improves the absorption of nitrogen, calcium and magnesium, and encourages the growth of fermentative rather than putrefactive bacteria. It is one of the factors in the lower incidence of gastrointestinal upsets and perianal dermatitis in breast-fed infants. Galactose is essential for the synthesis of galactosides and cerebrosides for myelin formation and for the synthesis of collagen.

Lipid

The most variable macronutrient in human milk is fat, as indicated by the wide range and high standard deviations in Tables 4.2 and 4.3. Some of the variation is due to sampling within a single nursing period or in different nursings of the day. A true picture of the lipid content can be obtained only by complete 24-hour milk collection and analysis. Fat supplies approximately 50 percent of the calories of breast milk, including five percent as essential fatty acids, primarily linoleic acid (18:2).[1] Maternal dietary intake affects the fatty acid composition of milk lipids but not total lipid content or volume. If maternal caloric intake is decreased, the fatty acid profile of breast milk reflects the mobilization of maternal fat stores.[62] Cow's milk contains slightly less total fat and significantly lower concentrations of essential fatty acids. In human milk 12 percent of fatty acids are unsaturated, in contrast to 4 percent in cow's milk.

Fat absorption is higher from human milk (85–90 percent) than from cow's milk (70 percent) due to its fine emulsification, the presence of active lipase, the higher degree of unsaturation, and the position of fatty acids on the glycerol base.[56] Pancreatic lipase hydrolyzes fatty acids in the 1 and 3 positions, allowing those to be absorbed as free fatty acids. The fatty acid esterified in the 2 position remains and is absorbed as monoglyceride. Widdowson[63] has shown that when palmitic acid is liberated it forms calcium soap, so both calcium and fat are lost in the stool. However, if palmitic acid is in the 2 position it is absorbed as the monoglyceride. In human milk 74 percent of the palmitic acid is in the 2 position, in contrast to only 39 percent in cow's milk.

Minerals

The mineral content of human milk responds less to changes in the maternal diet than does the vitamin content. Like protein, the concentration of some minerals decreases with later lactation, with compensation by a higher volume produced. The ash content of cow's milk is approximately three times that of human milk, resulting in a higher renal solute load. However, there are differences in the relative amounts of ash components. Cow's milk is four to six times higher in phosphorus, calcium, and sodium, and two to three times higher in potassium, magnesium, sulfur, chlorine, manganese, zinc, iodine, and selenium. However, copper is higher in human milk and iron slightly higher. The differences in ash components alter the ratios of nutrients, which may have physiological significance. For example, the ratio of nitrogen to phosphorus is approximately 20:1 in human milk and 6:1 in cow's milk. Human milk has a lower ratio of zinc to copper but a higher ratio of magnesium to phosphorus than cow's milk. Despite the relatively low iron content of both milks, the iron in breast milk is utilized more efficiently,[64,65] possibly enhanced by the higher copper content.

Calcium retention in infancy has been variously estimated between 50 and 70 percent from breast milk and between 10 and 55 percent from cow's milk.[66] The lower pH of intestinal contents of breast-fed infants may be a factor in their higher calcium absorption. Retention of phosphorus has been estimated as 90 percent or higher from human milk and between 25 and 37 percent from cow's milk. Although the content of both minerals is lower in breast milk, the infant utilizes them more efficiently. The ratio of calcium to phosphorus is approximately 2:1 in human milk and 1.5:1 in cow's milk. This difference may be related to the finding that infantile tetany occurs almost exclusively in formula-fed infants.[67] The importance of the calcium:phosphorus ratio has been controversial and is still unclear. The adequacy of vitamin D may be a factor in whether or not the ratio is critical.

Vitamins

Human milk contains approximately twice as much vitamin A and niacin, and four times as much ascorbic acid and tocopherol as cow's milk, but the range of variation is higher in human milk. Other vitamins of the B complex tend to be higher in cow's milk. The vitamin D content of human milk was reported to be low, despite the rarity of rickets in breast-fed infants. The finding of a water-soluble conjugate of vitamin D with sulfate[68] will necessitate re-evaluation, since previous determinations were done on only the lipid fraction of the milk. Vitamin K is low in human milk, and the sterile intestinal tract of the newborn prevents bacterial synthesis; the parenteral administration of 1 mg vitamin K to the neonate will protect against transient hypoprothrombinemia until the infant's intestinal flora synthesize vitamin K.

MATERNAL NUTRIENT REQUIREMENTS AND DIET DURING LACTATION

"Satisfactory lactation represents the greatest nutritional stress imposed by a physiological process on the human body."[62] However, the values now used for the nutrient requirements of the lactating woman contain a "high proportion of hypothesis to fact."[62] The major balance studies were those of Macy et al.[69] and of Coons and Blunt[70] in the United States in the 1930s. Since that time the only extensive studies on lactating women in westernized

198

countries have been done by Thomson, Hytten et al.[62] in Scotland and England, and recently by Lönnerdal and associates[44] in Sweden. Studies in developing countries have been based primarily on women with some degree of undernutrition. Therefore, the literature on lactation requirements includes studies with varying degrees of data on maternal intakes, size and weight changes of mother and infant, milk yield and content, and timing and techniques of milk sampling. This has led to a mass of calculations and recalculations of inadequate data. With each new interpretation changes are made in estimations of requirements and recommended dietary intakes.

A number of factors influence the dietary needs of the lactating woman, and these factors change with time. Breast milk contains energy and nutrients that are lost from the mother's body when milk is extracted. The process of synthesis of milk components requires additional energy and nutrients. The efficiency of the woman in converting dietary intake to milk nutrients is also a factor in estimating her needs. The volume of milk increases from the newborn period to at least the sixth month of lactation; nutrient needs change as volume increases, but are altered by progressive changes in milk composition. At least some of the nutrients in breast milk may be withdrawn from maternal tissues, so storage and availability of these nutrients must be taken into consideration. At the present time there is not universal agreement on the values to be assigned to any of these factors. Therefore, requirements and recommended allowances are only the best estimates at any given time.

The fact that chronically malnourished women in developing countries produce milk is ample evidence of the ability of the body to adjust to low intakes, but the physiological costs to the woman and her baby are difficult to estimate. Adaptation may include greater efficiency in absorption and utilization, depletion of body stores, restriction of maternal physical activity, lower volume of milk production, limitation of infant growth, and a longer period of amenorrhea following delivery. Lactation under such adverse nutritional circumstances is a remarkable tribute to human adaptation, and essential to the survival of infants in many areas of the world. Some writers have suggested that maternal adaptation makes it unnecessary to increase dietary intake during lactation, especially if the woman is well-nourished and healthy. A review of the costs of lactation, however, makes it clear that optimal long-term health of both mother and infant require an increase in maternal nutrient intake, even by women who were well-nourished before and during pregnancy.

Lactation allowances have usually been determined by the factorial method. Estimations are made of the volume and nutrient content of the milk produced, with addition of physiological needs of the mother for synthesis of the milk components; efficiency of maternal absorption may be factored into the calculation. These values are then added to the nonpregnant, nonlactating allowance. Table 4.4 lists the average content of 850 ml of human milk and the percentage increment to that allowance required to provide only the nutrients in the milk. The recommended allowances[71] for nonlactating and lactating women 19 to 22 years of age are listed, with the percentage increases in allowances for each nutrient. The allowances for energy and Vitamin A during lactation are lower than the theoretical total for nonlactating maintenance plus the content of milk. Other allowances equal or exceed the increment for milk content and provide a margin of safety for the efficiency of absorption and the metabolic needs for milk synthesis.

The higher needs of the young adolescent mother who nurses her infant include the sum of basic maintenance, nutrients for her own continued physical growth, and the increments for lactation. The nursing mother under 18 years of age should add 400 mg calcium, 400 mg phosphorus, and 15 µg iodine to the RDAs of the 19- to 22-year-old mother. Further increments of 200 kcal and 1 mg niacin should be allowed for the 11- to 14-year-old. The dietary recommendations for the adolescent who is breast feeding should err on the generous side. The combined stress of maintaining her own physical growth and providing nourishment for her infant results in the highest overall nutrient needs of her life.

ENERGY

Caloric requirements include the energy content of the milk (67–77 kcal/100 ml) and the energy required to synthesize the nutrients in milk from amino acids, glucose, fatty acids, and minerals. The efficiency of energy conversion must be taken into account. The RDA for lactation provides 500 kcal/day in addition to the needs of the woman in the nonpregnant, nonlactating state. The allowance provides for breast feeding a single infant for three months. If lactation continues longer than three months, if the woman's weight falls below ideal weight, or if more than one infant is nursed, the allowance should be increased.[71] Three assumptions have been made in this calculation and should be examined: (1) the conversion of maternal energy to milk energy is 90 percent efficient, so that 90 kcal would be required to produce 67 to 77 kcal for 100 ml milk; (2) the average milk volume is 850 ml/day; and (3) mobilization of maternal fat deposited during pregnancy supplies 200 to 300 kcal/day.

The conversion of maternal energy to milk energy was assumed in the 1958 RDA calculation to be 60 percent efficient. A recalculation of data by Hytten and Thomson[62] in 1961 raised the figure to 80 percent. Another recalculation by Thomson et al.[72] in 1970 produced an efficiency ratio of 97 percent, which they lowered to 90 percent because of potential errors.

200

Table 4.4 Nutrients in Breast Milk and Recommended Dietary Allowances

	Estimated Content of 850 ml Milk	Content as Percentage of Nonlactating RDA	Recommended Dietary Allowances		
			Woman 19–22 Years	Lactation 19–22 Years	Percentage Increase
Kilocalories	635	30	2100	2600	24
Protein, g	10	22	44	64	45
Calcium, mg	275	34	800	1200	50
Phosphorus, mg	120	15	800	1200	50
Iodine, μg	40	40	150	200	33
Iron, mg	0.4	2	18	[a]	[a]
Magnesium, mg	33	11	300	450	50
Zinc, mg	3	20	15	25	67
Vitamin A activity, μg R.E.	420	52	800	1200	50
Vitamin D, μg	0.5	5	7.5	12.5	67
Vitamin E, mg α T.E.	1.8	15	8	11	38
Ascorbic acid, mg	40	89	60	100	67
Folacin, μg	40	10	400	500	25
Niacin, mg	1.4	10	14	19	36
Riboflavin, mg	0.3	21	1.3	1.8	38
Thiamin, mg	0.1	9	1.1	1.6	45
Vitamin B_6, mg	0.1	5	2.0	2.5	25
Vitamin B_{12}, μg	0.2	7	3.0	4.0	33

[a]Iron needs during lactation are not substantially different from those of the nonpregnant woman, but continued supplementation for two to three months after parturition is advisable.

The second assumption is that average milk volume in the first three months is 850 ml/day. This is approximately the same volume used by Widdowson[43] for women in the second month, but is 100 ml higher than the volume reported by Lönnerdal et al.[44] for healthy Swedish women. Widdowson calculated that the daily energy cost of lactation increased from 446 kcal in the first month to 819 kcal in the sixth month.

The third assumption is that women who gain 11 to 12.5 kg during pregnancy store 2 to 4 kg of body fat which may be drawn upon to supply part of the energy for lactation. Healthy women gain up to 4 kg above the calculated total for fetal and maternal tissue increases (Chapter 3) and usually do not lose this weight by the end of the first postpartum week. High nitrogen retention found in the balance studies of pregnant women by Hunscher et al.[73] and by Coons and Blunt[70] led to the conclusion that the extra weight could be attributed to protein deposition. Later Hytten and Thomson[62] reasoned that the storage was fat, not protein. If the energy value of 2 to 4 kg of body fat is calculated as 25,000 kcal, it would provide 200 to 300 kcal/day for 100 days of lactation. This was taken into account in establishing the RDA.

The calculation of energy needs of the lactating woman, then, would be as follows: Milk supplies an average of 72 kcal/100 ml, requiring 90 kcal from the mother. A milk volume of 850 ml would provide the infant with 612 kcal but the mother would expend 765 kcal. If 250 kcal/day were available from mobilization of maternal body fat, the net dietary need would be slightly more than 500 kcal. However, additional nitrogen balance studies in pregnancy[74] confirm earlier studies that part of the unexplained weight gain may be due to protein storage; this would lower the amount of fat available for mobilization and raise the energy requirement in lactation.

To illustrate the changing concepts of energy needs, the provision of an additional 500 kcal for lactation in the 1974 and 1979 RDA is a reversion to the values for the 1943 and 1945 editions. In the interim, from 1953 to 1968, the increment for lactation was considered to be 1000 kcal/day.

The utilization of body fat during lactation is often accompanied by a natural decrease in body weight, subject, of course, to the balance with energy intake. However, deliberate greater weight reduction by limitation of caloric intake is not recommended, especially during the early phase of lactation, since it may decrease milk yield and compromise infant weight gain.[75]

PROTEIN

The extra allowance for protein in lactation is calculated from the amount in the milk produced, with a factor for the efficiency of conversion of dietary protein to milk protein and an added factor for the biological value of the protein in the woman's diet. Protein requirements are believed to in-

202

crease to a maximum in the fifth postpartum month and then remain stable. The RDA[71] and WHO[76] calculations are similar in their consideration of factors.

Breast milk contains an average of 1.1 to 1.2 g protein/100 ml, although there is wide individual variation, as shown in Table 4.2. A milk yield of 850 ml would provide approximately 10 g protein; the RDA committee considered 15 g an upper limit. The efficiency of conversion of dietary protein to milk protein is unknown. Hytten and Thomson[62] cited a range of 50 to 100 percent reported in the literature; they proposed that it was similar to the 80 percent efficiency for energy. The RDA is based on an efficiency of 70 percent. Therefore, to produce 10 g protein in milk, the lactating woman would need 16 to 17 g of the same high quality protein in her diet. Because most of the dietary protein is of lower quality, a factor of 1.25 was deemed applicable for the Western diet in which 60 percent of the protein is of animal origin. Therefore, approximately 20 g of protein above the woman's nonlactating allowance should be provided.

The protein allowance should be increased if milk yield exceeds 850 ml/day or if the dietary protein is of poorer quality. On a vegetarian diet protein should be increased by a factor of 1.6 instead of 1.25 to compensate for the lower protein score. If caloric intake is inadequate, the protein allowance should be increased to adjust for diversion of protein to energy. The protein content of human milk is little affected by changes in maternal intake, but milk volume may be decreased when dietary protein is inadequate.

Over a period of years the RDAs for protein have decreased for all individuals. In addition, the differential allowed for lactation has decreased. Between 1943 and 1963 an addition of 40 g above nonlactating allowances was recommended, except in 1953, when the figure was 45 g. In 1968, 1974 and 1979 the additional protein allowance for lactation was lowered to 20 g. The earlier figures had been based on the evidence of higher needs from nitrogen balance studies and on an efficiency conversion of 50 percent.

MINERALS

The mineral content of human milk varies more with maternal intake than macronutrient content but less than vitamin content. However, to protect the mother's reserves, her diet should be adjusted to provide the minerals lost in milk, with an added factor for absorption rate.

Calcium content of human milk is approximately 30 mg/100 ml. It is estimated that the infant obtains a total of 250 mg/day in early lactation, increasing to 300 mg/day after three months. The mammary glands withdraw this amount from maternal blood. Since the plasma calcium is homeostatically controlled, it must be replaced either from absorption of dietary calcium or from maternal bone storage. If the maternal diet provides inadequate calcium, the calcium level of milk will be maintained at the expense of the mother. Total calcium secreted in milk during six months of lactation would range between 50 and 70 g. Although this is a small amount relative to the estimated 1000 g in the mother's body, repeated cycles of pregnancy and lactation in a woman with low calcium intake would produce cumulative losses which might be detrimental.[62]

The absorption rate of calcium varies widely. In part, it is dependent on the availability of food calcium and on the presence of vitamin D. Adaptation to long-term low intakes of calcium has been demonstrated, indicating the ability of the body to conserve calcium. X-ray studies of the size and cortical thickness of bone showed that Bantu mothers accustomed to low calcium intakes had significantly lower mean values than Caucasian mothers. However, within the Bantu group, values of mothers with more than six children did not differ from those with two or fewer children,[77] suggesting the persistence of adaptation through repeated periods of increased requirement. Even in well-nourished women there is little agreement about the absorption rate of dietary calcium. The RDA for adults is based on 40 percent absorption. During lactation, various estimates have been used in the literature, ranging from 20 to 50 percent.[43,62,78]

As shown in Table 4.4, the RDAs for calcium and phosphorus have been set at 50 percent above the woman's nonlactating allowances. The iron allowance is not specified, but is not substantially different from that of the nonpregnant woman. The iron content of milk is relatively low, and amenorrhea during part of the lactation period would offset the iron needed for milk production. The zinc allowance for lactation is relatively higher than other minerals when compared to nonlactating allowances, but this value must be considered tentative in view of the limited knowledge of zinc in human nutrition.

VITAMINS

An increased allowance of 25 to 38 percent is provided in lactation for all vitamins except three. For vitamin A, ascorbic acid, and vitamin D the increment is 50 to 67 percent. In breast milk the vitamin A activity is primarily in the form of retinol and is relatively high. Because the maternal dietary allowance is based on the assumption that half the vitamin A activity is provided as carotenoids, the allowance has been increased to provide for conversion. The concentration of ascorbic acid in breast milk reflects maternal intake, so a generous amount of this vitamin should be included in the mother's diet to maintain a high level in milk.

Several changes in vitamin allowances were made in the 1979 revision. The differentials between allowances for the nonpregnant woman and for the lactating woman were increased for absorbic acid, thiamin, and niacin and decreased for folacin.

FLUIDS

Approximately 87 percent of the volume of breast milk is water. Nearly 750 ml is excreted in 850 ml of milk. A generous fluid intake, probably close to 3 liters per day, is essential to avoid dehydration. In most women natural thirst is a guide to fluid requirement. Many experience thirst during a nursing period; sitting quietly while breast feeding provides an opportunity for extra fluid consumption.

DIET DURING LACTATION

Allowances for many nutrients during lactation are the same as for pregnancy, so the diet during pregnancy (Chapter 3) is an excellent basis for diet during lactation. The additional leeway of 200 kcal/day in lactation should be provided by foods that meet the higher needs for vitamin A, ascorbic acid, niacin, riboflavin, and zinc. At least one quart of milk daily provides excellent protection for meeting the allowances for protein and calcium as well as other minerals and vitamins. Women with lactose intolerance may be able to take buttermilk and yogurt without discomfort. For the woman who cannot or will not take milk or milk products, a supplement of at least 1 g calcium daily is recommended to prevent or minimize loss of bone calcium, but will not provide the other nutrients of milk. The lactating woman should also increase her intake of citrus fruits and green leafy and yellow vegetables above her prenatal diet. Salt should be iodized to meet the higher iodine allowance.

REFERENCES

1. American Academy of Pediatrics Committee on Nutrition. Commentary on breast feeding and infant formulas, including proposed standards for formulas. *Pediat.* 57:278-285, 1976.
2. Jelliffe, D. B., and E. F. P. Jelliffe. Adaptive suckling. *Ecol. Food Nutr.* 5:249-253, 1976.
3. Grulee, C. G., H. N. Sanford, and P. H. Herron. Breast and artificial feeding. *JAMA 103*:735-748, 1934.
4. Hirschman, C., and J. A. Sweet. Social background and breast feeding among American mothers. *Soc. Biol. 21*:39-57, 1974.

5. Bain, K. The incidence of breast feeding in hospitals in the United States. *Pediat. 2*:313–320, 1948.
6. Meyer, H. F. Breast feeding in the United States: Extent and possible trend. A survey of 1,904 hospitals with two and a quarter million births in 1956. *Pediat. 22*:116–121, 1958.
7. Robertson, W. O. Breast feeding practices: Some implications of regional variations. *Am. J. Pub. Health 51*:1035–1042, 1961.
8. Meyer, H. F. Breast feeding in the United States: Report of a 1966 national survey with comparable 1946 and 1956 data. *Clin. Pediat. 7*:708–715, 1968.
9. Eppright, E. M., H. M. Fox, B. A. Fryer, G. H. Lamkin, V. M. Vivian, and E. S. Fuller. Nutrition of infants and children in the North Central region of the United States of America. *World Rev. Nutr. Dietet. 14*:269–332, 1972.
10. Jelliffe, D. B. World trends in infant feeding. *Am. J. Clin. Nutr. 29*:1227–1237, 1976.
11. Fomon, S. J. *Infant Nutrition,* Second Edition. W. B. Saunders, Philadelphia, 1974.
12. Aykroyd, W., and J. Kevaney. Mortality in infancy and early childhood in Ireland, Scotland, England, and Wales, 1871–1970. *Ecol. Food Nutr. 2*:11–17, 1973.
13. Brown, R. E. Breast Feeding in modern times. *Am. J. Clin. Nutri. 26*:556–562, 1973.
14. Latham, M. C. Infant feeding in national and international perspective: An examination in human lactation, and the modern crisis in infant and young child feeding practices. *Ann. N. Y. Acad. Sci. 300*:197–209, 1977.
15. Berg, A. *The Nutrition Factor.* The Brookings Institution, Washington, D.C., 1973.
16. Berg, A. The crisis in infant feeding practices. *Nutr. Today 12*:18–23, 1977.
17. Salber, E. J., P. G. Stitt, and J. G. Babbott. Patterns of breast feeding. I. Factors affecting the frequency of breast feeding in the newborn period. *N. Engl. J. Med. 259*:707–713, 1958.
18. Salber, E. J., and M. Feinleib. Breast feeding in Boston. *Pediat. 37*:299–303, 1966.
19. Guthrie, H., and G. Guthrie. The resurgence of natural child feeding. *Clin. Pediat. 5*:481–484, 1966.
20. Cole, J. P. Breast feeding in the Boston suburbs in relation to personal-social factors. *Clin. Pediat. 16*:352–356, 1977.
21. Jackson, E. B., L. C. Wilkin, and H. Auerbach. Statistical report on incidence and duration of breast feeding in relation to personal-social and hospital maternity factors. *Pediat. 17*:700–715, 1956.

22. *The Womanly Art of Breast Feeding.* La Leche League International, Franklin Park, Ill., 1963.

23. Kon, S. K. and A. T. Cowie (Eds.) *Milk: The Mammary Gland and Its Secretions.* Academic Press, New York, 1967.

24. Cowie, A. T., and J. S. Tindal. *The Physiology of Lactation.* Edward Arnold, Ltd., London, 1971.

25. Josimovich, J. B., M. Reynolds, and E. Cobo (Eds.) *Lactogenic Hormones, Fetal Nutrition, and Lactation.* John Wiley and Sons, New York, 1974.

26. Wolstenholme, G. E. W., and K. Knight (Eds.) *Lactogenic Hormones.* Churchill Livingstone, Edinburgh, 1972.

27. Laupus, W. E. Feeding of Infants. In: Vaughan, V. G., III, R. J. McKay, and W. E. Nelson (Eds.) *Nelson Textbook of Pediatrics,* Tenth Edition. W. B. Saunders, Philadelphia, 1975.

28. Johnson, J. D. Neonatal nonhemolytic jaundice. *N. Engl. J. Med. 292*:194–197, 1975.

29. Jelliffe, D. B., and E. F. P. Jelliffe. How breast feeding really works. *J. Trop. Pediat. 17*:62–64, 1971.

30. Tyson, J. E., N. Khojandi, J. Huth, and B. Anfreassen. The influence of prolactin secretion on human lactation. *J. Clin. Endocrinol. Metab. 40*:764–773, 1975.

31. Fournier, P. J. R., P. D. Desjardins, and H. G. Friesen. Current understanding of human prolactin physiology and its diagnostic and therapeutic applications: A review. *Am. J. Obstet. Gynecol. 118*: 337–343, 1974.

32. Sala, N. L., E. C. Luther, J. C. Arballo, and J. C. C. Funes. Oxytocin reproducing reflex milk ejection in lactating women. *J. Appl. Physiol. 36*:154–158, 1974.

33. Cobo, E. Effect of different doses of ethanol on the milk-ejecting reflex in lactating women. *Am. J. Obstet. Gynecol. 115*:817–821, 1973.

34. Thoman, E. B. Development of synchrony in mother-infant interaction in feeding and other situations. *Fed. Proc. 34*:1587–1592, 1975.

35. Otte, M. J. Correcting inverted nipples—an aid to breast feeding. *Am. J. Nurs. 75*:454–456, 1975.

36. Brown, M. S., and J. T. Hurlock. Preparation of the breast for breastfeeding. *Nurs. Res. 24*:448–451, 1975.

37. Barnes, G. R., Jr., A. N. Lethin, Jr., E. B. Jackson, and N. Shea. Management of breast feeding. *JAMA 151*:192–199, 1953.

38. Timiras, P. S. *Developmental Physiology and Aging.* Macmillan, New York, 1972.

39. Newton, N. Psychologic differences between breast and bottle feeding. *Am. J. Clin. Nutr. 24*:993–1004, 1971

40. Egli, G. E., N. S. Egli, and M. Newton. Influence of number of breast feedings on milk production. *Pediat. 27*:314–317, 1961.

41. Illingworth, R. S., and D. G. H. Stone. Self-demand feeding in a maternity unit. *Lancet 1*:683–687, 1952.

42. Salber, E. J. Effect of different feeding schedules on growth of Bantu babies in the first week of life. *J. Trop. Pediat. 2*:97–102, 1956.

43. Widdowson, E. M. Nutrition and lactation. In: Winick, M. (Ed.) *Nutritional Disorders of American Women.* John Wiley and Sons, New York, 1977.

44. Lönnerdal, B., E. Forsum, and L. Hambraeus. A longitudinal study of the protein, nitrogen and lactose contents of human milk from Swedish well-nourished mothers. *Am. J. Clin. Nutr. 29*:1127–1133, 1976.

45. Delgado, H., A. Lechtig, R. Martorell, E. Brineman, and R. E. Klein. Nutrition, lactation and postpartum amenorrhea. *Am. J. Clin. Nutr. 31*:322–327, 1978.

46. Rosa, F. W. Resolving the "public health dilemma" of steroid contraception and its effect on lactation. *Am. J. Pub. Health 66*:791–792, 1976.

47. Guiloff, E., A. Ibarro-Polo, J. Zanartu, C. Torcanini, T. W. Mischler, and C. Gomez-Rogers. Effect of contraception on lactation. *Am. J. Obstet. Gynecol. 118*:42–45, 1974.

48. Goldman, A. S., and C. W. Smith. Host resistant factors in human milk. *J. Pediat. 82*:1082–1090, 1973.

49. Gerrard, J. W. Breast feeding: Second thoughts. *Pediat. 54*:757–764, 1974.

50. Oseid, B. J. Breast-feeding and infant health. *Clin. Obstet. Gynecol. 18*:149–173, 1975.

51. Knowles, J. A. Breast milk—A source of more than nutrients for the neonate. *Clin. Toxicol. 7*:69–82, 1974.

52. Stirrat, G. M. Prescribing problems in the second half of pregnancy and during lactation. *Obstet. Gynecol. Surv. 31*:1–7, 1976.

53. Macy, I. G., H. J. Kelly, and R. E. Sloan. *The Composition of Milks.* Publ. 254, National Academy of Sciences, Washington, D.C. 1953.

54. Macy, I. G. The composition of human colostrum and milk. *Am. J. Dis. Child. 78*:589–603, 1949.

55. Macy, I. G., and H. J. Kelly. Human milk and cow's milk in infant nutrition. In: Kon, S. K., and A. T. Cowie (Eds.) *Milk: The Mammary Gland and Its Secretion,* Vol. II. Academic Press, New York, 1961.

56. Burman, D. Nutrition in early childhood. In: McLaren, D. S., and D. Burman (Eds.) *Textbook of Paediatric Nutrition.* Churchill Livingstone, Edinburgh, 1976.

57. Hytten, F. E. Clinical and chemical studies in human lactation. III.

Diurnal variation in major constituents of milk. *Brit. Med. J.* *1*:179–182, 1954.

58. Hall, B. Changing composition of human milk and early development of an appetite control. *Lancet 1*:779–781, 1975.

59. Hytten, F. E. Clinical and chemical studies in human lactation. II. Variations in major constituents during a feeding. *Brit. Med. J.* *1*:176–179, 1954.

60. Emery, W. B., Jr., N. L. Canolty, J. M. Aitchison, and W. L. Dunkley. Influence of sampling on fatty acid composition of human milk. *Am. J. Clin. Nutr. 31*:1127–1130, 1978.

61. György, P. Biochemical aspects of human milk. *Am. J. Clin. Nutr. 24*:970–975, 1971.

62. Hytten, F. E., and A. M. Thomson. Nutrition of the lactating woman. In: Kon, S. K., and A. T. Cowie (Eds.) *Milk: The Mammary Gland and Its Secretion.* Academic Press, New York, 1961.

63. Widdowson, E. M. Nutrition. In: Davis, J. A., and J. Dobbing (Eds.) *Scientific Foundations of Paediatrics.* Heinemann, London, 1974.

64. Coulson, K. M., R. L. Cohen, W. F. Coulson, and D. B. Jelliffe. Hematocrit levels in breast-fed American babies. *Clin. Pediat. 16*:649–651, 1977.

65. Woodruff, C. W., C. Latham, and S. McDavid. Iron nutrition in the breast-fed infant. *J. Pediat. 90*:36–38, 1976.

66. Beal, V. A. Calcium and phosphorus in infancy. *J. Am. Dietet. Assoc. 53*:450–459, 1968.

67. Baum, D. J. Nutritional value of human milk. *Obstet. Gynecol. 37*:126–130, 1971.

68. Lakdawala, D. R., and E. M. Widdowson. Vitamin-D in human milk. *Lancet 1*:167–168, 1977.

69. Macy, I. G. *Nutrition and Chemical Growth in Childhood,* Vol. I. Charles C Thomas, Springfield, Ill., 1942. (Contains a complete list of publications of the Children's Fund of Michigan.)

70. Coons, C. M., and K. Blunt. Retention of nitrogen, calcium, phosphorus and magnesium by pregnant women. *J. Biol. Chem. 86*:1–16, 1930.

71. *Recommended Dietary Allowances,* Eighth Edition. National Academy of Sciences, Washington, D.C., 1974.

72. Thomson, A. M., F. E. Hytten, and W. Z. Billewicz. The energy cost of human lactation. *Brit. Med. J. 24*:565–572, 1970.

73. Hunscher, H. A., F. C. Hummell, B. N. Erickson, and I. G. Macy. Metabolism of women during the reproductive cycle. VI. A case study of the continuous nitrogen utilization of a multipara during pregnancy, parturition, puerperium and lactation. *J. Nutr. 10*:579–597, 1935.

74. King, J. C. Protein metabolism during pregnancy. *Clin. Perinatol.* 2:243–254, 1975.
75. Wichelow, M. J. Caloric requirements for successful breast feeding. *Arch. Dis. Child. 50*:669, 1975.
76. Food and Agriculture Organization/World Health Organization. *Protein Requirements.* Report of a Joint FAO/WHO Expert Group. WHO Tech. Rept. Series No. 301. World Health Organization, Geneva, 1965.
77. Walker, A. R. P., B. Richardson, and F. Walker. The influence of numerous pregnancies and lactations on bone dimensions in South African Bantu and Caucasian mothers. *Clin. Science 42*:189–195, 1972.
78. Davidson, S., R. Passmore, and J. F. Brock. *Human Nutrition and Dietetics,* Fifth edition. Williams and Wilkins, Baltimore, 1972.

5

INFANCY
(BIRTH
TO
ONE
YEAR)

The first year of life is one of remarkable change. After being in a warm and protected environment, provided with oxygen, predigested nutrients, and other materials required for growth and survival, the newly born infant is thrust into a world in which he* must immediately carry out essential functions on his own. He must be capable of respiration, changes in circulation, all metabolic processes, temperature control, and other physiological functions as an independent organism. With the first feeding, he is responsible for his own digestion, absorption, and assimilation. The high mortality rate among infants in the first 24 hours attests to the trauma of the transition and the importance of providing for adequate growth, development, and maturation during gestation. The full-term infant whose prenatal environment has endowed him with a healthy body, free from congenital defects, and sufficiently large and mature to be able to make the transition to independent existence faces much less risk than the infant whose intrauterine environment has been suboptimal.

During the first year the infant continues to undergo stress, both in physical growth and in many aspects of maturation. Per unit of body size, the need for nutrients to synthesize new tissue is greater than at any later age. In the first 12 months, the infant will probably triple his weight and increase his length by 50 percent. The increase in weight is due both to increment in lean body mass and to fat deposition. His body fat will rise to approx-

*I recognize that human beings are either male or female. However, I also feel that the repeated use of he/she, the conversion of singular to plural, and other nonsexist wording interfere with the easy reading of a text. Therefore, in this text "he" is used during infancy and childhood for either sex to distinguish the child from the mother, who is obviously "she."

imately one-fourth of body weight. At the same time, body water decreases during the year. The rate of growth during the year is not linear, but is rapid during the first few months and then tapers off.

While somatic growth occurs, the infant is also maturing, with stabilization of physiological and metabolic functions. Born with immature renal function and poor ability to concentrate solutes in urine, the infant rapidly increases in maturity, and by six weeks his ability to concentrate solutes is closer to adult levels. Stomach capacity increases more than tenfold during the year, from 10 to 20 ml at birth to approximately 200 ml by 12 months. Digestive ability is enhanced with more efficient production of enzymes and greater tolerance of a variety of foods.

Neuromuscular development is also rapid. The central nervous system becomes more stable. Control of muscular contraction and relaxation gradually evolves. Head lag and newborn reflexes are replaced by voluntary control of the trunk and neck, as well as of the extremities. Progression to head control, sitting erect, crawling, and standing erect lead to the first tentative efforts to walk. Fine motor ability improves, and by the end of the year, the infant has accomplished hand manipulation with thumb-finger prehension. The muscles of the jaw and tongue come under voluntary control with greater ability to chew and swallow. Purposive movements of all parts of the body increase markedly during the first year.

Social and psychological development is also rapid. The interaction between the infant and mother during the early weeks and months is critical to his well-being. In the past few years there has been increased appreciation of the importance of closeness of mother and infant immediately after delivery to the bonding between them. The infant needs tactile, auditory, and visual stimulation as well as physical care and feeding; inadequate social and psychological contact may lead to failure to thrive, just as undernutrition can. The infant learns to react with people in his environment and gradually develops a sense of self as different from others. Social responses and the acquisition of skills of communication by body movement, vocalizations, and words evolve during the year.

By the end of the first year, the infant is not only larger, but also more mature, more capable, and more adaptable. Body functions and muscular control are well advanced. Personality characteristics and socialization have become more pronounced. The year-old child is far more independent, both physically and emotionally, than the newborn. He is more aware of people and objects in his surroundings. He has learned to distinguish his needs and to express them. With such rapid development in a short time, the importance of health care, nutritional adequacy, and psychosocial attention during the first year cannot be overemphasized. When growth is most rapid the organism is most vulnerable to any deficiencies in the environment. The first year is second only to the gestational period as a determinant of health throughout life.

PHYSICAL GROWTH

The rate of gain in both weight and length is faster during the first year than at any later age. This was shown in Figure 1.6 in Chapter 1. The very rapid growth of the first few months is followed by a gradual deceleration toward the end of the year, but even then the growth rate is more rapid than in adolescence.

It has been speculated that the early phase of postnatal growth is still under the influence of prenatal hormonal control, and that the child's own physiological control gradually comes into play. However, when constraining influences during pregnancy are released, some small infants grow at a faster rate beginning early in the neonatal period; this is especially seen in infants who were small for gestational age. There are wide individual differences in growth during early infancy, and it is not uncommon for the infant to change percentile channels during the early months.

WEIGHT AND ITS COMPONENTS

The neonate loses weight immediately after delivery, due largely to loss of body water, but partially also to catabolism of body tissue. Birth weight is usually regained by 7 to 10 days. Thereafter weight gain is rapid, and birth weight is usually doubled in the first 4 months. For many years pediatric textbooks stated that birth weight could be expected to double by 6 months, but at the present time most infants double their weight by the fourth or early fifth month. The faster growth has been attributed to changes in infant feeding, and particularly to the earlier introduction of solid foods. Lack of comparable studies before and after the marketing of puréed foods for infants makes such a conclusion speculative. The simultaneous improvement in health care and control of infectious diseases may also be factors. The present faster gain in weight early in life may reflect potential growth under optimal conditions. However, the quality of growth is important, since there may ultimately be many disadvantages to the excessive deposition of body fat. The chubby baby, although admired by many parents and relatives, especially among some cultural groups, may actually represent a lesser degree of health than his leaner counterpart.

The initial doubling of weight, from an average of 3.0–3.5 kg to 6–7 kg, takes about four months. The slowing of the rate of growth is evident from the fact that the second addition of 3.0 to 3.5 kg requires approximately 8 months more, and is reached at approximately 1 year. The third addition of

3.4 kg will not be accomplished until about 2½ years of age. Expressed in another way, two-thirds of the weight gain for the first year occurs in the first 6 months, and only one-third in the final 6 months of the year. Daily weight gain toward the end of the first month may average 35 to 40 g, but by the end of the year the gain is closer to an average of 11 to 12 g/day.[1]

The increase in weight is due to both lean body mass and fat deposition. As the body grows in length and all organs increase in size, the increment of body mass adds to weight. However, the proportion of fat to lean body mass also changes. At birth, fat comprises 11 to 16 percent of body weight[1,2]; by four to six months the proportion of body fat reaches a peak, and then declines to a level of 25 percent of body weight at one year. This is consistent with measurements of skinfold thicknesses by caliper[3] and fat widths by X rays,[4] which show a peak at 6 months followed by a plateau and then a decrease. Fomon has estimated that approximately 42 percent of the weight gained in the first four months by the "male reference infant" is accounted for by lipid, but that between 4 and 12 months only 19 percent of the weight gain is due to lipid.[1] Greater accumulation of fat occurs on the extremities than on the trunk. Triceps skinfold measurements are approximately 75 percent greater at one year than at birth, but subscapular thicknesses have increased only 25 percent.

Total body water increases with the accretion of tissue, but its increase is not proportional to weight increase, so that it comprises a smaller percentage of body weight. At birth, water contributes approximately 75 percent of body weight, but at one year only 60 percent. The change is due primarily to a decrease in extracellular fluids.

Sex differences in weight are relatively small at birth, but become larger by the end of the year. Boys tend to be slightly heavier at birth and gain more weight. The percentiles of the National Center for Health Statistics growth charts,[5] which were derived from the infant data of the Fels Research Institute, show a difference of 150 g in median weights at birth and of 530 g at 1 year. The increments during the year at each percentile level range between 5.5 and 7.5 kg for girls and between 6 and 8 kg for boys. The median weights at 1 year were 9.57 kg for girls and 10.10 kg for boys. However, the composition of gain differs, since girls tend to increase more in body fat and boys more in lean body mass.

SKELETAL GROWTH

Median lengths of boys in the Fels series increased from 49.9 cm at birth to 76.2 cm at 1 year, an increase of 26.3 cm. Medians of girls were 49.3 cm and 74.4 cm, a gain of 25.1 cm.[5] Therefore the increase in the boys' median was 53 percent and in the girls' median 51 percent during the year. As with weight, approximately two-thirds of the gain in stature was accomplished in the first 6 months of the year.

Bone widths also increase about 50 percent during the year, as measured from X rays of the humerus, radius, femur, and tibia.[4] The concentration of calcium in the femur, estimated as 89.4 g per kg bone at birth, decreases to 87.8 g/kg at 4 months, then increases to 94.0 g/kg at one year. However, with the increase in bone length and width, the total gain in bone calcium is assumed to be 18.9 g (155 mg/day) between birth and 4 months, and 31.7 g (130 mg/day) between 4 and 12 months.[1] In summary, bones increase in length, width, and density during the first year.

Head circumference, however, increases less than other bones during the first year. Major growth in the skull occurs prenatally, and growth is slower in the postnatal period. Head circumference increases approximately 36 percent in males and 33 to 34 percent in females during the first 12 months.

PHYSIOLOGICAL DEVELOPMENT RELATED TO NUTRITION

The maturation of function during the first year affects how the infant is fed and his ability to tolerate various types of foods. As Schick[6] expressed it, "Nature is very kind to the pediatrician and to the child, in that it gave the infant an excellent tolerance." Over the centuries young infants have been given a wide variety of milks, of milk substitutes, and of semisolid foods. Each new era has brought changing concepts of what foods should be given to infants and at what ages, some resulting in improved growth and health, and some revised or withdrawn when they proved to be harmful or impractical. The adaptability of the infant has sometimes disguised the negative aspects of practices, and it is only with greater understanding of infant physiology than we now possess that practices can be adapted to the capability of the infant rather than imposing a feeding regime which stresses neuromuscular or physiological function.

NEUROMUSCULAR DEVELOPMENT

The neonate has a number of reflexes that work together to permit the ingestion and swallowing of food. Primary among these are the rooting, sucking, and swallowing reflexes. The rooting reflex causes the infant to turn his head in the direction of a touch on the face, and to seek the nipple with his mouth. This is of particular importance to the breast-fed infant, who roots with any contact of the nipple or breast to his cheek. Sometimes the mother, a nurse, or other person trying to be helpful during the first day or two of breast feeding may attempt to push the infant's face toward the breast. The reflex of rooting brings the opposite response, and the infant turns toward the touch rather than toward the breast. The rooting reflex gradually diminishes and is lost in the second or third month, replaced by voluntary movement (Table 5.1).

The sucking reflex is also present at birth, but the strength of the reflex varies from one infant to another. The infant with a strong sucking reflex provides an excellent stimulus to the neurohormonal sequence essential to successful lactation, as described in Chapter 4. The sucking may be so vigorous, however, that the mother may find it uncomfortable until her nipples become accustomed to it. The bottle-fed infant with a strong sucking reflex is also likely to take a relatively short time in obtaining enough milk to satisfy his hunger. At first the sucking reflex involves only up-and-down motions of the tongue in concert with the mandible, but gradually the tongue becomes capable of motion forward and back, increasing its efficiency and adding licking motions to the sucking motions. Around three to four months, the reflex aspect of the sucking diminishes and it comes under voluntary control.

When the young infant takes the nipple into the mouth, it fits well back on the tongue, and swallowing follows. The swallowing reflex at first involves the posterior part of the tongue, and later develops to include the whole tongue.

A reverse type of reflex, in terms of its action, is the extrusive, or protrusive, reflex. Anything that is put on the anterior third of the tongue is

Table 5.1   Pattern of Development of Feeding Skills in the First Year

Age (Months)	Behavior
0–1	Rooting reflex—turns head to seek with mouth object touching cheek
	Sucking reflex—vertical movements of tongue and mandible to create negative pressure
	Swallowing reflex—initially involves posterior part of tongue
	Extrusion reflex—pushes food out of mouth when placed on anterior part of tongue
	Poor motor control of head, neck, trunk. Cannot localize; uses whole body in response
1–2	Pump sucking—tongue moves down with mandible to create negative pressure to pull food into pharynx
	Position awareness for feeding; begins mouthing and sucking when placed in that position

2-4	Primitive reflexes diminishing; voluntary control increasing
	Rooting reflex—little or none by 3 months
	Extrusion reflex gradually decreases; lost by 4 months
	Lick sucking develops, with tongue motion forward and backward
	Lip closure still poor; loss of fluid from corners of mouth to 4 months
	Better motor control of head and neck; better sitting balance
	Beginning coordination of eye-body movements; learning to reach for objects and carry them to mouth
	Greater tolerance in waiting for food
4-6	Sucking becomes voluntary
	Lateral motions of jaws begin
	Increased use of hands in reaching; able to grasp objects with thumb and palm at 5 months; finger sucking and transport of objects to mouth by 6 months
	Biting and chewing added to sucking by 6 months
	Sits erect with support by 6 months
6-9	Easier sitting balance; may need support to 8 to 9 months
	Good closure of mouth by 8 months; can drink from cup with help and little loss of liquid by 9 months
	Chewing motions vertical, not grinding
	Reaches; grasps with pincer motion; carries food to mouth; finger-feeding by 7 to 8 months; transfers items hand to hand
9-12	Sits erect without support; good head control
	Variety of lip and tongue movements; tongue movement independent of jaws; tongue lateralization within mouth; can move food from one cheek to the other
	Rotary chewing motion of jaws beginning
	Holds own bottle; proficiency with cup increasing but some wrist rotation
	Finger-feeding proficient, with thumb-finger opposition and grasp; puts fingers into food on plate
	Reaches for spoon to hold, play, or move food, but not usually to carry food to mouth

pushed out of the mouth. This may be evident first to the mother who squirts a vitamin supplement from a dropper onto the infant's tongue; the baby attempts to push it out, and the mother attributes the reaction to a dislike of the supplement rather than to a reflex motion. The early introduction of spoon feeding is likely to have the same response. An infant with a weak extrusion reflex may accept food from the spoon with little resistance, but an infant with a strong reflex spits the food out.

The extrusion reflex is usually strong in the first 8 to 9 weeks, then gradually diminishes and is lost around 3 to 4 months. Attempts to feed solid foods before this age are often frustrating. As Bakwin[7] expressed it, "The proper time to introduce solids is determined by a change in the behavior of the oral musculature. When a solid object like a spoon or a tongue depressor is introduced between the lips of a young baby, he purses his lips, raises his tongue, and pushes against the object vigorously. By 3 months, sometimes a little earlier, sometimes a little later, the behavior changes. Now when the spoon is inserted between the lips, the lips part, the tongue depresses, and food placed in the mouth is thrown to the back of the pharynx and swallowed. This marks the proper time to begin feeding solids."

The gradual development of control over the lips, tongue, and mandible must be understood in order for the feeding of the infant to keep pace with his physiological capabilities. The newborn who is gestationally mature is able to suck from the nipple and to swallow the fluid. Until primitive reflexes are replaced by voluntary control mechanisms, the wise mother or health professional should respect the cues offered by the infant. Only when the infant progresses to the stage of control over functions of his mouth and of his neck and back can he easily and successfully manage being fed by other than a nipple. Readiness for chewing requires maturation of the neuromuscular system, with vertical chewing motions followed by rotary chewing. Illingworth and Lister[8] have speculated that there is a critical or sensitive period when the child is ready for progress. Forcing an activity before the critical period, or delaying the introduction of the stimulus past the critical period may produce difficulties. Readiness for chewing is evident in normal children at about six months. In retarded children, slower maturation delays readiness.

Control of the mandible, tongue, and especially the lips is essential to ability of the infant to drink from a cup. Until good lip closure can be accomplished, at about 8 months, poor control over the lateral parts of the lips allows fluid to drip from the corners of the mouth. The cup may be offered for fluids at an earlier age, primarily for practice, since the amount consumed is small.

Large and fine muscular maturation are important to the development of self-feeding. The ability to control neck and back muscles develops gradually, and the infant is usually able to sit erect with support by 4 to 6 months, and without support between 6 and 8 months. Use of the hands becomes progressively more efficient, changing from indiscriminate reaching to purposeful motion, and from reaching or grasping with the palms and whole hand to more precise thumb-finger opposition. Ability to pick up food and carry it to the mouth begins around 7 to 8 months, becoming more proficient within the next few months. Although the infant may reach for the spoon and play with it or put it into the food, efficiency in self-feeding with a spoon depends on proper wrist rotation, which may not be accomplished until after 1 year.

DIGESTION AND ABSORPTION

The digestive ability of the newborn is different in some respects from that of the older child or adult, and the infant with low birth weight, whether prematurely born or small for gestational age (Chapter 3), is different from the full-term infant. However, the wide range of tolerance of all infants has been shown by generally satisfactory growth and health even as marked changes have been made in the formulation of substitutes for breast milk and as the infant's gastrointestinal tract has been subjected to semisolid foods as early as the second day of life.

Carbohydrate

Lactase, sucrase, and maltase have all been shown to be present in the fetus in the first trimester of gestation. Sucrase and maltase production are well established by the eight month *in utero*. Lactase production reaches its peak shortly before delivery, but has been found to be present in the 1000 g fetus. Lactase activity in the full-term infant is high at birth and remains high throughout infancy and early childhood, even in populations in which adults have a high incidence of lactose intolerance.[1]

There are conflicting data in the literature on the ability of the young infant to digest starch. Salivary amylase begins the hydrolysis of starch, but is inactivated by gastric acidity. Pancreatic α-amylase may be low in the young infant, especially under 6 months, and then rises. However, there is no evidence of adverse effects as a result of feeding starch to young infants.[9]

Lipid

There is evidence that gastric juice in the infant contains a lipase that is different from pancreatic lipase. Gastric lipase hydrolyzes medium-chain triglycerides which may be absorbed without the necessity of micelle formation; therefore bile acids are not essential for this hydrolysis. Gastric lipase is inactivated by trypsin when the food enters the duodenum, and further hydrolysis is accomplished by pancreatic lipase in the presence of bile acids. Lipase activity in the premature infant has been reported to be lower than in the full-term infant during the first week, but thereafter higher than in the term infant.

Newborns, even full-term, seem to digest and absorb lipid with more difficulty than either protein or carbohydrate. It has been speculated that their less efficient handling of fats may be due to the activity of pancreatic lipase, the concentration of bile acids, or the composition of the bile salts, possibly of taurine or glycine conjugates. Triglycerides of medium-chain fatty acids (8:0, 10:0, and 12:0) are more easily hydrolyzed and absorbed than those of long-chain fatty acids, especially stearic acid. Unsaturated fatty acids are better absorbed than saturated. It is an interesting inconsistency that colostrum has a smaller proportion of medium-chain fatty acids, although it contains a higher percentage of unsaturated fatty acids than mature milk.

The fat in human milk is better absorbed than either butterfat or vegetable oils. This may be due to the fact that the triglycerides of human milk contain a higher proportion of palmitic acid in the 2 position, and 2-monopalmitin is more readily absorbed than other monoglycerides.

Despite the evidence that infants digest lipids less efficiently than other macronutrients, they tolerate a wide range of intake. The Committee on Nutrition of the American Academy of Pediatrics[10] has recommended that infant formulas should be within the range of 3.3 to 6 g fat/100 kcal (30 to 54 percent of total calories).

Protein

Although there are some differences in the production of proteolytic enzymes of premature infants in contrast to full-term infants, there are no differences of practical significance in the digestion of proteins by infants and adults. Digestion is somewhat slower in the infant, possibly because the smaller stomach capacity of the infant results in faster passage to the duodenum, and the slower action of trypsin. However, since stomach capacity, which at birth is only 10-20 ml, rises rapidly to 80 ml after 2 weeks and to 100 ml at the end of the first month,[11] the limited capacity rapidly ceases to be an inhibiting factor. Protein continues to be absorbed more slowly than either lipid or glucose.

KIDNEY FUNCTION

From time to time pediatricians have been concerned about the relative immaturity of the ability of the newborn's kidneys to concentrate urine. The renal solute load has sometimes been used as a basis for trying to define optimal protein intake. The literature on this subject reflects a great deal of controversy. Calculations for renal solute load have been based on nitrogen (urea), sodium, potassium, chloride, and phosphate, and on the obligatory water associated with their excretion. It is generally agreed that renal mechanisms for conserving and excreting salt are well developed by one month[12] and that the full-term infant can maintain water and electrolyte balance at that age almost as efficiently as the adult.

Human milk has a calculated solute load of 79 mOsm/liter, in contrast to a load of 221 mOsm/liter for whole cow's milk and 308 mOsm/liter for boiled skim milk.[1] Limitation of renal solute load was part of the rationale for reducing protein and electrolyte content of cow's milk in the marketing of commercially premodified formulas based on cow's milk. However, the high renal solute load of cow's milk obviously has been well tolerated for years by healthy infants, and studies have demonstrated no significant difference in the rate of renal water excretion in infants fed high or low protein diets.[13] Fisher et al.[14] have suggested that the lack of urine concentration in the neonatal period may be merely a correction of the relative excess of body water that exists at birth.

Problems of renal solute load and water balance rarely occur in healthy infants who are growing rapidly, since the high requirements for tissue synthesis limit the amount of nitrogen and electrolytes to be excreted.[1] This is also true of small infants, both premature and small for gestational age, during their rapid catch-up growth. Protein requirements of the premature infant have been extensively studied, and the best growth in both weight and length is observed when protein intake is higher than that estimated to be required by the full-term infant. The premature infant not only tolerates but thrives on a high-protein intake.

There are situations that require attention to fluid intake and to concentration of electrolytes in the urine. These include fever, diarrhea, renal pathology or other disease affecting kidney function, and restricted fluid intakes, especially during hot weather. The mistaken recommendation for use of boiled skim milk in therapy of infants with diarrhea compounds the problem, since a high renal solute load is superimposed on excessive loss of body water, thereby risking dehydration and electrolyte imbalance.

PSYCHOSOCIAL-BIOLOGICAL INTERACTIONS

The confluence of specialists from many fields of study on the relationship between nutritional status and cognitive behavior and personality development has been strongly emphasized within the past decade. Research workers in nutrition, biochemistry, medicine, cultural and physical anthropology, psychology, psychiatry, sociology, and education have found a common ground in analysis of factors in the mother-infant relationship as these factors affect mental development and learning. Malnutrition in the mother and/or infant is an index of multiple environmental disadvantages, all of which combine to limit both the somatic and mental development of the infant. The interdependence of factors has been more pronounced in developing countries where the disadvantages are most acute, but a number of studies in technologically advanced countries have also supplied understanding of some of the complexities of the mother-infant relationship.

Thirty years ago Spitz and Wolf[15] described a syndrome in infants and young children who were deprived of their mothers by institutionalization. These children responded with depression, withdrawal, and apathy, and suffered permanent damage to their physical growth, mental ability, and emotional status. A number of studies in the United States and Europe showed that, despite adequate dietary intake, children failed to grow well or were in negative biochemical balance when interpersonal relationships were lacking in gratification. Birch and Gussow[16] reviewed school failure in relation to maternal and child nutrition. The circumstantial evidence was strong that negative economic, social, cultural, and environmental factors, mediated through nutrition, interfered with healthy development of personality and cognitive ability.

Inadequate functioning of infants born to malnourished mothers was shown to be related to limitation of cell replication, leading to deficits in both physical size and brain growth. Infants who died of marasmus had smaller than normal brain weights, with low content of DNA, RNA, protein, and lipids.[17,18] Infants who survived early malnutrition showed improvement with nutritional rehabilitation, and recovery was more complete when environmental stimulation was also provided.[19] Dietary supplementation, either during pregnancy or during infancy, resulted in increased birth weight or infant weight gain, and presumably in better growth of all organs, including the brain.

The concept of "matroenvironment," encompassing all aspects of the physical and biochemical environment of the fetus and infant, as well as the sociocultural factors which include nutrition, economic status, education, and medical care provided by the mother and other caregivers, is being increasingly recognized as critical to the total functioning of the infant.[20] For many years emphasis has been placed on preconceptional and prenatal nutrition as a determinant of fetal growth (Chapter 3). Breast feeding has recently come back into favor with both mothers and physicians as the ideal source of nutrients and immunological substances for the infant (Chapter 4). However, the interrelationship of mother and infant and the psychological advantages of breast feeding were denigrated by many professionals because they could not be quantified. The recent work of Klaus and associates[21] and of many other workers interested in early psychological development of the infant has led to clarification of the mother-infant bonding, which is greater with the close physical contact of the nursing mother and child than when the infant is bottle-fed. These studies have also led to a re-evaluation of the effects of the contact of mother and infant within the first 24 hours and especially within the first hour after delivery.

The feeding situation has been the basis for many studies of the neonate and mother because it is the time of greatest interaction between them during early postnatal life. Neonates vary in their feeding characteristics, as described in Chapter 4. Mothers show equal variation in their response to infants. As a generalization, primiparous mothers are less certain of their own ability, more tense in their handling of the infant, and less sensitive than multiparous mothers to cues of infant behavior. However, mothers and fathers tend to be more attentive to the firstborn, more directive, more interfering, and more inconsistent in handling and training. Primiparous mothers spend more time in feeding their newborn infants, but part of the time is spent in burping and talking. Multiparous mothers tend to be more relaxed, but also more sensitive to infant needs and more effective in feeding.[22]

Through most of history the mother has had immediate and continuous contact with her infant from delivery on. The relatively recent use of hospitals for deliveries led to the routine postpartum separation of mother and infant and to limited contact between them during the hospital stay. This has been considered one of the factors in the decline in the practice of breast feeding, and there is now evidence that the separation and the delay of the first nursing are associated with earlier cessation of breast feeding.[21] There is increasing concern that the behavioral interaction of mother and infant during the first few hours after birth may be essential to the organization and development of the infant. Animal studies have shown that handling and stimulation of the newborn offspring result in better growth and in more desirable behavioral characteristics of the young, and there are indications that the same may be true of humans.

The interplay between prenatal and postnatal nutrition, growth, and behavior is complex. Intrauterine malnutrition may restrict fetal growth. The small newborn is likely to be slower in development, less active, and less demanding of maternal attention than a large, vigorous newborn. This results in less contact and less socialization between mother and infant. The malnourished mother may also lack energy herself. Therefore, the relationship between them is more apathetic. If the undernutrition continues in the infant during early life, growth is slow, activity is restricted due to caloric inadequacy, and the infant is more lethargic. This causes even further aloofness between mother and infant, and the infant does not get the tactile, physical, and emotional stimuli necessary for good development.

In contrast, a large infant is developmentally more advanced, physically more active, more demanding of attention and food, and initiates socialization in the process. In addition, the pride of parents in a healthy, large, active, and responsive infant leads them to initiate contact. Expectations of performance are higher with the large, mature infant, who is likely to be given more stimulation and help in achievement.

The complexity of trying to delineate the part that nutrition plays in behavior and cognitive development is further confused by epidemiological data that malnutrition and smallness of infants occur most often when income and educational level of the parents is low. The environment itself is less stimulating; there is less desire for achievement and usually less time for the parents to spend with the child.

The inability of the infant or child to maintain his own channel of growth when there is no apparent organic dysfunction has been termed failure to thrive. In some cases the slow growth occurs when the parent-child interactions are distorted or there is family disruption even though there is a history of seemingly adequate dietary intake. Many of these children resume normal growth when they are hospitalized or removed from the home environment.[23] Some observers have speculated that failure to thrive may be a less obvious form of child abuse.

The complexity of these studies illustrates the interrelatedness of nutrition with the socio-psychological environment and the multiplicity of factors that influence physical growth, mental achievement, and adaptation to society.

NUTRIENT REQUIREMENTS AND RECOMMENDED DIETARY ALLOWANCES

There is little definitive information about the nutrient requirements of infants. Extensive nitrogen balance studies have been done on very young infants, as well as fecal analyses for fat and calcium on various formulas or other milk feedings, but for practical reasons few other balance studies have been attempted. The estimations of requirements are, for the most part, based on observed intakes of infants with satisfactory growth and on calculations of probable nutrient intakes of breast-fed infants. The higher absorption and utilization of nutrients from breast milk, when compared to cow's milk, has led to some adjustments of requirements when cow's milk is the basis of the infant's diet. The lack of consensus over the years, particularly about protein and iron requirements, attests to the uncertainty about determining real needs.

During the first year the marked changes in growth, body composition, physical activity, and sleep result in greater alterations in the needs of the infant than in any single year later in life. The one-month-old infant spends most of the day sleeping, and physical activity is comparatively low. However, growth is very rapid and body surface area is relatively large. In contrast, the ten-month-old infant is growing less rapidly, spends far more time awake and physically active, and is depositing less body fat. Most of the tables of recommended allowances have, for convenience, divided the first year into six-month segments, despite the fact that within each half-year the changes in physiological need are great.

ENERGY

The caloric requirement during the first year gradually increases, but the caloric requirement per kilogram of body weight is very high during the first few months and then decreases as the year progresses. Table 5.2 shows the ranges of intakes observed in the longitudinal studies of the infants in the Child Research Council.[24] Only formula-fed infants were included in the dietary calculations, so the number of subjects increased during the year. These values represent voluntary intakes of healthy infants, calculated from extensive nutrition histories which included both the types of foods and the quantities consumed during the time intervals noted.

The sex difference in intake, although relatively small at this age, is evident from the first month. The individual variation within each age and sex group is large. For boys the 90th percentile is 300 to 350 kcal/day higher than the 10th percentile at most ages, and the 90th percentile for girls is 200 to 300 kcal/day higher than the 10th percentile. Between 9 and 12 months, the 90th percentile for each sex is more than 400 kcal/day higher than the 10th percentile. All children grew at acceptable rates and were healthy, but showed the usual variations of any group of children in activity and, probably, in food utilization. It is obvious that a single figure for total caloric requirement in any one month during the year cannot apply to all infants, and that using a single value for a six-month span is even more impractical.

Recommended allowances during the first year are usually expressed as kcal/kg to allow for the changing weight with growth. For example, the mean RDA is 115 kcal/kg (0.48 MJ/kg) during the first six months and 105 kcal/kg (0.44MJ/kg) during the last half of the year. However, as shown in Table 5.2, median intake per kilogram rose to a peak of approximately 130 kcal (0.54 MJ) in the second month, decreased to 100 kcal (0.42 MJ) by 6 months, and remained close to that level during the final six months of the year. The wide range of variation is evident also in intake per kilogram, with a difference of 50 kcal/kg between the 10th and 90th percentiles in the last trimester of the year.[24]

It would be helpful to calculate caloric needs of the infant on a factorial basis, but changes in activity and basal heat production, in addition to the alteration in growth rate, result in differences from one month to another.

Table 5.2   Daily Energy Intakes of Healthy Infants

Age Range (months)	Number of Cases	kilocalories/day							kcal/kg/day			kcal/cm/day		
		mean	S.D.	Percentiles					Percentiles			Percentiles		
				10	25	50	75	90	10	50	90	10	50	90
Males														
0–1	33	405	110	275	315	400	480	580	88	115	150	5.7	7.7	10.7
1–2	39	575	86	465	515	565	635	680	108	131	157	8.7	10.3	12.0
2–3	42	630	107	505	545	625	715	795	93	116	139	8.4	10.8	13.3
3–4	44	655	97	550	590	640	715	785	90	103	124	9.1	10.4	12.7
4–5	46	710	124	550	625	675	810	885	88	101	122	8.9	10.5	13.5
5–6	45	760	138	615	670	740	850	960	81	100	122	9.4	11.0	14.3
6–9	46	845	135	710	760	820	895	1020	82	100	123	10.1	11.8	14.5
9–12	49	985	196	795	845	925	1070	1230	81	101	137	10.6	12.5	17.7
Females														
0–1	23	385	86	290	310	375	440	510	84	115	144	5.8	7.7	9.7
1–2	30	530	105	415	445	510	580	700	100	131	160	7.6	9.6	13.0
2–3	32	565	90	455	510	580	645	675	98	115	133	8.0	10.1	11.4
3–4	34	620	84	515	575	615	665	730	97	111	130	8.8	10.5	12.1
4–5	37	665	85	540	615	675	725	775	89	104	120	8.8	10.7	12.5
5–6	38	715	93	610	635	690	770	840	89	104	127	9.6	10.8	12.7
6–9	41	770	122	620	690	760	825	915	76	97	122	9.2	11.1	14.3
9–12	44	885	149	705	755	890	950	1125	80	97	129	9.8	12.0	15.8

Source: Beal, V. A. Nutritional Intake. In: McCammon, R. W. (Ed.) *Human Growth and Development.* Charles C Thomas, Springfield, Ill., 1970.

In infancy, as in any period of growth, measurement of basal metabolic rate includes growth, since they cannot be separately measured except by gross estimation. Figure 5.1 is a schematic representation of the relative changes in caloric needs during the first year. The early months are characterized by a relatively high need of energy for growth, and more than one-third of the calories may be used for this purpose. Fomon[1] has estimated that 7.5 kcal are required to synthesize 1 g of protein and 11.6 kcal to synthesize 1 g of fat. In calculating needs for the synthesis of body tissues, WHO[26] has used a requirement of 5.0 kcal for each gram of body weight gained. As the rate of growth slows, a smaller proportion of energy intake is needed for growth and a larger proportion for maintenance of the greater body mass.

Energy requirements for activity increase during the year as the infant spends more time awake and in motion. Wide individual variations in caloric needs for physical activity are easily evident, even in very young infants. Some are placid and sedentary; others seem to be in perpetual motion when they are awake. Crying increases caloric needs sharply, especially if rapid total body movements accompany the crying. Rose and Mayer,[27] in a study of infants at 4 to 6 months of age, found that the measured amount of activity of the arms and legs was highly correlated with caloric intake above basal metabolic needs.

As observed at all ages, the use of body weight as a basis for assessing requirements or evaluating intake results in distortion in fat and lean individuals. It is a foregone conclusion that most fat people consume fewer calories per kilogram and most thin people consume more calories per kilogram, simply because of the magnitude of the divisor. Adipose tissue has little energy requirement for maintenance in contrast to lean body mass. Ideally, caloric requirement should be based on the weight of lean body tissue, but estimations of lean and adipose tissue in body composition have large margins of error, as shown in Chapter 1. If observed weight of an individual is used in calculating energy allowance, the value will be underestimated for the thin person and overestimated for the obese. It is better to use desirable weight for sex, age, and height.

Height, or length of infants and young children, is related to lean body mass and therefore to the major components of the basal metabolic requirement. Intake per centimeter is, in this respect, a more meaningful concept than intake per kilogram of body weight.

The limited gastric capacity of the low-birth-weight infant presents a problem of feeding because the rapid growth rate necessitates a high intake of nutrients. Therefore, a formula with high caloric density is indicated. The standard premodified formula contains 67 kcal/100 ml (20 kcal/oz), but the low birth weight infant may do better with a formula of 81 to 91 kcal/100 ml (24 to 27 kcal/oz).[28] An evaporated milk formula can be

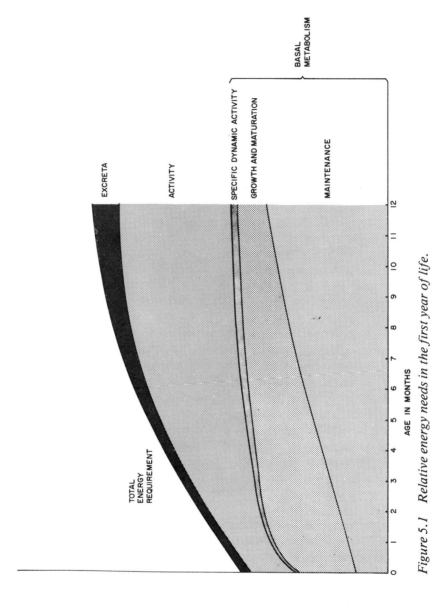

Figure 5.1   Relative energy needs in the first year of life.

228

adapted easily to energy needs, and at the same time provides the higher mineral requirements of the small infant.

CARBOHYDRATE

No requirement or allowance has been set for carbohydrate. In early infancy diets of healthy children may range from 28 to 63 percent of calories from carbohydrate.[24] In human milk, 37 to 38 percent of calories are supplied by lactose, and in cow's milk without added carbohydrate, 27 to 29 percent of calories. Most commercial formulas have carbohydrate added so that 40 to 50 percent of calories are supplied by lactose or other disaccharides.

Lactose has particular significance for the small infant, since it is the only dietary source of galactose. Galactose and glucose are incorporated in cerebrosides and therefore are vital to brain and other central nervous system development. In addition they are components of the glycoprotein of collagen and are needed for the conjugation of bilirubin and also for the detoxication of ammonia, thereby combatting acidosis. In experimental animals lactose has been shown to increase the absorption of calcium, magnesium, and strontium; whether this applies also to human infants is not clear, but it may be a factor in the high rate of absorption of calcium from human milk.

The need for very early feeding of the newborn, especially the infant with low birth weight and the infant born to a diabetic mother, has been stressed in recent pediatric literature. These infants are especially susceptible to hypoglycemia in the neonatal period. The risk is increased when feeding is withheld for 24 hours or more, as has sometimes been customary. A constant supply of monosaccharides to the brain is also essential since this is a period of rapid brain growth.

Malabsorption of specific sugars, including those that result from inborn errors of metabolism, require individual attention.

LIPIDS

Little attempt has been made to determine recommendations for total fat in the diet, but calculations are usually made on the contribution of fat to total calories. Fat contributes 50 to 55 percent of the calories of human milk, and slightly less in whole cow's milk. In commercially premodified infant formulas fat ranges from 35 to 50 percent of calories. The Committee on Nutrition of the American Academy of Pediatrics[10] recommended in 1976 that the Food and Drug Administration standard of a minimum of 15 percent of calories from fat in infant formulas should be raised to a minimum of 30 percent, with a maximum of 54 percent.

As a carrier of fat-soluble vitamins and a source of essential fatty acids, fat is essential in the diet. When milk is the sole source of food for the young infant, skim milk is not advisable. The practice of some mothers and the recommendation by some pediatricians to feed the young infant skim milk should be discouraged. The low calorie content of skim milk requires a high volume intake to satisfy energy needs, a volume that may exceed the capacity of the infant and result in undernutrition. If fat intake is low, carbohydrate and protein intake are high. The added renal solute load, especially if total fluid intake is not increased, may lead to dehydration and hypernatremia. If the carbohydrate is primarily mono- and di-saccharides, the elevated osmolality of the formula may result in diarrhea,[1] further exacerbating dehydration. Under three years of age there is impaired ability to form cholesterol and fatty acids from glucose and pyruvate.[29] The low intake of cholesterol from skim milk may compromise the synthesis of myelin, steroid hormones, and bile acids.

Essential fatty acids contribute five percent of the calories in human milk; linoleic acid is in greatest concentration. It has been recommended[10] that infant formulas should contain a minimum of three percent of calories as linoleate (300 mg/100 kcal). Deficiency symptoms reported in infants have included an eczema-like dermatitis and depressed growth.

An excess of dietary fat may lead to obesity unless calories are limited, thereby lowering protein intake as well. However, bulk of the stool is likely to be increased on a high fat intake, lowering the percentage of fat absorbed. The saponification of fat for excretion may cause excessive calcium excretion. If the diet is high in fat and low in carbohydrate, ketosis may result. Therefore, a diet that contains more fat than that in whole cow's milk should not be recommended.

In recent years interest has been centered on the hypothesis that feeding a high cholesterol intake in early life may make the adult better able to cope with dietary cholesterol. This was postulated from animal studies. However, the fact that human milk, ostensibly ideally designed for the human infant, has a higher concentration of cholesterol than cow's milk presented a dilemma which several workers have tried to explain. Infants fed human or cow's milk tend to have similar levels of plasma cholesterol, higher than those of infants fed commercially premodified formulas in which the butterfat has been replaced by vegetable oils. Recently an increasing number of studies have shown that the effect on plasma cholesterol of early milk feeding has disappeared by one year of age or later.[30] Whether adult levels of plasma cholesterol are affected by infant feeding has not yet been determined.

Type II hyperlipoproteinemia (familial hypercholesterolemia), which is associated with premature vascular disease, can be diagnosed in infancy. A

230   INFANCY (BIRTH TO ONE YEAR)

fall in plasma cholesterol can be accomplished by a diet low in cholesterol and saturated fat and high in polyunsaturated fat.[31] Infants whose family history suggests a risk should have blood determinations done; if the condition is confirmed, dietary intervention with alteration of lipid intake is indicated for these infants.

PROTEIN

The Food and Nutrition Board of the National Research Council[25] has had greater difficulty in determining allowances for protein in infancy than for most other nutrients. Table 5.3 traces the changes in the allowances since 1943. The allowances over this span of time have reflected protein contents of formulas in common use at the time the allowances were established. Since there is no consensus on the amount of protein needed for healthy growth if the infant is not breast fed, there are no clear guidelines for establishing an allowance. Infants in the United States and other technologically advanced countries commonly use cow's milk or some modification of cow's milk for bottle feeding. Cow's milk contains approximately three times the protein concentration of breast milk (Table 4.2). However, the percentage absorption of nitrogen from human milk is higher than from cow's milk. It is generally agreed that infants fed cow's milk need a higher protein intake than infants who are breast fed. However, there is little agreement on how much higher the protein intake should be.

From the 1920s until the 1950s, evaporated milk formulas were the most commonly used substitutes for breast milk. The marketing of powdered commercially premodified formulas with some of the protein of cow's milk removed began in 1915, but it was during the 1950s that liquid concentrates

Table 5.3   N.R.C. Recommended Dietary Allowances for Protein in Infancy

Year of Publication		Protein
1943	Under 1 year	3–4 g/kg
1945, 1948, 1953	Under 1 year	3.5 g/kg
1958	No allowance given for first year	
1963	Under 1 year	2.5 ± 0.5 g/kg
1968	0–2 months	2.2 g/kg
	2–6 months	2.0 g/kg
	6–12 months	1.8 g/kg
1974, 1979	0–6 months	2.2 g/kg
	6–12 months	2.0 g/kg

of prepared formula were marketed and began to be used more commonly because they are easier to mix than the powdered product. By 1962, the prepared liquid concentrates were being used as often as evaporated milk formulas,[1] and at the present time physicians rarely recommend evaporated milk formulas. The easy availability and widespread use of the commercial formulas, which are lower in protein than evaporated milk, influenced decisions about the level of the protein allowances.

From the first edition of the RDAs in 1943 through the fourth edition in 1953, the recommendation was 3.5 or 3 to 4 g protein/kg body weight. Each of the first three editions contained a statement that dietary requirements of protein and calcium were less for infants who were breast fed. Usual intakes of breast-fed infants would be closer to 1.5 to 2.5 g/kg. The fourth edition, in 1953, retained 3.5 g/kg on the table, but the text suggested that if the milk from which the formula is made "has been treated to render it more digestible, the allowance may be in the range of 2 to 3 g/kg." In 1958 a committee established to determine the allowance of protein for infants could reach no decision; some wished to retain the 3.5 g recommendation,[32] and some thought it should be lowered.[33] In the 1958 edition, therefore, there was no allowance on the table for protein in the first year. Instead, there was an extensive discussion in the text of the questions addressed by the committee.

The 1963 edition of the RDAs equivocated by offering an allowance of 2.5 ± 0.5 g/kg. Again the text had a lengthy discussion on the range of protein intakes observed among healthy infants and the reasons for recommending a higher or lower level. By 1968 the problem had been resolved, and the RDA was lowered to 2.2 g/kg in the first 2 months of life, 2.0 g/kg between 2 and 6 months, and 1.8 g/kg in the latter half of the year. This allowance was qualified in the text, however, with a statement that the estimate was based on "protein of optimum quality" and that "if proteins of lower quality than those of human milk are fed, the intake should be proportionately higher." They recognized the fact that proteins of lower quality are progressively introduced into the infant's diet and recommended a quality correction factor of 100/70 to the figures that were based on milk protein. However, the factor was included in calculating the allowance for 1 to 2 years and "this explains the apparent discrepancy between the daily allowance for this age (25 g) compared with the one-half- to one-year group (16 g)." It might be pointed out that the 1.8 g/kg allowance from 6 to 12 months provided a level of 7.2 percent of calories, although the text emphasized that protein requirements could not be met if dietary protein fell significantly below 8 percent of calories.

In the 1974 edition,[25] 2.2 g/kg was the allowance for the first half of the year, and 2.0 g/kg for the second half. However, the caloric allowance was

232

raised from 100 to 108 kcal/kg, so the allowance for protein still supplied only 7.4 percent of calories in the last half of the year. In 1979 the caloric allowances were lowered slightly and the protein allowances were unchanged, so protein supplied 7.6 percent of calories (Appendix 1).

The observed protein intakes of the infants enrolled in the Child Research Council study[24] between 1946 and 1966 ranged between 2.3 and 6.9 g/kg (10th to 90th percentiles), with medians close to 5 g/kg in the first 3 months, dropping to 4.3 g/kg during the final 3 months of the year for both sexes. Most of the infants in this series were fed evaporated milk formulas early in the year and undiluted whole cow's milk by the end of the year. These values were typical of the era before widespread use of premodified formulas. In contrast, the protein intakes were consistently lower in a group of female infants in western Massachusetts, studied by the same dietary methodology in 1976.[34] During the first six months the 10th to 90th percentiles ranged from 1.8 to 5.9 g/kg, with medians rising from 2.5 to 4.1 g/kg. Most of the infants in this later study were fed premodified formulas, and the highest intakes from the third month on were observed for infants who were changed from formula to low-fat or skim milk.

It is clear that healthy breast-fed infants grow well on protein intakes that are lower than those usually recommended for bottle-fed infants. It is equally clear that infants adapt to varying levels of protein intake. During the three decades when evaporated milk formulas were fed to the majority of bottle-fed infants, protein intakes of 4 to 6 g/kg were common, were well tolerated, and produced good growth. As Gordon[32] pointed out, one practice that should be avoided is feeding an excessive amount of undiluted whole cow's milk without added carbohydrate to a very young infant, since the content of electrolytes, especially phosphate, is high; the proper addition of water and carbohydrate to evaporated milk results in a formula with 15 percent of calories from protein, providing 3.5 g/kg/day.

The lower protein intakes of infants on commercially premodified formulas also demonstrate physiological adaptation. Holt[33] stated that there was no evidence of difference in health when protein supplied 10 percent of calories (2 g/kg) or 15 percent. The questions raised by the 1958 committee unable to reach a decision about protein allowances are still unanswered. The answer may lie in the fact that even when the whey:casein ratio of cow's milk is altered to approach that of human milk, there are still marked differences in amino acid content. However, the RDA levels since 1968, in which protein supplies less than 8 percent of calories, need further justification.

Extensive studies of protein requirements of premature infants have shown that the best gains in weight and length occur on intakes of 3 to 5 g/kg/day, with caloric intake 120 kcal/kg/day or higher. Poor growth and increased incidence of edema often result when protein is at a level of 2.25 g/kg or less. Levels above 6 g/kg are probably excessive. The low protein content of premodified formulas may not be adequate for optimal growth of the small and premature infant. Fomon et al.[36] recommended a cow's milk formula with 2.54 g protein/100 kcal for the infant gaining 20 g/day, and higher levels for infants with more rapid gain. Premature infants seem to utilize protein better than full-term infants, perhaps related to accelerated growth during the catch-up phenomenon which is characteristic of these infants.

Balance studies have shown that histidine is essential as a dietary component for infants, in addition to the eight amino acids essential for older children and adults. Although there is evidence that infants can synthesize histidine, the amount may not be adequate to meet their physiological requirements. The premature infant may, in addition, require a dietary source of tyrosine and possibly arginine and taurine.

MINERALS

Appendix I contains the table of Recommended Dietary Allowances. The allowances for magnesium, first included in the 1968 edition, and for zinc, first included in the 1974 edition, may be considered tentative until further studies clarify the requirements and safety margins to be included in the allowances. However, calcium and iron have been included in the allowances since the first edition in 1943, and the changes in their levels have reflected both increased knowledge and differences in interpretation over time.

Calcium

From 1943 to 1948 the RDA for calcium in the first year was 1.0 g/day. In 1953 the allowance was lowered to 0.6 g for 1 to 3 months and 0.8 g for 4 to 9 months, with the 1.0 g level maintained only at 10 to 12 months. In 1958 and 1963 the allowances were 0.6 to 0.8 g (or 0.7 g) for the entire year. The lowering of levels was based on observed intakes of healthy children who were growing well, as explained in the text.

In 1968, with no further explanation in the text, the allowances were lowered further to 0.4 g in the first month, 0.5 g from 1 to 6 months, and 0.6 g from 6 to 12 months. In the 1974 and 1979 editions, the allowance was lowered still further to 0.36 g in the first 6 months and 0.54 g in the last half of the year. Those figures are lower than the calcium recommendation of 0.5 to 0.6 g per day for infants under 1 year of age by FAO/WHO.[35]

Calcium requirements are difficult to establish. The adaptation of individuals to various levels of intake has long been recognized, and no clear-cut deficiency disease has been identified. Calcium balance studies have not been easy to interpret because of the physiological adaptation to experimental levels and the dependence of absorption and retention on previous intakes. Absorption of dietary calcium has been reported to range from 25 percent to nearly 70 percent. The Food and Nutrition Board assumed a retention of two-thirds of the calcium in breast milk; the retention from cow's milk was assumed in 1963 to be 35 to 50 percent, but in 1974 this was revised to 25 to 30 percent at the same time the allowance was lowered.

Adequate retention and utilization of calcium depends on the presence of vitamin D. A number of other factors are believed to affect the absorption and utilization of calcium, including the level of phosphorus. For some time the calcium:phosphorus ratio has been in and out of style as a major concern in nutrition. The ratio in human milk is approximately 2:1, and in cow's milk 1.2:1. It has been recommended by the Academy of Pediatrics[10] that the ratio of calcium to phosphorus should be no less than 1.1:1 and no greater than 2:1.

At birth, the premature infant has a lower body calcium content than the term infant and therefore has higher calcium requirements. Fomon et al.[36] calculated that the premature infant requires 132 mg calcium per 100 kcal of formula for adequate bone mineralization when weight gain is 20 g/day. Proprietary infant formulas contain 60 to 102 mg/100 kcal. An evaporated milk formula more readily meets the higher needs of the premature infant for both protein and calcium.

Iron

At birth the hemoglobin concentration of the healthy full-term infant is usually within the range of 18 to 20 g/100 ml blood. Much of the fetal deposition of iron occurs during the last trimester of gestation (Chapter 3). Fetal erythrocytes have an average life span of 70 days, in contrast to 120 days in adult erythrocytes.[37] Therefore, the destruction of red blood cells in the first two months after birth results in a hemoglobin level of 10 to 12 g/100 ml. The iron that is released from the cells is stored and used in the synthesis of new hemoglobin as blood volume expands with growth of the body mass. It has been estimated that the iron storage provides for needs in the first 4 to 6 months, after which exogenous iron is needed for maintenance of hemoglobin formation. If sufficient iron is not supplied, the risk of iron deficiency followed by anemia increases after 6 months, reaches a peak at 18 months, and then declines.

The premature infant has not accumulated the iron normally deposited in the last few months of gestation, and storage may be depleted some time after 2 months of age. "Although greater need for iron by the low-birthweight infant has been interpreted to indicate that iron-fortified formulas be given as early as possible, recent findings show that iron-supplemented formulas increase the susceptibility of infants to vitamin E deficiency and hemolytic anemia, especially when formulas are high in polyunsaturated fatty acids. These studies leave unresolved the question of whether supplementary iron should be started at two months of age or shortly after birth."[28] They also suggest that formulas with high levels of polyunsaturated fatty acids should contain no more iron than is found in human milk.

Both breast milk and cow's milk contain relatively little iron, ranging from 0.4 to 1.0 mg/liter. However, the absorption of iron from breast milk has been determined as 49 percent,[38] in contrast to 4 to 10 percent from cow's milk. Infants who are exclusively breast fed rarely have iron-deficiency anemia. The higher absorption of iron from breast milk may be related to the lower protein and phosphorus content, or the higher lactose and ascorbic acid content.[39]

The ability of the term infant to absorb dietary iron in the first three months has been questioned, although some data indicate that iron retention may occur and augment iron storage. However, the premature infant and the infant with low birth weight for gestational age or limited hemoglobin mass at birth for some other reason seem to be capable of more efficient absorption at an earlier age; the greater need of these infants for a supply of exogenous iron not later than 2 months seems well established.[28]

The iron requirement in infancy has been the subject of intensive debate and changing concepts during the past 25 years, and there is still no consensus. As shown in Table 5.4, a requirement of 0.8 mg/kg/day had been generally accepted for many years. During the 1950s a few studies and some hypothetical calculations suggested a higher requirement. As a result, the Committee on Nutrition of the American Academy of Pediatrics in 1960[40] recommended an intake of 1.5 mg/kg. A later review, in 1969,[41] lowered the

Table 5.4 Recommended Iron Intakes for Full-term Infants

	NRC Recommended Dietary Allowance	American Academy of Pediatrics
	mg/kg	mg/kg
1943–1958	0.8	
1960		1.5
1963	1.0	
1968	1.67a	
1969		1.0
1974	1.67a	
1976		1.0
1979	1.67a	

aSee text

level to 1.0 mg/kg for full-term infants, while stating that 2.0 mg/kg/day was advisable for low birth weight infants, for infants with low initial hemoglobin values, and for those who have experienced significant blood loss. The level of 1.0 mg/kg was reaffirmed in 1976.[42]

The RDA for iron in infancy rose in 1960 to 1.0 mg/kg. The 1968 and 1974 editions stated in the text that full-term infants could maintain optimal hemoglobin levels on intakes of 1 mg/kg/day starting about the third month of life, but infants with birth weights under 2500 g, or with significant reduction in hemoglobin mass require 2 mg/kg/day. "The recommended allowance is based on an average need of 1.5 mg/kg/day during the first year of life." However, the values in the table (10 mg for a weight of 6 kg, and 15 mg for a weight of 9 kg) are 1.67 mg/kg/day.

The RDA levels of 10 mg in the first 6 months and 15 mg in the last half of the year are higher than the recommendations from other countries. The Canadian recommended allowance[43] in the first year is 7 mg/day. The Caribbean allowance[44] is 5 mg/day. The FAO/WHO[35] recommendation is 5 to 10 mg/day. Fomon[1] estimated that 7 mg/day is the requirement in the first year.

The changing recommendations and the uncertainty of which level to aim for has resulted in a series of problems for physicians and nutritionists giving advice to mothers. The major sources of iron in infant diets are iron-enriched cereals and iron-enriched formulas. The bioavailability of iron added to infant products was subjected to further study, and since 1972 baby cereals have contained iron of small particle size. However, the absorption of iron from both infant cereals and iron-enriched formulas has been reported as 4 percent. In 1971 a statement of the American Academy of Pediatrics[45] recommended that iron-fortified formulas should be fed by bottle or by cup for the first 12 months. This recommendation brought strong objections both from physicians and from nutritionists. Studies had repeatedly shown that the use of proprietary formulas was often discontinued before 6 months of age, and the recommendation would have required "a program of public education to convince American mothers," just as the A.A.P. statement said.

A later statement of the committee (1976) provided a more reasonable approach.[42] It recognized that "most children in middle-income families have little or no anemia" and that the highest incidence is found among infants and children in lower socioeconomic populations and in small preterm infants. Therefore, recommendations for iron supplementation "must be flexible and should emphasize the needs of low-birthweight infants and normal-birthweight infants in lower socioeconomic populations." The use of iron-fortified cereals for both breast- and formula-fed infants was recognized as the most convenient source of iron and should be urged past the age when they are commonly discontinued. For the bottle-fed infant, the iron-fortified formula is also a convenient method of including iron, and may be a more predictable source if the mother feeds solids only sporadically. Because fresh cow's milk may cause gastrointestinal blood loss, heat-treated milk, such as evaporated milk or proprietary formulas, is preferable. The problems of iron drops necessitate caution since medicinal iron was designed for treatment of iron deficiency rather than for prevention, the concentration of iron is high, and it is difficult to give a dose as small as 1 mg/kg; larger doses may cause gastrointestinal side effects, and there is the hazard of accidental poisoning when large quantities are consumed. The committee also recommended screening term infants between 9 and 12 months and low-birthweight infants between 6 and 9 months, using hemoglobin levels < 11 g/100 ml and hematocrit < 33 percent as criteria of anemia.

Zinc

The requirements for zinc have not been established with any certainty, and recommended allowances may be accepted as only tentative. Studies of absorption of zinc from various types of milk fed to rats resulted in higher absorption from human and cow's milk than from a zinc-supplemented proprietary formula.[46] The removal of protein from cow's milk resulted in a proportional decrease in zinc content of the commercial formulas most commonly used[47]; concern about the low level led to fortification of the formulas with zinc. Soy-based formulas gave the lowest absorption rate, due perhaps to the high phytate content. Zinc deficiencies have been related to impaired growth, appetite, and sense of taste.

VITAMINS

The Recommended Dietary Allowances for vitamins are shown in Appendix 1. However, some of the vitamins deserve particular attention, especially for the preterm infant.

Ascorbic Acid

The RDA for the first year of life is 35 mg/day. This is a higher level than the 20 mg/day recommended by the Canadian Dietary Standard,[43] the Caribbean Allowances,[44] and the FAO/WHO.[35]

Breast milk from a well-nourished mother contains approximately 50 mg/liter. Cow's milk formulas are low in ascorbic acid unless they are fortified. Orange juice is an excellent source and is widely used. An ascorbic acid supplement should be given if the infant is not being given breast milk, a fortified formula, or at least two ounces of orange juice a day.

Vitamin D

A daily intake of 100 I.U. (2.5 μg) of vitamin D prevents rickets in the full-term infant, but a level of 300 to 400 I.U. (7.5 to 10 μg) per day provides better growth and calcium absorption. The RDA and other standards recommend 400 I.U. (10 μg)/day. This level may be obtained from one liter of fortified milk or formula. Rickets have rarely been observed in the breast-fed infant, despite a reported low vitamin D content. However, the finding of a water-soluble conjugate of vitamin D with sulfate in breast milk in addition to the previously reported vitamin D in the lipid fraction suggests that the intake of the breast-fed infant may be appreciably higher than has previously been believed. Because of poor fat absorption, the premature infant may need a higher intake of vitamin D, although this may be supplied by the formula if ad libitum feeding results in consumption of more than 120 kcal/kg.[28]

No benefit is derived by the term infant from an intake of more than 400 I.U. Intakes above 2000 I.U./day have sometimes been associated with hypercalcemia and nephrocalcinosis in infants.

Vitamin E

The infant with birth weight below 2000 g may absorb vitamin E poorly and be at risk of hemolytic anemia, especially on a diet high in polyunsaturated fats and iron.[48] A high intake of polyunsaturated fatty acids causes a change in the fat composition of the red blood cell membrane, which becomes more susceptible to damage by lipid peroxidation. Iron is a co-factor which catalyzes the oxidative breakdown of red cell lipids *in vitro,* increasing need for the antioxidant protection of vitamin E. Therefore vitamin E supplementation has been recommended for the low-birth-weight infant.[28] However, this is a self-limited problem that requires treatment only during the first 2 to 3 months.[48]

Vitamin K

A deficiency of vitamin K may occur in the newborn prior to the establishment of intestinal flora. The concentration of prothrombin is low at birth and during the first few weeks, rising gradually through the first year. Hypoprothrombinemic hemmorhagic disease of the newborn is therefore a risk, but the coagulation abnormality can be corrected by the administration of 0.5 to 1.0 mg phytylmenaquinone (vitamin K_1) parenterally. This is recommended as a routine procedure. For the normal infant, a single injection is adequate; for the infant with fat malabsorption or bleeding due to hypoprothrombinemia, continued administration may be necessary.[1]

Breast milk contains less vitamin K than cow's milk, so prophylactic vitamin K is especially important for the breast-fed infant. Formulas with soy or meat base were low in vitamin K, but are now fortified.

WATER

The recommended allowance of water in infancy is 150 ml/100 kcal/day.[25] Water expenditure in the first year has been estimated to range between 400 and 800 ml/day.[1] Intakes of healthy children are generally in excess of the requirement for water. Close to 90 percent of the volumes of milks and formulas of typical dilution is water, supplying more than is needed for growth and to replace water lost through lungs, skin, urine, and feces.

There are, however, situations in which water balance may be of concern. Evaporative losses from skin and lungs account for two-thirds of body water loss in the infant; under normal conditions this may range from 30 to 70 ml/kg/day. High environmental temperatures may increase evaporative losses 50 to 100 percent, so infants should be given extra fluids during hot weather. Evaporative losses may also increase with any illness involving fever. Fecal losses increase with diarrhea. Vomiting, if persistent, may also jeopardize water balance. In each of these situations, care should be taken to replenish water supply. If the infant is taking a highly concentrated formula or skim milk, with high solutes, water balance may become critical. The recommendation of boiled skim milk for diarrhea and other infectious diseases exacerbates the problem of water balance and may lead to further dehydration and hypernatremia.

MEETING NUTRIENT NEEDS

MILKS AND FORMULAS

Breast milk is designed by nature as the food for the infant. It is ideally suited to meet nutritional needs completely for the first 6 months, and provides a high degree of immunity to E. coli and other gastrointestinal organisms. The closeness of breast feeding and its stimulation of all of the neonate's senses provide greater opportunity than bottle feeding for maternal-infant bonding, which is now recognized as critical to the socio-psychological development of the infant. The nutrient content of breast milk and the contrast with cow's milk was presented in Chapter 4 and will not be repeated in detail here.

When a mother is unable or unwilling to breast-feed her infant, a number of substitute milks are available. When bottle-feeding is bacteriologically safe and nutritionally adequate, and the mother warm and responsive to her infant's needs, the formula-fed infant thrives. These conditions can be met in technologically advanced nations where availability of cow's milk, sanitation, education, and health care make the feeding of formulas safe.

In developing countries, even when milks or grain mixtures are available for infant feeding, the safety of their use is usually restricted to high income families. The tragically high rate of infant morbidity and mortality attests to the hazards associated with the decline in breast feeding. The use of polluted water and lack of sterilizing techniques in mixing formulas too often cause gastrointestinal disease with diarrhea. The high cost of the formula in relation to family income leads to over-dilution, resulting in undernutrition. The incidence of protein-energy malnutrition is high. The synergism of malnutrition and infection creates a cycle in which the malnourished infant has lowered resistance to disease, the mother treats diarrhea by withholding or further diluting the formula, and the malnutrition becomes acute. The increasing incidence of marasmus in the first year of life is closely associated with the decline in breast feeding. While the causative factors in this decline are complex, a reversal of the trend is vital to the health and lives of countless infants.

The history of infant feeding has been recounted in a number of reports, and is closely related to the social, cultural, and economic characteristics of a population. Milk of various animals has been used since earliest antiquity, but usually only when it became necessary to wean an infant from breast milk before the end of the first year. During the sixteenth century nursing by the mother herself declined in Europe, and the use of animal's milk rose, but the employment of wet nurses was more common (Figure 5.2). Desir-

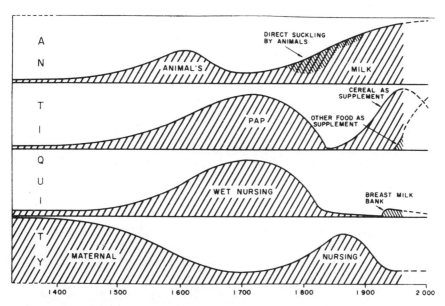

Figure 5.2 Schematic outline of principal means of infant nutrition. (Source: Levin, S. S. A Philosophy of Infant Feeding. Charles C Thomas, Springfield, Ill., 1963.)

able qualities in a wet nurse included youth, health, sobriety, a moral and chaste outlook, a placid and pleasant disposition, and large breasts with a good supply of milk. Wet nursing was so widespread and so profitable that young girls contrived to have illegitimate babies—which were conveniently "overlaid"—in order that they might obtain employment as wet nurses. Wet nursing fell into disrepute early in the nineteenth century, and the use of animal milks increased, sometimes by direct suckling, and nursing by the mother herself also became more customary.[49]

The feeding of semisolid foods to infants is often thought to be a phenomenon of the present era. However, "pap" was often given during the period when wet nursing was common. This usually consisted of some variety of bread, flour, or grains mixed with fluids such as water, milk, beer, wine, or broth. Food prechewed by an adult has been used for feeding infants and young children in many societies.

Before the manufacture of glass bottles and rubber nipples, a variety of utensils have been adapted for feeding the infant. Leather bags, clay pottery, animal horns, and containers of wood, pewter, or porcelain have been used as containers for milk. Although glass had intermittently been used earlier, it did not become popular until after 1800. Since glass can be sterilized, this solved one problem of contamination. Recently disposable plastic containers have partially replaced glass bottles. Means of getting milk from the container into the infant have also varied. Linen or other cloth, glove fingers, sponges, leather, parchment, and even prepared teats of heifers have been used. The first rubber nipple was patented in 1845, providing a sterilizable material that could be firmly attached to the top of the bottle. By 1900, glass bottles, rubber nipples, chlorination of water, and pasteurization of milk combined to make substitutes for breast feeding compatible with bacteriological safety.[1,49]

The gradual recognition of the chemical differences between human and cow's milk has led to a series of adaptations of cow's milk. The word "formula" is indicative of the complexity of many of the mixtures, including those in common use today. At first the complexity was handled by the physician and the mother; now it is handled by the commercial producers before the products are marketed. Some of the formula mixtures were so intricate that the kitchen must have resembled a laboratory. Each new development in the adaptation of cow's milk was hailed as a major advance, but history shows that styles in infant formulas have been nearly as changeable as styles in clothing. In documenting the "built-in additives and subtractives" to cow's milk in the past century, Levin[49] pointed out that the number of permutations and combinations is large and that "the final conclusions to the art and science of infant feeding have not, as yet, been recorded."

242

One of the first sources of concern was the high protein content of cow's milk. Acidification of human milk in the stomach produces small, flocculent curds which are readily digestible. Cow's milk, with its higher casein content, produces large rubbery curds containing calcium. The size and high tension of the curds limits accessibility to digestive enzymes, lowering absorption. Curd tension can be lowered by heat treatment, homogenization, alteration of the casein:lactalbumin ratio, or addition of lactic acid or enzymes.

Dilution with water to lower the protein concentration resulted in a decrease of caloric value, so carbohydrate was added. In many early formulas cereal was the carbohydrate recommended, but the low level of pancreatic α-amylase in the small intestine of the very young infant may limit starch digestion. A change was made to disaccharides and hydrolysates, including dextrin, maltose, and sucrose. Corn syrup or sucrose is most commonly used now in formulas made at home. Lactose, alone or in combination with other sugars, is used in most commercially produced formulas.

The fat of formulas has been equally subject to change. Some early recommendations included addition of cream, increasing the lipid content. Concern about the melting point and iodine number of butterfat led to its replacement by a mixture of beef fat and vegetable oils in the first commercially premodified formula, marketed in 1915. More recent commercial formulas have replaced butterfat with various combinations of oils, including corn, coconut, soy, and sometimes safflower. Recent concerns about obesity and heart disease in the population have led to use of low-fat or skim milk, recommended by some physicians or voluntarily selected by mothers.

Micronutrient alterations have been both "additives" and "subtractives." Some changes have been the result of increased knowledge about food components and nutritional requirements. However, some have been necessitated by deficiencies or imbalances of nutrients created by progressively more intensive manipulation and processing of cow's milk. Lowering the protein, calcium, and phosphorus concentrations also lowered the levels of other minerals, including zinc.[47] Increase in the polyunsaturated:saturated fat ratio increases the requirement of vitamin E. A change in the heat treatment of one commercial formula led to destruction of pyridoxine and symptoms of deficiencies in infants.[50] As a result, the final product in the can purchased by the mother is far removed from the cow's milk on which it is based.

The varieties of milks and formulas available for infant feeding in the United States are diverse. Although the common practice at the present time is the recommendation of commercially premodified formulas for infants who are not breast fed, many mothers discontinue their use and substitute other types of milk, often without professional guidance. Reasons for the change may be the expense of commercial preparations, adverse reactions of the infant, or greater convenience of giving the baby whatever milk is used in the home. Since there are advantages and disadvantages to each type of milk, the physician, nutritionist, or other professional who has contact with the mother should be aware of them.

Whole Cow's Milk

During the first 4 to 6 weeks, when some infants may have difficulty in concentrating urine, the high nitrogen and mineral content of whole milk may provide too great a solute load. Dilution with water and addition of carbohydrate decreases the concentration of nitrogen and electrolytes, but there are other disadvantages to whole milk. The hard curd formation on acidification in the stomach may result in digestive upsets and poor absorption of nutrients. Enteric blood loss, with occult blood in the stool and increased incidence of anemia, has been reported in infants who were fed whole milk. Heat treatment eliminates the hazard, and this phenomenon has not been observed in the same infants when fed evaporated milk or premodified formula.[51] Fomon[1] has reported that infants who are given cow's milk as the sole source of calories have large fecal loss of fat, which may amount to 15 percent of caloric intake. When fat is decreased from 50 percent of calories, as observed with whole milk, to 35 percent by the addition of carbohydrate, fecal loss of calories is not excessive. He recommended that the transfer to whole milk should be delayed until the infant is consuming two jars of infant foods or its equivalent.

Skim Milk

Despite the current trend toward limitation of fat, and especially butterfat, for the population in general, skim milk is not an appropriate food for the infant. The low fat content results in a greater concentration of carbohydrate and protein. Due to its low satiety value and low caloric content, the infant must either take frequent feedings or consume a larger volume at each feeding in order to meet energy requirements, thereby increasing the total intake of protein and minerals. Skim milk does not provide essential fatty acids and places greater stress on the absorption of fat-soluble vitamins. Fat should constitute a minimum of 30 to 35 percent of total calories. It is recommended that milk or formula should contain a minimum of 3.3 g fat/100 kcal and 300 mg linoleic acid/100 kcal.[10]

A number of reports from Great Britain have indicated that there is great variation in the measurement of powdered formula when mothers reconstitute it at home, with the hazard of high osmolality. Since powdered commercial formulas are rarely used in the United States, powdered skim milk is one of the few feedings in which an excessive concentration may be used.

The high solute concentration of skim milk may lead to dehydration and hypernatremia; the problem would be intensified by the addition of extra skim milk powder.

Condensed Milk

Although rarely used at the present time, sweetened condensed milk had a brief period of popularity in infant feeding. The practice led to obese infants with a high incidence of diarrhea and was soon discontinued. Occasionally mothers, particularly those who are poorly educated, use condensed milk instead of evaporated milk, and the health professional working with mothers should be aware of this possibility. Condensed milk has seven times the carbohydrate content of evaporated milk, with other nutrients thereby lowered. Undiluted sweetened condensed milk contains 21 g carbohydrate and 120 kcal/oz. It is not suitable for infant feeding.

Commercially Premodified Milk-based Formulas

The commercial formulas were first marketed as a powdered concentrate, which was difficult to dissolve in water to a smooth consistency. When liquid concentrates were made available around 1950 and vigorously promoted, sales increased. By 1965, 90 percent of formulas recommended at hospital discharge were commercially premodified, replacing evaporated milk formulas.[1] In the late 1960s the ready-to-feed formulas became available, with water already added before canning so that no further dilution was necessary. By 1973, one-third of the premodified formulas sold were ready-to-feed.[1] The cost of premodified formulas is higher than for evaporated milk formulas, and the ready-to-feed mixtures cost two to three times as much as evaporated milk in most retail markets.

Table 5.5 shows the content of the formulas in common use in the United States, in contrast to human milk, whole cow's milk, and evaporated milk formulas. Changes are intermittently made in the content of these formulas, necessitating up-dating of information when precise values are required. Although the contents and methods of preparation vary from one to another, some basic concepts are common to all.

The protein concentration of cow's milk is decreased about 50 percent so that it more nearly resembles the concentration of human milk, although there are still large differences in the amino acid ratios of the two milks. Calcium and phosphorus also are lowered approximately 50 percent, as are other minerals. The lower value of zinc led to questions about its adequacy,[47] and fortification with zinc followed.

Butterfat has been replaced by vegetable oils with an increase in the unsaturated fatty acids to the level of breast milk. Carbohydrate is added; at

Table 5.5 *Average Nutrient Content of Milks and Infant Formulas (per 100 ml)*

| | R.D.A. 0-6 mos. | Mature Human Milk | Premodified Formulas | | | Evap. Milk, 13 oz. Water, 18 oz. Corn Syrup, 2 Tbsp. | Evap. Milk, 13 oz. Water, 13 oz. | Whole Cow's Milk 3.5% Fat |
			Enfamil	Similac	SMA			
Energy, kcal	115/kg	75	67	68	67	72	73	67
Protein, g	2.2/kg	1.1	1.5	1.55	1.5	3.0	3.7	3.6
Fat, total, g		3.8–4.5	3.7	3.6	3.6	3.4	4.2	3.6
Saturated, g		1.7–2.2	1.2	1.4	1.6	2.1	2.6	2.2
Unsaturated, g		2.3–2.6	2.5	2.2	2.0	1.3	1.6	1.3
Type of fat		Human	Soy, coco-nut	Coconut, soy	Oleo, coco-nut, soy, safflower	Cow	Cow	Cow
Cholesterol, mg		14	1.4	1.6	3.3	9	11	11
Carbohydrate, g		7.0	7.0	7.2	7.2	7.4	5.2	5.0
Type of carbohydrate		Lactose	Lactose	Lactose	Lactose	Lactose, sucrose	Lactose	Lactose
Ash, g		0.2	0.4	0.4	0.3	0.6	0.7	0.7
Calcium, mg	360	34	55	51	44a	110	134	122
Phosphorus, mg	240	14	46	39	33	89	109	96
Iron, mg	10	0.05	0.15a (1.27)b	Trace (1.2)b	(1.3)b	0.14	0.06	0.04

Continued

Iodine, μg	40	3–6	46	10[a]	7	4	5	5.2
Copper, μg	50	50	63[a]	41[a]	48[a]	24	30	30
Magnesium, mg		3.5–4.0	4.7	4.1	5.3	10	12	12
Zinc, mg	3	0.1–0.5	0.42[a]	0.50[a]	0.37[a]	0.3	0.4	0.4
Sodium, mg		16–19	28	22	15	53	63	52
Potassium, mg		50–55	70[a]	78[a]	56[a]	131	162	148
Vitamin A activity, I.U.	1400	190	251[a]	250[a]	264[a]	139	171	149
Vitamin D, I.U.	400	2	42[a]	40[a]	42[a]	34[a]	42[a]	42[a]
Vitamin E, mg	3	0.2	1.3[a]	1.5[a]	1.0[a]	0.2	0.2	0.2
Vitamin K, μg		1.5	7[a]	9[a]	6[a]	5	6	6
Ascorbic acid, mg	35	4–5	5.5[a]	5.5[a]	5.8[a]	0.5	0.6	1.1
Thiamin, μg	300	16	53[a]	65[a]	71[a]	17	21	31
Riboflavin, μg	400	36	63[a]	100[a]	106[a]	148	182	175
Niacin equiv., mg	6	0.1–0.2	0.8[a]	0.7[a]	1.0[a]	0.1	0.1	0.1
Pyridoxine, μg	300	10–18	42[a]	40[a]	42[a]	33	40	60
Pantothenic acid, mg		0.18–0.25	0.32[a]	0.30[a]	0.21[a]	0.3	0.3	0.34
Vitamin B$_{12}$, μg	0.5	0.03	0.21[a]	0.15[a]	0.11[a]	0.3	0.4	0.4
Folacin, μg	30	5.2	10.6[a]	5.0[a]	5.3[a]	4	5	4–5.5

[a] Including nutrients added to the product in processing.
[b] Sold as "Iron Fortified Formula."

247

first a variety of disaccharides were used, but more recently lactose has been the carbohydrate of choice.

Fortification with vitamins and minerals has varied over the years. The addition of vitamin D was made early in the history of these products. A number of cases of megaloblastic anemia led to the incorporation of ascorbic acid, and the formulas were then advertised as complete feeding for the infant. In the early 1950s, a new method of heat treatment of one formula led to destruction of pyridoxine, causing convulsive seizures in many infants,[50] so pyridoxine is now routinely added. Concern about the increased need for vitamin E on high intakes of polyunsaturated fats led to the addition of vitamin E.

Since cow's milk is a poor source of iron, fortification of formulas with iron was begun, and now each brand may be purchased with or without added iron; approximately one:third of the formulas sold contain added iron. A statement of the Committee on Nutrition of the Academy of Pediatrics in 1971[45] that more than 70 percent of the proprietary formulas prescribed by physicians did not contain added iron, and strongly recommending that iron-supplemented formulas should be used routinely was followed by a series of letters to the editor of *Pediatrics* in the next several months from physicians in practice who expressed contrary opinions. A report of the committee in 1976[42] recognized the fact that formula is discontinued for most infants by six months of age, prior to the period of greatest risk of iron deficiency, and suggested flexible recommendations for iron supplementation, with special attention to those at greatest risk, infants in low socioeconomic families and those with low birth weight.

The small infant who has no other source of nutrients than formula is uniquely vulnerable to the adequacy of that single food. Changes in formulation and processing have not always been adequately tested, as shown by the development of pyridoxine deficiency. Many of the additions have been the result of the realization that the level or balance of nutrients was less than optimal. Jelliffe and Jelliffe,[52] strong advocates of breast feeding, stated that the formulas "are constantly changing mixtures based on dried skim milk. Their record shows a stumbling from one formula-derived metabolic upset to another (e.g., pyridoxine, vitamin E, linoleic acid, sodium overload, etc.). Each adaptation leads to further disbalance and uncertainty. It may be confidently predicted that problems with deficiencies of cystine, taurine, arachidonic acid, or other nutrients, are likely to be forthcoming, as are unsuspected ill-effects from compounds currently used in processing, such as carrageenan."

As knowledge of the nutritional requirements of infants becomes more detailed, changes in the content of formulas may be expected. The Committee on Nutrition of the Academy of Pediatrics[10] in 1976 recommended revision of the 1971 regulations of the Food and Drug Administration on the nutrient levels of infant formulas. These revisions are shown in Table 5.6, based on the minimum and maximum levels per 100 kcal of the formulas.

At the present time, commercially premodified formulas are most often prescribed for infants on hospital discharge. However, many mothers, especially in low income families, discontinue their use and substitute less expensive milks, often without professional advice.[53,54] Some of these milks may be ill-suited to the young infant, and may be given until the first visit to a physician or clinic, often at 4 to 6 weeks. One of the major gaps in the nutritional supervision of infants is the lack of advice to mothers who do not intend or cannot afford to continue feeding commercial formulas. Since evaporated milk formulas are less expensive, they are commonly used, and are certainly preferable to skim or low-fat milk, which is often the alternative. Unfortunately, the teaching in pediatric courses in medical schools rarely covers instructions for making formulas at home, which used to be a routine part of those courses. However, many mothers are averse to use of premodified formulas, and they need advice in preparing a substitute formula.

Evaporated Milk Formulas

For 3 to 4 decades following its introduction in the 1920s, evaporated milk was the basis for most infant formulas. In the process of evaporation, the heat treatment results in an increase in digestibility and a decrease in curd tension and allergenicity. Approximately 50 percent of the water of whole cow's milk is removed. Therefore dilution of 1 part of evaporated milk with 1 part of water provides essentially the same food value as whole milk. It is a standardized, pooled product, and there is little or no difference between brands.

Adaptation of evaporated milk for infant feeding includes dilution with water and addition of carbohydrate. During the first month the formula may be made with 1 ounce of evaporated milk and 2 ounces of water per pound of body weight, with 2 to 3 tablespoons of corn syrup or sucrose added to the total day's mixture. For example, the day's formula for an 8-pound infant would be 8 ounces of evaporated milk, 16 ounces of water, and 2 to 3 tablespoons of carbohydrate. The water may be gradually decreased after the first month. A common intermediate mixture is 13 ounces (one can) of evaporated milk, 19 ounces of water, and 2 tablespoons of carbohydrate; this is simple for the mother, who can pour one can of evaporated milk into a quart container and then fill it with water. By six months the infant can be taking equal parts of evaporated milk and water.

An advantage of mixing this formula at home is that the sugar can be decreased as semisolid foods are added to the diet. In contrast, when premodified formulas are fed in addition to semisolid foods, the total carbohydrate

Table 5.6   *Nutrient Levels of Infant Formulas (per 100 kcal)*

Nutrient	FDA 1971 Regulations: Minimum	CON 1976 Recommendations: Minimum	Maximum
Protein (gm)	1.8	1.8	4.5
Fat			
(gm)	1.7	3.3	6.0
(% cal)	15.0	30.0	54.0
Essential fatty acids (linoleate)			
(% cal)	2.0	3.0	—
(mg)	222.0	300.0	—
Vitamins			
A (IU)	250.0	250.0 (75µg)[a]	750.0 (225µg)[a]
D (IU)	40.0	40.0	100.0
K (µg)	—	4.0	—
E (IU)	0.3	0.3 (with 0.7 IU/gm linoleic acid)	—
C (ascorbic acid) (mg)	7.8	8.0	—
B$_1$ (thiamine) (µg)	25.0	40.0	—
B$_2$ (riboflavin) (µg)	60.0	60.0	—
B$_6$ (pyridoxine) (µg)	35.0	35.0 (with 15µg/gm of protein in formula)	—
B$_{12}$ (µg)	0.15	0.15	—

Continued

250

Niacin		
(μg)	—	—
(μg equiv)	800.0	250.0
Folic acid (μg)	4.0	4.0
Pantothenic acid (μg)	300.0	300.0
Biotin (μg)	—	1.5
Choline (mg)	—	7.0
Inositol (mg)	—	4.0
Minerals		
Calcium (mg)	50.0[b]	50.0[b]
Phosphorus (mg)	25.0[b]	25.0[b]
Magnesium (mg)	6.0	6.0
Iron (mg)	1.0	0.15
Iodine (μg)	5.0	5.0
Zinc (mg)	—	0.5
Copper (μg)	60.0	60.0
Manganese (μg)	—	5.0
Sodium (mg)	20.0 (6 mEq)[c]	60.0 (17 mEq)[c]
Potassium (mg)	80.0 (14 mEq)[c]	200.0 (34 mEq)[c]
Chloride (mg)	55.0 (11 mEq)[c]	150.0 (29 mEq)[c]

[a]Retinol equivalents.
[b]Calcium to phosphorus ratio must be no less than 1.1 nor more than 2.0
[c]Milliequivalent for 670 kcal/liter of formula

Source: American Academy of Pediatrics Committee on Nutrition. Commentary on breast-feeding and infant formulas, including proposed standards for formulas. *Pediat. 57:278–285,* 1976.

251

in the diet may be high. Recent concern about "nursing bottle caries" as a result of prolonged bottle feeding, particularly when the bottle is propped or taken to bed at night or nap times, suggests that sugar should not be included in the formula once teeth have erupted.[55]

Both evaporated milk and premodified formula are fortified with vitamin D. Evaporated milk contains little or no ascorbic acid, however, so either orange juice or a vitamin C supplement should be given to the infant.

Nonmilk Formulas

For the infant who is allergic to or intolerant of cow's milk, formulas are available with a basis of goat's milk, soybean milk, or meat. These commercial formulas have been fortified so that they have nutrient content similar to premodified formulas. There are, however, basic differences in amino acid composition and in other respects. The least allergenic milk for the infant is breast milk, and breast feeding should be stongly urged for the infant whose family history includes allergy.

INTRODUCTION OF SEMISOLID FOODS

The offering of food other than milk, formula, or juice to the infant has been influenced more by society and culture than by physiological and developmental needs. As shown in Figure 5.2, pap was commonly fed during the seventeenth and eighteenth centuries. This practice then lost favor and infants were seldom given foods other than fluids until after the age of one year, and in some cultures not until after three years. In the present century it has become customary to offer semisolids at progressively early ages. This may be related to the decline of breast feeding, and one may speculate about the subtle differences in the pyschological approach to feeding between the nursing mother and the mother who feeds formula by bottle. Mothers of the present generation who breast feed tend to start solid feeding later than has been the practice in recent years. Whatever the reasons, the trend during the twentieth century has been toward earlier introduction of semisolids, although recently there are indications that even with bottle-feeding mothers there seems to be a growing tendency to delay solids.

Prior to 1920, mashed potato or cooked cereal was sometimes offered after 9 months, and mashed table foods after 12 months. Commercially prepared infant cereals, which needed only the addition of milk or formula, and puréed foods, which might be fed at room temperature or warmed, became available in the 1920s. Until 1950 pediatric textbooks were recommending that solids should be started at 6 months. However, in actual practice, babies were being given solids much earlier. A survey[56] of 2,000 pediatricians in 1954 showed that 66 percent of infants under the care of physicians

252

in private practice were receiving solids by 2 months, and 99 percent by 3 months. Younger pediatricians tended to recommend starting solids earlier than those who had been in practice longer, citing pressure of mothers as a major influence. In a companion survey of "a group of pediatricians somewhat protected from the pressures of practice and permitted the luxury of scholarly objectivity" who were asked to comment on the results of the survey, typical responses included the following: "I know of no important nutritional benefits to be gained by adding solids under the age of 3 to 4 months"; "The fact that most infants accept and tolerate such food well is a credit to both the human structure and the manufacturer's ability, but it does not prove that the practice is necessarily good"; "This is not at all necessary for the proper nutrition of the infant—it simply happens to be the fashion"; "It is the result of empiricism and competition, not of sound nutritional principles." Similar comments may be found even to the present time by those who respect the physiological and developmental characteristics of young infants.

Reports were published in the 1940s and 1950s of feeding cereal to infants as young as 2 to 3 days of age, with a variety of other foods following soon after. While the eagerness of mothers who were competitive and expressed pride in the early ability of their infants to take solids was one factor in the initiation of the trend, it became a common pediatric recommendation to introduce solids no later than one month of age. The refusal of some infants to accept solids at such a young age has been documented,[57] and several gadgets appeared on the market to help mothers—a plunger with a nipple on the end, a squeezable polyethylene container with a tube or spoon to be put directly into the infant's mouth, and a nipple with an attached trough through which the mother could force food into the infant's mouth. Many conscientious mothers, trying to follow the physicians' recommendations, simply put the solids into a bottle with large holes in the nipple and added enough water so that the infant could suck the food. These devices are all aimed at by-passing the extrusive reflex, and they represented an era of incorrect but well-intentioned infant feeding.

Physiologically, the full-term infant's nutritional needs can be met by breast milk or a proper formula, with attention to ascorbic acid and vitamin D intake, until close to 6 months. Thereafter sources of iron should be added to the diet because of depleted stores. Pancreatic amylase production may be inadequate for proper digestion of starch until 4 to 5 months. Early feeding of solids may result in allergy because of absorption of unaltered protein by an immature gastrointestinal wall.

Developmentally, the disappearance of the primitive extrusion reflex is an essential preliminary to the willing acceptance of spoon feeding. Neuromuscular control of the head and the ability to sit in an upright position are usually accomplished at 3 to 4 months. Therefore, the ability of the infant seems timed in several ways to reach a stage of maturity to handle spoon feeding some time after 4 months.

One of the reasons often cited for the early introduction of solids was to encourage the infant to sleep through the night. However, several studies have shown that feeding solids has no effect. In two studies,[58,59] the average age of omitting one night feeding, providing an 8-hour span without food, was between 4 and 6 weeks, and in one study[60] it was 9 weeks. This seems to be a developmental stage with wide individual variation unrelated to feeding of solids. In one study,[58] there seemed to be a relationship with birth weight, since smaller infants continued night feedings somewhat longer than larger infants.

The negative psychological aspects of early solid feeding are more difficult to document or assess. Age cannot be used as a sole criterion for acceptance, since some infants accept and are even eager for spoon feeding at an early age. However, if the infant resists, as many do before 3 months,[57] feeding time may become unpleasant if the mother persists and a battle of wills results. This places stress on the mother-child relationship. Early feeding experiences influence the development of responses to appetite cues. The baby who is forced to take a food he does not want may suffer some distortion of the hunger-satiety mechanism, just like the infant who is urged to take more formula than he wants.

There is little evidence of harm to infants as a result of the early introduction of semisolid foods, but delaying spoon feeding until 4 to 6 months seems more consistent with many aspects of development.

The earliest nutritional need, aside from milk, ascorbic acid, and vitamin D, is for iron. Therefore, iron-fortified cereals are the logical first foods. Infant cereals are bland foods which can be diluted with milk or formula to varying degrees of thickness, and most infants accept them well. The replacement of poorly absorbed forms of iron by small particle electrolytic iron in the enrichment of infant cereals has ensured better utilization. Infant cereals should be continued throughout the first year as a source of iron. Meat is also an excellent source of iron; heme iron is well absorbed and increases the absorption of nonheme iron as well. However, many physicians prefer to delay the introduction of meat into the diet of the infant fed cow's milk because of its high protein content. Since the breast-fed infant needs an additional source of protein for optimal growth after 6 months, meat is an excellent food to supplement nursing, in addition to cereal.

The order of other foods is a matter of choice. Fruit may be offered as the second semisolid food in the diet, but some physicians prefer to offer vegetables before fruit because they are less sweet. Meat and egg yolks are usually offered after fruits and vegetables. The vegetable-meat mixtures, both soups and "dinners," contain varying amounts of meat; while they are convenient and offer variety, feeding plain strained or junior meats in addition to vegetables enables the mother to monitor meat intake more readily.

Only one new food should be offered at a time, and the amount should be not more than one teaspoon at first. This allows easier identification of any food that might cause an allergic reaction or digestive upset. After the first few days of offering a limited amount of a new food, the amount per serving can be governed by the infant's appetite. Rigid rules about size of servings should be avoided, allowing individual variation in intake. The infant should not be forced to take more than desired. The sensitive mother soon learns to distinguish between satiety and playfulness when the child stops eating. Respect for appetite in the healthy infant as an indicator of his caloric needs provides a better basis for prevention of obesity than urging extra food.

The content of commercially prepared infant foods has changed in response to increased knowledge of benefits and risks.[61] As previously noted, the type of iron now used for fortification has a higher level of bioavailability. Addition of sucrose has been sharply limited or discontinued. Salt addition has been curtailed. The addition of salt had been largely to suit the mothers' tastes; mothers who found some infant foods too bland tended to buy those that were saltier, but studies of infants showed no difference in acceptance whether foods were salted or not.[62] The possibility that a high salt intake during infancy might predispose to hypertension in later life or to the cultivation of a taste for well-salted foods led to a recommendation[63] that salt should be restricted to 0.25 percent in infant foods, and some manufacturers have eliminated salt completely from their products. As a result, the infant at the end of the first year obtains more salt from home-prepared foods than he obtained from infant foods at earlier ages. Monosodium glutamate, sodium nitrate, sodium nitrite, and some modified food starches have also been eliminated from products for infants.[61]

SUPPLEMENTARY VITAMINS AND MINERALS

It is difficult to make a standard rule for all infants as to whether or not they should be given separate supplements of vitamins and/or minerals. Factors that influence the decision include birth weight and degree of maturity; type of milk or formula; use of iron-fortified cereal or formula; presence of fluorine in water and amount consumed by the infant plain or in formula; exposure to sunshine; and inclusion of juices containing ascorbic acid. If the recommended allowances are met by the foods consumed, additional supplements are unnecessary.

FEEDING PROGRESS DURING THE YEAR

The number of feedings in a 24-hour period during infancy is influenced by age, individual needs, and whether or not a time schedule of feedings is imposed. The rigidity of time scheduling, which was typical a few decades ago, has been relaxed, and many infants now are fed on demand. Breast-fed infants may prefer to be fed every 2 to 3 hours during the neonatal period, while formula-fed infants are more likely to be satisfied with an interval of 3 to 4 hours between feedings. By the end of the first month infants who are fed on demand have usually established a fairly predictable time pattern.

Figure 5.3 shows the distribution of the number of feedings per day at each age in the first two years of children enrolled in the longitudinal studies of the Child Research Council. The arbitrary definition of "feedings" included offerings of breast or formula and solids considered by the mothers to constitute a meal; excluded were snacks and fluids by cup which mothers viewed as between-meal foods. During the first month, one-third of the in-

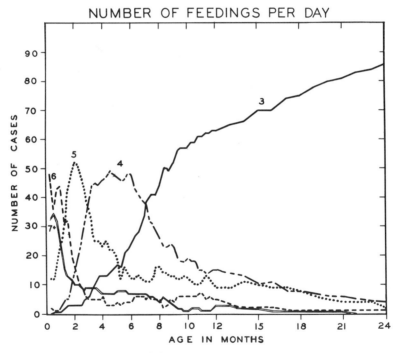

Figure 5.3 Number of feedings per 24 hours, Child Research Council series.

INFANCY (BIRTH TO ONE YEAR)

fants took 7 or more feedings a day, half took 6 feedings, and the remainder were satisfied with fewer. By two months the majority took 5 feedings in a 24-hour period. From the fourth to the seventh month, 4 feedings were most common, and thereafter the number of infants on 3 feedings a day increased. However, some children continued to take 4 or more feedings through the second year. The extra feeding was usually a bottle or nursing at naptime or bedtime.

The semisolid foods offered to the infant may be either home-prepared or commercially puréed. If home-prepared, no salt or other spices should be added, and care taken to avoid bacterial contamination, especially if the foods are to be refrigerated or frozen for later feeding. Many fresh ripe fruits and cooked vegetables may be mashed or cut finely. Cooked egg yolks may be given, but egg white is a potential allergen and is best avoided during the early months of life. Without a blender, meat is difficult to make fine enough for the infant to manage easily, and many mothers who prepare other foods find it simpler to purchase strained meats. Sweetened desserts should be used only in moderation for variety.

Foods to be chewed should be offered when the infant begins to make chewing motions, usually around 6 months. Care must be taken that such foods can be easily dissolved or softened in the mouth to avoid choking. The transition from strained to junior or table foods may be accomplished gradually in the last half of the first year or early in the second year. The texture can be made progressively more coarse by chopping instead of mashing. During the last month or two of the year, the infant often prefers foods that can be picked up and eaten by hand.

The value of milk for growing children has been stressed repeatedly, but milk intake should not exceed 32 ounces daily except under unusual circumstances. Some mothers, aware of the nutritive values of milk or lacking the patience required when a baby is learning to manage solid foods, may find it easier to give a bottle in preference to other foods. Excessive milk intake and inadequate intake of solid foods increases the hazard of iron-deficiency anemia. In addition, the developmental value of providing foods for chewing when the infant is at the proper stage of readiness must be considered. As Illingworth and Lister[8] stated, after the sensitive period has passed, it is more difficult to learn a particular pattern of behavior. If a baby is not given solid foods shortly after he has learned to chew, there may well be considerable difficulty in getting him to take solids later. During the last half of the first year a varied diet should be offered in addition to milk, with daily servings of iron-fortified cereal, meat, egg yolk, citrus and other fruits, vegetables, potato, and possibly some desserts high in nutritive value. Toasted bread is less likely to cause choking than soft bread. Toward the

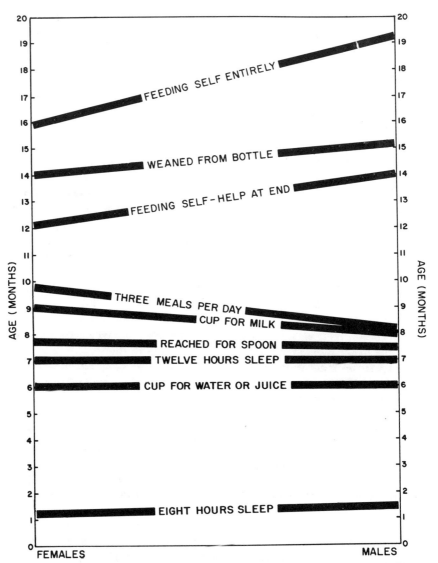

Figure 5.4   Median ages of feeding landmarks of boys and girls, Child Research Council series.

last few months of the year, most infants voluntarily decrease milk intake; this will be discussed in more detail in Chapter 6.

Figure 5.4 shows the stages of progress toward independent feeding of children in the Child Research Council series. The mothers in this series used the cup for water or juice at an average of six months, and for milk between eight and nine months. Weaning from the bottle was accomplished at an average of 14 to 15 months. When mothers breast fed past 7 to 8 months, transition was often directly to the cup; earlier weaning from the breast usually was followed by bottle feeding for a period of time.Individualization was necessary, since some infants were proficient enough with a cup to obtain enough milk while others took very little by cup and therefore the mother fed milk by bottle. Most infants were completely on table foods between 12 and 15 months, although many mothers continued to use junior foods for lunch or dinner when family meals were not suitable. In this group, boys were somewhat slower than girls in feeding themselves entirely.

A SIMPLE SAGA OF INFANT FEEDING

"In our progress upward, whether in religion, in economics or in the science and art of infant feeding, we advance by epochs, and often the gospel of one epoch becomes the heresy of the next, only to become again the gospel in the light of some newer truth." That statement of Joseph Brenneman[64] in 1916 is still applicable more than half a century later.

In view of the changing concepts in infant feeding over the ages, it seems fitting to end this chapter with a verse that Meyer[65] used as a frontispiece in his book, *Infant Foods and Feeding Practices*. Most of the verse was written by John Ruhrah (1872–1935). The stanzas in italics were added by Meyer "to bring to light the more recent episodes of this quaint thumbnail history."

A Simple Saga of Infant Feeding

Soranus, he of ancient Rome,
He had a simple trick
To see if milk was fit for sale,
He merely dropped it on his nail
To see if it would stick;
Yet 'spite of this the babies grew,
As any school boy'll tell to you.

Good Metlinger in ages dark
Just called milk good or bad.
No acid milk to vex his soul;
He gave it good, he gave it whole,
A method very sad;
Yet babies grew to man's estate,
A fact quite curious to relate.

Time sped, and Science came along
To help the human race;
Percentages were brought to fame
By dear old Rotch, (of honored name)
We miss his kindly face;
Percentages were fed to all—
Yet babies grew, both broad and tall.

The calories now helped us know
The food that is required.
Before the baby now could feed
We figured out his daily need—
A factor much desired;
Again we see with great surprise
That babies grow in weight and size.

The vitamin helps clarify
Why infants fail to gain;
We feed the baby leafy food
Which for the guinea pig is good—
A reason very plain;
And still we watch the human race
Go madly at its usual pace.

We have the baby weighed today;
The nursing time is set,
At last we find we are so wise
We can begin to standardize—
No baby now need fret;
In spite of this the baby grows,
But why it does God only knows!

Away with all such childish stuff!
Bring chemists to the fore!
The ion now is all the rage.
We listen to the modern sage

With all his latest lore;
And if the baby fret or cry,
We'll just see how the ions lie!

The pendulum swings back again—
Great-grandmas have their say.
"Feed any hour or any time,"
To let them cry is now a crime—
It's 'ad lib' feeding's day!
"Security"—The Clarion Call
From Ivory Towers, stern and tall!

A controversy shows its head—
Shall early solid foods win out?
Feed them meat and feed them bread—
It's a gastronomic race instead!

Nutrition's rules—"To Route!"
Yet fewer babies seem to die
And more and more they multiply.

Science to the front once more!
Solute loads are scanned;
The carbohydrate is at bay—
In babies' milk it is passe
And oft' may be completely banned!
Synthetic mixtures hold sway now,
And soon they'll say—"Who needs a
  cow?"

Amino acids are "the rage";
'N balance' is in fashion;
Which Fats are best—do all agree
With neonates' gastronomy?
What is a balanced ration?
Yet Man continues to succeed
In making Him the leading breed.

Breast Feeding! Ah—that ancient art
Is losing out, it seems—
"The female breast is for display!"
"Utility be damned!"—they say,
(It may be just a dream).
While no one asks the babies' choice—
Proprietary firms rejoice!

A hundred years will soon go by;
Our places will be filled
By others, who will theorize
And talk as long and look as wise
Until they too are stilled;
And I predict no one will know
What makes the baby gain and grow!

Source: Meyer, H. F. *Infant Foods and Feeding Practices.* Charles C Thomas, Springfield, Ill., 1960

REFERENCES

1. Fomon, S. J. *Infant Nutrition,* Second Edition. W. B. Saunders, Philadelphia, 1974.
2. Widdowson, E. M. Growth and composition of the fetus and newborn. In: Assali, N. S. (Ed.) *Biology of Gestation,* Vol. II. Academic Press, New York, 1968.

3. Karlberg, P., I. Engström, H. Lichtenstein, and I. Svennberg. The development of children in a Swedish urban community. A prospective longitudinal study. III. Physical growth during the first three years of life. *Acta Paediatr. Scand.* (Suppl. 187): 48–66, 1968.

4. Maresh, M. M. Measurements from roentgenograms. In: McCammon, R. W. (Ed.) *Human Growth and Development.* Charles C Thomas, Springfield, Ill., 1970.

5. Hamill, P. V. V., T. A. Drizd, C. L. Johnson, R. B. Reed, and A. F. Roche. *NCHS Growth Curves for Children Birth–18 Years.* DHEW Publ. No. (PHS) 78-1650. Supt. of Documents, U.S. Government Printing Office, 1977.

6. Schick, B. Pediatrics in Vienna at the beginning of the century. *J. Pediat. 50*:114-124, 1957.

7. Bakwin, H. Feeding program for infants. *Fed. Proc. 23*:66-68, 1964.

8. Illingworth, R. S., and J. Lister. The critical or sensitive period, with special reference to certain feeding problems in infants and children. *J. Pediat. 65*:839-848, 1964.

9. Food and Nutrition Board Food Protection Committee. *Safety and Suitability of Modified Starches for Use in Baby Foods.* National Academy of Sciences, 1970.

10. American Academy of Pediatrics Committee on Nutrition. Commentary on breast-feeding and infant formulas, including proposed standards for formulas. *Pediat. 57*:278-285, 1976.

11. Timiras, P. S. *Developmental Physiology and Aging.* Macmillan, New York, 1972.

12. American Academy of Pediatrics Committee on Nutrition. Salt intake and eating patterns of infants and children in relation to blood pressure. *Pediat. 53*:115-121, 1974.

13. Edelman, C. M. Jr., and H. L. Barnett. Role of the kidney in water metabolism in young infants. *J. Pediat. 56*:154–179, 1960.

14. Fisher, D. A., H. R. Pyle, Jr., J. C. Porter, A. G. Beard, and T. C. Panes. Control of water balance in the newborn. *Am. J. Dis. Child. 106*:137–146, 1963.

15. Spitz, R., and A. M. Wolf. Hospitalism: An inquiry into the psychiatric conditions in early childhood. *Psychoanal. Study Child 1*:53–58, 1946.

16. Birch, H. G., and J. D. Gussow. *Disadvantaged Children, Health, Nutrition, and School Failure.* Harcourt, Brace and World, and Grune and Stratton, New York, 1970.

17. Winick, M. (Ed.) *Nutrition and Development.* John Wiley and Sons, New York, 1972.

18. Food and Nutrition Board, National Research Council. *The Relation*

of Nutrition to Brain Development and Behavior. National Academy of Sciences, Washington, D.C., 1973.

19. Graham, G. G. Environmental factors affecting the growth of children. *Am. J. Clin. Nutr. 25*:1184–1188, 1972.

20. Gordon, J. E. Nutritional individuality. *Am. J. Dis. Child. 129*: 422–424, 1975.

21. Lozoff, B., G. M. Brittenham, M. A. Trause, J. H. Kennell, and M. H. Klaus. The mother-newborn relationship: Limits of adaptability. *J. Pediat. 91*:1–12, 1977.

22. Thoman, E. B. Development of synchrony in mother-infant interaction in feeding and other situations. *Fed. Proc. 34*:1587–1592, 1975.

23. Whitten, C. F. T.L.C. and the hungry child. *Nutr. Today 7*:10–14, 1972.

24. Beal, V. A. Nutritional Intake. In: McCammon, R. W. (Ed.) *Human Growth and Development.* Charles C Thomas, Springfield, Ill., 1970.

25. *Recommended Dietary Allowances,* Eighth Edition. National Academy of Sciences, Washington, D. C., 1974.

26. World Health Organization. *Energy and Protein Requirements.* WHO Tech. Report Series, No. 522. World Health Organization, 1973.

27. Rose, H. E., and J. Mayer. Activity, calorie intake, fat storage, and the energy balance of infants. *Pediat. 41*:18–29, 1968.

28. American Academy of Pediatrics Committee on Nutrition. Nutritional needs of low-birth-weight infants. *Pediat. 60*:519–530, 1977.

29. Burman, R. D. Nutrition in Early Childhood. In: McLaren, D. S., and D. Burman. *Textbook of Paediatric Nutrition.* Churchill Livingstone, Edinburgh, 1976.

30. Jensen, R. G., M. M. Hagerty, and K. E. McMahon. Lipids of human milk and infant formulas. A review. *Am. J. Clin. Nutr. 31*:990–1016, 1978.

31. Glueck, C. J., and R. C. Tsang. Pediatric familial type II hyper-lipoproteinemia: Effects of diet on plasma cholesterol in the first year of life. *Am. J. Clin. Nutr. 25*:224–230, 1972.

32. Gordon, H. H., and A. F. Ganzon. On the protein allowances for young infants. *J. Pediat. 54*:503–528, 1959.

33. Holt, L. E., Jr. The protein requirement of infants. *J. Pediat. 54*:496–502, 1959.

34. Ferris, A. M. The effect of feeding pattern on weight gain and fat deposition in early infancy. Unpublished doctoral dissertation, University of Massachusetts, 1978.

35. FAO/WHO Handbook on Human Nutritional Requirements, 1974. *Nutr. Rev. 33*:147–157, 1975.

36. Fomon, S., E. Ziegler, and H. Vazquez. Human milk and the small premature infant. *Am. J. Dis. Child. 131*:463–467, 1977.

37. Pearson, H. A. Life-span of the fetal red blood cell. *J. Pediat. 70*:166–171, 1967.

38. Saarinen, U. M., M. A. Siimes, and P. R. Dallman. Iron absorption in infants: High bioavailability of breast milk iron as indicated by the extrinsic tag method of iron absorption and by the concentration of serum ferritin. *J. Pediat. 91*:36–39, 1977.

39. McMillan, J. A., S. A. Landaw, and F. A. Oski. Iron sufficiency in breast-fed infants and the availability of iron from human milk. *Pediat. 58*:686–691, 1976.

40. American Academy of Pediatrics Committee on Nutrition. Trace elements in infant nutrition. *Pediat. 26*:715–721, 1960.

41. American Academy of Pediatrics Committee on Nutrition. Iron balance and requirements in infancy. *Pediat. 43*:134–142, 1969.

42. American Academy of Pediatrics Committee on Nutrition. Iron supplementation for infants. *Pediat. 58*:765–768, 1976.

43. *Dietary Standard for Canada.* Bureau of Nutritional Sciences, Department of National Health and Welfare, Ottawa, 1976.

44. *Recommended Dietary Allowances for the Caribbean.* Caribbean Food and Nutrition Institute, Kingston, Jamaica, 1976.

45. American Academy of Pediatrics Committee on Nutrition. Iron-fortified formulas. *Pediat. 47*:786, 1971.

46. Johnson, P. E., and G. W. Evans. Relative zinc availability in human breast milk, infant formulas, and cow's milk. *Am. J. Clin. Nutr. 31*:416–421, 1978.

47. Hambidge, K. M. The role of zinc and other trace metals in pediatric nutrition and health. *Pediat. Clin. No. Amer. 24*:95–106, 1977.

48. Dallman, P. R. Iron, vitamin E, and folate in the preterm infant. *J. Pediat. 85*:742–752, 1974.

49. Levin, S. S. *A Philosophy of Infant Feeding.* Charles C Thomas, Springfield, Ill., 1963.

50. Coursin, D. B. Convulsive seizures in infants with pyridoxine-deficient diets. *JAMA 154*:406–408, 1954.

51. Lahey, M. E., and J. F. Wilson. The etiology of iron-deficiency anemia in infants—A reappraisal. *J. Pediat. 69*:339–342, 1966.

52. Jelliffe, D. B., and E. F. P. Jelliffe. Breast feeding *is* best for infants everywhere. *Nutr. Today 13*:12–16, 1978.

53. Fomon, S. J., and T. A. Anderson (Eds.) *Practices of low-income families in feeding infants and small children with particular attention to cultural subgroups.* Proceeding of a National Workshop. Maternal

and Child Health Service, U.S. Dept. of Health, Education, and Welfare, Rockville, Md., 1972.

54. Ferris, A. G., L. B. Vilhjalmsdottir, V. A. Beal, and P. L. Pellett. Diets in the first six months of infants in western Massachusetts. *J. Am. Dietet. Assoc. 72*:155–160, 1978.

55. Shelton, P. G., R. J. Berkowitz, and D. J. Forrester. Nursing bottle caries. *Pediat. 59*:777–778, 1977.

56. Butler, A. M., and I. J. Wolman. Trends in the early feeding of supplementary foods to infants. *Quart. Rev. Pediat. 9*:63–85, 1954.

57. Beal, V. A. On the acceptance of solid foods and other food patterns of infants and children. *Pediat. 20*:448–457, 1957.

58. Campbell, J. R. Duration of night feeding in infancy. *Lancet 1*:877, 1958.

59 Beal, V. A. Termination of night feeding in infancy. *J. Pediat. 75*: 690–692, 1969.

60. Grunwaldt, E., T. Bates, and D. Guthrie, Jr. The onset of sleeping through the night in infancy. *Pediat. 26*:667–668, 1960.

61. Anderson, T. A. Commercial infant foods: Content and composition. *Pediat. Clin. No. Amer. 24*:37–47, 1977.

62. Fomon, S. J., L. N. Thomas, and L. J. Filer, Jr. Acceptance of unsalted strained foods by normal infants. *J. Pediat. 76*:242–246, 1970.

63. Food and Nutrition Board Food Protection Committee. *Safety and Suitability of Salt for Use in Baby Foods.* National Academy of Sciences, Washington, D. C., 1970.

64. Brennemann, J. The use of boiled milk in infant feeding and elsewhere. *JAMA 67*:1413–1418, 1916.

65. Meyer, H. F. *Infant Foods and Feeding Practices.* Charles C Thomas, Springfield, Ill., 1960.

6

THE
PRESCHOOL
YEARS
(ONE
TO
SIX)

In contrast to the rapid and usually smooth growth in the first year, the period from one to six years is characterized by a slower rate of increase in both stature and weight. During the first year the average infant triples birth weight and adds 50 percent to length. If this rate of growth were to continue, the child would be 96 feet tall and weigh more than 200 tons by the tenth year. Instead, it will take the entire span from one to six years to increase height by 50 percent again, and to double the weight attained at one year. The deceleration in growth rate which began in the first year (Figure 1.6) continues throughout childhood until the second acceleration in adolescence.

Maturation of function, control of the body, and development of social and cognitive abilities are more pronounced than somatic growth during the preschool years. In infancy the world was brought to the child; the preschooler ventures out into the world. The child becomes proficient in walking, running, and many other physical skills. He learns a language and can express needs and reactions. The environment widens as a result of mobility, and interests expand. The child develops a sense of self as different from others and progresses rapidly toward independence in many respects. Exploration at this age includes not only investigation of the environment, but also exploration of the reactions of others to various types of behavior. The child learns the limits of behavior that are acceptable in his milieu by experimenting with many kinds of activity.

Relationships with others in the family develop. In our present culture, the mother or a substitute mother figure is dominant in the care of the young infant, although fathers increasingly are taking responsibility for

265

some aspects of infant care. During the preschool years the father and other family members become more important to the child and dependence on mother lessens. In the present era, nearly 50 percent of mothers with preschool children are employed outside the home, and primary care of the children may rest in other family members, sitters, day care centers, or preschools. More fathers have assumed the responsibilities of child care as single parents. As a result, social development progresses rapidly and the child learns to relate to a wide variety of people, both young and adult.

PHYSICAL GROWTH

In the first year, the infant may have had an increment of 25 cm in length. During the second year, the increment is more likely to be 11 to 13 cm. In the third year, height increases only 8 to 9 cm, and in the next three years approximately 7 cm/year. Body proportions change, with faster growth of the trunk and legs than of the head. The average increase in head circumference in the first year is close to 12 cm, but in the second year it is only 2 to 2.5 cm, in the third year approximately 1.2 cm, and thereafter less than 1 cm increment per year.[1,2] As a result, the general conformation of the preschool child gives progressively less an impression of a disproportionately large head on a short body. By the end of the preschool period the head will have attained 90 percent of its adult size. In contrast, although growth of the rest of the body is now more rapid than head growth, by six years the child will have attained only 65 to 70 percent of adult height.

Extremities grow at a more rapid rapid rate than the trunk during the preschool years as well as throughout childhood. At the end of the first year crown–rump length accounted for 65 percent of total height, but by six years sitting height accounts for only 55 percent of total height.[2] Therefore, by the end of the sixth year the child is taller, but with a smaller head and longer legs relative to total size.

Weight gain in the second year is less than half of the gain in the first year, averaging close to 2.5 kg instead of 6 to 7 kg. Through the rest of the preschool period, average weight increment per year is approximately 2 kg/year.[1,2] As with all measurements, there is wide individual variation. Weight gain may become erratic during this period. Some children may have a temporary loss in weight, which is not surprising in view of the increased physical activity and some degree of anorexia commonly seen at this age.

Skinfold thickness measurements decrease during the preschool period in both boys and girls, although the decrease is less in girls. The pattern of wider layers of subcutaneous fat in females becomes more evident in the second year (Figure 1.15). One must remember, however, that the narrower

THE PRESCHOOL YEARS (ONE TO SIX)

layers of fat cover progressively longer body segments, so that total body fat is not decreased as much as the skinfold measurements suggest.

Individualism becomes apparent in respect to the channel of growth followed by each child. It has been speculated that the impetus for fetal growth, whatever hormonal or genetic factors are involved, continues postnatally for a period of time, and then is gradually replaced by growth factors developed within the child. At any rate, there are marked changes in patterns of growth during the post-infancy period. In the longitudinal studies of the Child Research Council, nearly two-thirds of the children changed in percentile rank for bone lengths of the extremities relative to height, as well as in percentile rank for sitting height, by four years of age.[3] Smith et al.[4] speculated that an upward shift in percentile position for length occurs primarily in the first year for those infants who presumably were limited in fetal growth and have a catch-up period after delivery, but that the downward shift from tall to average height is more likely to occur after one year of age, reflecting the influence of genetic factors from both parents rather than only maternal size, which was a dominant influence during gestation. Tanner[5] found a correlation coefficient of only 0.20 to 0.25 between birth length and adult height, but the coefficient increased to more than 0.70 between height at two years and adult height (Figure 1.11).Change in percentile position for body measurements may occur at any age, but the high frequency of its occurrence in the first four years of life suggests that the controlling mechanisms have altered from those in effect during gestation.

Sex differences in growth in height and weight are not remarkable during the preschool period, but there are changes in body composition.[6] Girls tend toward greater subcutaneous fat widths and boys toward wider bones. Muscle widths are similar for both sexes (Figure 1.15).

Eruption of deciduous teeth progresses relatively rapidly during the second and third years. At one year the infant may have all 8 incisors and possibly the mandibular first molars. By 2½ years all 20 deciduous teeth have probably erupted.[7] However, there is wide individual variation, both in the order of appearance of teeth and in the timing of eruption. During the preschool years the face and mandible grow more rapidly than the rest of the head.

Racial differences in growth rates have been documented in a number of studies.[8-10] At birth, black infants tend to be smaller than white infants (Chapter 3), and the incidence of low birth weight is approximately twice as high among black infants. However, by two years, black children are taller and heavier, with more ossification centers and more advanced tooth eruption than white children. In contrast, blacks have less subcutaneous fat. It is obvious, then, that black children grow more rapidly in stature and skeletal maturation during the early postnatal period. This difference is maintained throughout childhood. However, Hamill et al.[1] concluded that the differences were not great enough to warrant separate growth curves for these two ethnic groups in the United States. Habicht et al.[11] determined that environmental factors, including income, had greater influence than ethnic background on growth, especially after six months of age, justifying the use in developing countries of growth standards derived from middle-class children in the United States. Robson et al.,[12] on the other hand, proposed that errors in evaluation of growth of black children would be made unless race-specific standards are developed. The need for separate racial standards remains unresolved.

PHYSIOLOGICAL DEVELOPMENT RELATED TO NUTRITION

NEUROMUSCULAR DEVELOPMENT

Mobility and body control are accomplished during the second year. The child can usually walk alone by 15 months, climb stairs with help at 18 months, and run by 18 to 24 months.[7] With this development of gross motor skills, the child acquires greater access to the environment and becomes less dependent on others.

Fine motor coordination also progresses rapidly, and manipulation of objects, including food, becomes more proficient. Although familiar with the cup for fluids, the infant needs to have the cup held and guided; early in the second year the child can usually manage to hold and direct a cup with fair precision, but spilling may be common. Wrist control is a prerequisite to efficiency in self-feeding, since the spoon must be filled with food and then carried to the mouth in an upright position. Most children accomplish this skill between 12 and 18 months, but usually need some help, especially toward the end of a meal when they may become tired. In the Child Research Council series, girls were feeding themselves without help at a median age of 18 months and boys at 19½ months, but individual children were as young as 8 to 9 months or as old as 3 years when they reached that stage of independence. Lateness in self-feeding by healthy children is more likely to be related to unwillingness of the mother to allow the child to feed himself than to the child's inability. Mentally retarded children are slower in learning feeding skills as well as many other skills, but wide variation is observed even among healthy children.

HEMATOLOGICAL DEVELOPMENT

As the body grows, an expanded blood supply is necessary to supply the new tissues. The large hemoglobin mass of the healthy full-term neonate

268

supplies iron for formation of new hemoglobin for the first six months. Thereafter a supply of exogenous iron is essential to maintain adequate hematopoiesis. When dietary supplies of iron are adequate in the last half of the first year, the child enters the preschool period with a hemoglobin concentration of perhaps 12 g/100 ml. Hemoglobin concentration rises slowly, and by 6 years the median is 12 to 13 g/100 ml.[8,13]

Standards for acceptable hemoglobin levels in the ages from 1 to 6 years are not firmly established, but vary from one health center to another. Lower levels of "normal" may be 11 or 10 g/100 ml, but in some centers 12 g/100 ml is used as a criterion. Data from the Preschool Nutrition Survey (PNS)[8] were analyzed in relation to the saturation of transferrin. On the assumption that when serum transferrin saturation is maintained at a level greater than 15 percent, iron is not a limiting factor in the production of hemoglobin, statistical analysis showed that the lower limit of "normal" hemoglobin level for children with 16 percent transferrin saturation or higher was 10.5 g/100 ml.

When the diet during the last half of the first year and early in the second year is composed largely of milk and other foods with low iron content, a sequence of biochemical and hematological events may result in iron-deficiency anemia, which becomes apparent early in the second year. Tissue iron stores are depleted. Serum iron decreases to less than 50 μg/100 ml and iron-binding capacity increases to more than 350 ug/100 ml, as the percent transferrin saturation drops to 15 percent or less. As the deficiency progresses, newly formed red cells become progressively more microcytic and hypochromic.

The peak prevalence of iron-deficiency anemia, identified usually by a hemoglobin level lower than 10 to 11 g/100 ml and hematocrit less than 31 to 34 percent, is at approximately 18 months. The prevalence of iron-deficiency anemia has been reported to vary from 10 to 65 percent of children in low income families, but is rarely as high as 10 percent of children in middle income families.

After the peak age, the prevalence of anemia in preschool children declines, even without therapy, in population groups where it has been most common.[14-16] After 3 years the risk of anemia is relatively small. In the PNS,[8] mean transferrin saturations, which ranged from 13 to 18 percent in the second year, increased with age until approximately 47 months, when they stabilized at 23 to 24 percent, reflecting iron stores. Therefore, the period of greatest risk is in the second year, and thereafter is much less common.

Racial differences in hematological indices have been reported in all three national surveys at all ages and at all income levels.[17] Black children have mean hemoglobin levels 0.5 g/100 ml lower than white children.[18] In the PNS,[8] the difference in hemoglobin concentration persisted even when transferrin saturation was held constant. There is increasing awareness that different criteria for the diagnosis of anemia should be used for the two ethnic groups. Since there is a disproportionate number of blacks in the lower socioeconomic group, the use of a different standard of hemoglobin for blacks would result in a lower figure for the prevalence of anemia.

In the Ten-State Nutrition Survey,[10] children with higher hemoglobin levels tended to be taller and heavier than children with lower hemoglobin levels. A similar relationship between size and hemoglobin levels was found for boys, but not for girls, in the PNS.[8] This suggests that a dietary intake high enough to support rapid growth also contains sufficient protein, iron, and other nutrients for good blood formation.

PSYCHOSOCIAL-BIOLOGICAL INTERACTIONS

The preschool period is a time of increasing independence, ability, and socialization. It is also a time when many of the effects of social, economic, and educational disadvantages of the environment become manifest. The interplay of the child's increasing capabilities, the encouragement and support of parents and others in the child's environment, and the degree of stimulation determine to a large measure whether development progresses at an optimal rate or is inhibited. As the child becomes more independent, the type of guidance provided in relation to physical activity, foods and feeding practices, and psychological and social handling is critical to health and function throughout life.

The slowing of the rate of growth results in a less pressing demand for nutrients than was observed in the first year. The widening of the child's environment and curiosity about the expanding world place food in a secondary position of importance. Learning to talk allows expression of likes and dislikes, acceptance and refusal, and pleasure and displeasure. The need for assertion of independence is applied to eating as well as to other activities. As a result of this combination of developments, food may become the focus of dissension between preschool children and their parents.

APPETITE

Toward the end of the first year, the infant begins to show some disinterest in food. Refusal of the bottle is common; many mothers discontinue use of the bottle because the child no longer wants it. The decrease in milk consumption is often the first sign of the onset of the typically poor appetite of the preschooler. The change from eager acceptance of food during most of the first year to indifference or refusal may be traumatic to parents of a first-born, since they seldom anticipate the change; many become concerned, and some feel a sense of guilt that somehow they themselves are to blame. In contrast, the parents of later-born children accept anorexia as a normal and expected phase of development and know that it will run its course and pass.

Changes in appetite as reported at successive ages by mothers of the children enrolled in the longitudinal studies of the Child Research Council[19] are shown in Figure 6.1. Although these ratings are subjective and undoubtedly based on different criteria by different mothers, the ratings are from the same mother-child combinations at each age and reflect changes over this span of time. At six months, 85 percent of the children had good or ex-

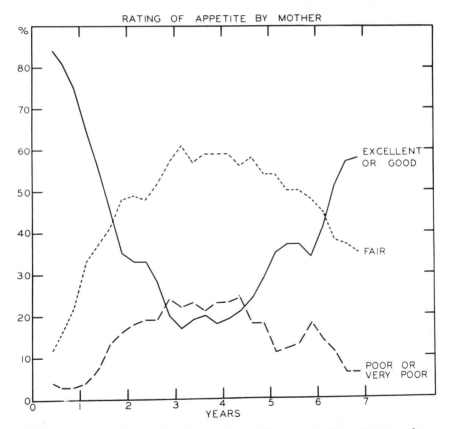

Figure 6.1   Percent of children at each age from 6 months to 7 years whose appetites were rated by their mothers as excellent or good, fair, or poor or very poor, Child Research Council series. (Source: Beal, V. A. On the acceptance of solid foods, and other food patterns of infants and children. Pediat. 20:448–457, 1957.)

cellent appetites, 10 percent fair, and 5 percent poor or very poor. By three years, only 20 percent of the children still had good or excellent appetites, the poor ratings had increased to 20 percent, and the majority of children (60 percent) had appetites that their mothers considered to be only fair. The nadir was between 3 and 4½ years, and thereafter appetites improved; by the age of school entry, a majority of the children were eating well again.

Analysis of the dietary histories showed that, although few children had a real decrease in caloric intake, there were distinct differences in acceptance of specific foods. Figure 6.2 shows the median calories from various food groups and their pattern of alteration. The most marked decrease in consumption was observed with milk; only 5 percent of the children in this series did not have a decrease in milk consumption. Vegetable consumption decreased, although the substitution of more fruit lessened the nutritional impact. During this interval, desserts, sweets, and starches were the only foods that were consumed in progressively larger amounts. Meat, eggs, and fats maintained a relatively stable caloric contribution.

Figure 6.3 shows the pattern of milk consumption of children in the Child Research Council series. Expressed both as grams of calcium and ounces of milk, these values were based on only the milk consumed as a beverage, excluding milk in soups, desserts, and so on. The median intake of milk decreased from 26 ounces daily at the end of the first year of life to 16 ounces

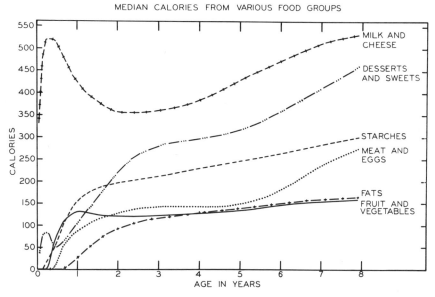

Figure 6.2   *Median calories from various food groups in first 8 years of life, Child Research Council series.*

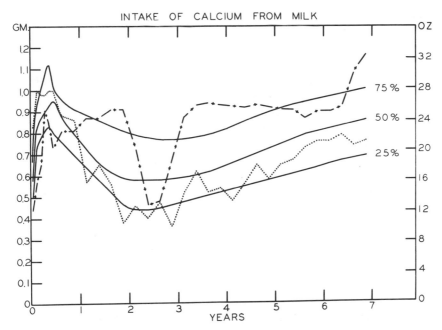

Figure 6.3 *Intake of calcium from milk consumed as a beverage. Patterns of two children are compared with group percentiles, Child Research Council series. (Source: Beal, V. A. On the acceptance of solid foods, and other food patterns of infants and children. Pediat. 20:448–457, 1957.)*

at two to three years, then increased to 24 ounces by school age. The range of variation among children was wide, both in timing and degree of change in intake. In the third year of life the lowest observed intake during any three-month interval covered by the dietary history was an average of 3 ounces/day, and the highest more than 32 ounces/day. Individual patterns of two children, selected to show early and late decreases in milk consumption, are plotted against the group quartiles. Decrease in milk intake during the preschool period has been reported in other studies.[8, 21-23]

In addition to the changes in consumption of specific foods, eating behavior may follow a common pattern. The child prefers five small meals to three larger meals per day. He does not eat a large amount at a time, and as a result becomes hungry more often. The evening meal is often the most difficult. By the end of the day the child is tired and may be fussy. His mother or other caretaker may be busy preparing the meal or paying more attention to other members of the family who have come home, and the preschooler gets less individual attention. There is more noise and confusion in the home, and therefore more diversion than has been true earlier in the day. If the child is then confronted with a large meal, rebellion may result in refusal to eat, irritability, or tantrums.

The child's reaction to food may be closely related to striving for independence. In addition to wanting to dress without help or to perform other tasks independently, refusal of food is also an expression of independence, particularly when parents express concern. The power of language is another area of development, and the child may say "no" when offered a food usually liked, presumably because the satisfaction of self-expression is greater than the satisfaction of eating a favorite food.

Specific types of foods may be accepted or rejected for seemingly irrational reasons. Some children refuse to eat broken cookies or crackers. Most casseroles are unpopular, although spaghetti with tomato sauce and macaroni with cheese are often favorites. The child may object when foods are mixed or even touch each other on the plate when served, despite the fact that he may stir the food together himself. Egg yolk or egg white may be refused for a period of time, and the child may change suddenly in acceptance of either part of the egg. Hamburgers, frankfurters, and chicken are most likely to be accepted, and meats that require more chewing may be rejected. Favorite vegetables of most children are peas, corn, and green beans, but in general raw vegetables are better accepted than cooked vegetables. Most fruits are well liked.

Hunger of the child varies from day to day and foods that might be refused one day are eaten with pleasure the next day. There is also a tendency for the beginning of the separation of breakfast eaters and noneaters at this age. Some children who refuse breakfast shortly after rising will eat willingly after being allowed to play for a while; others are content to skip breakfast but become hungry and want food at mid-morning.

Although there is a common pattern of food acceptance and rejection, there are wide individual variations in the timing, the degree, and the duration of anorexia. Many mothers are convinced that their children are eating less, but a careful dietary history usually reveals that caloric intake has plateaued and that only for a short time do children actually decrease their total food consumption. More common is a replacement of some foods at meals by snacks and foods high in carbohydrate, thus maintaining energy intake.

Lower milk consumption is usually of long duration, and an increase may not occur until school age. Intakes of other foods are variable from day to day or from month to month. Overall enthusiasm for food may be low for only a few months or may continue to be low through most of the preschool years. Therefore, the usual rules for stimulation of a child's appetite are helpful, but may not be very effective. A comfortable arrangement of table and chair, utensils that are easy to manipulate, colorful foods cut to a size that the child can manage easily, and small first servings with additional servings as the child wishes may elicit greater willingness to eat, but the anorexia may be little affected. Permissiveness or rigidity of the parents seems to have little influence on the duration of the problem.

Since the poor appetite and disinterest in food shown by the preschool child are self-limiting, they need not be of major concern with most children, although it is wise to be sure that foods of high nutrient density are given priority. If the preschool child appears healthy, is normally energetic, and grows at an acceptable rate, the parent may accept the change in eating pattern as an expected characteristic of this age group. On the other hand, if the child is lethargic, has repeated and persistent infections, or has a prolonged period without weight gain, a physical examination and appropriate laboratory tests should be done.

DEVELOPMENT OF ATTITUDES TOWARD FOOD

From the first feeding in the newborn period, the infant associates food with relief from discomfort. Confidence in mother or other adults develops when hunger needs are met promptly, and the infant learns to wait when sounds and movement indicate that food will be forthcoming. Throughout the first year, natural appetites as a result of growth needs are large enough to ensure a willing acceptance of food.

With the curtailed demands for growth and the wider interests and abilities of the preschool child, food is of secondary importance. Decreasing appetite, increasing independence, and transition to family foods create a very different situation. Being able to choose whether to accept or reject foods, the child learns he has control that he did not have previously. The reactions of parents and others in the household affect both standards of behavior and attitudes toward eating which may set a pattern for his lifetime. Although food tastes will change, the general approach of the child to food and its meaning to him are based to a large extent on his experiences during the preschool years.

Patterns of eating behavior may be set during this period.[24] Mealtimes that are pleasant and satisfying create a positive attitude. When parents become anxious, irritated, or angry about the messiness, dawdling, and spilling that accompany self-feeding, or when reluctance to eat ends in forcing, tantrums, or banishment, meals become an unpleasant part of the day. Insistence on the child's cleaning his plate or eating more than he wants may distort the natural development of the appetite-satiety balance and may be a factor in later obesity. Impatience of parents with self-feeding may lead to continued spoon feeding and interrupt the sequence of developmental progress by not allowing acquisition of a skill at a time of readiness.

Food has many meanings that are not biological. The child soon learns that food is one of the few weapons he can use against his parents. Refusal of food may attract wanted attention. Equally, it can be a means of expression of independence and proof that he is a separate person with a mind of his own. Behavior during meals may sometimes be a matter of testing what permissible limits are set by parents. Parents also use food and feeding in a variety of ways. When food is offered with pleasure and enjoyment, parents express satisfaction and pride in their offspring and in their ability to interact with love and understanding. When parents force children to eat, it may be out of desire to do what is best, but it also may be a symptom of dominance. Food is used as a bribe for good behavior, and withholding of food as a punishment for unacceptable behavior. Foods most commonly used as rewards and punishment are sweets, which then become more desirable than other foods. In many cultural groups, particularly those in which a plump child is a source of pride, food is often used as a means of providing special attention and privilege.

Socioeconomic level, as reflected by income, education, and occupation, influences behavior of parents toward their children. In the PNS,[8] mothers in lower socioeconomic ranks tended to be more lax with their children, were more likely to cater to food preferences, allowed their children to eat meals or snacks at any time of day, more often used food for rewards and withheld food for punishment, and were less concerned about poor eating. In contrast, mothers in the higher levels were more rigid and demanding, had a more established daily eating pattern, and less often used food as a reward or punishment. However, at all income levels catering to food preferences was more common with the younger preschool child and decreased as the child grew older, but the giving or withholding of food as a response to behavior increased.

PICA

Most children begin mouthing objects in the middle of the first year as part of the normal hand-to-mouth stage of development. This type of activity usually subsides early during the second year. Its persistence past 18 months, especially when it involves a craving for particular non-food substances, may be considered abnormal.[25] Pica in children has been reported to include the eating of dirt, paint chips, plaster, paper, crayons, and other objects. The highest incidence is between 1½ and 2 years and then the practice decreases, but may persist up to 4-6 years in some children. It has been most commonly reported in low income children, and in blacks and Spanish-Americans more than whites. It persists longer when parents are tolerant of the practice and the cultural pattern accepts it. The women themselves may eat dirt, clay, laundry starch, or other nonfood items, particularly during pregnancy.

The highest incidence of pica occurs at ages when iron-deficiency anemia is common, and a causal relationship has been investigated. Some have contended that anemia causes pica by creating a desire for those substances. Others have proposed that pica limits the consumption of nutritious foods or inhibits iron absorption and therefore results in anemia. Treatment with iron has been reported to be effective in curing pica, but such studies have usually been done without controls. In controlled studies, Gutelius et al.[26,27] found that either oral iron or intramuscular injection of iron was no more effective than placebos or saline solution and suggested that the reported cure was related more to the spontaneous improvement in pica with increasing age than to the therapy.

The relationship of pica to lead poisoning and its resulting brain damage has been of particular concern in cities with substandard housing where small children eat paint chips. Paint is the primary source of lead for these children, and campaigns to identify children wtih pica have been used in finding children who need to be screened for lead poisoning.[28]

PROTEIN-ENERGY MALNUTRITION

International attention on child health and nutrition in the past 30 years has focused on protein-energy malnutrition which, directly or indirectly, is the leading cause of death of children under five in developing countries.[29,30] The symptoms of the disease may be seen at any age in populations with chronic undernutrition, but morbidity and mortality rates are highest in infants and young children. Marasmus is most common in young infants, with absence of adipose tissue, emaciation, dehydration, and electrolyte imbalance following growth retardation, as a result of total inadequacy of food intake, whether by breast or substitute feedings. Kwashiorkor is more often seen in the infant or young child after weaning from the breast to inadequate foods. Growth retardation is often the first sign that is recognized. The deficit in lean body mass and adiposity may be masked by overhydration, especially of extracellular space. Distortion of metabolic functions involves not only energy and protein, but also carbohydrate, lipid, minerals, and vitamins. The synergism of malnutrition and susceptibility to disease, especially diarrhea, exacerbate the problems of both. The incidence, symptomatology, and age distribution vary from one country to another.

When the magnitude of the problem became evident, programs were instituted for treatment and prevention. At first the emphasis in kwashiorkor was on the protein deficit, and programs for food supplementation with total proteins or fortification with specific limiting amino acids were conducted, with disappointing results. The debate about the relative importance of protein or calories in the diet has not yet been clarified; [31,32] both are deficient in most diets, and the clarification is important primarily in giving direction to preventive programs on the massive scale required to eradicate the disease. It has become increasingly evident that direct supplementary feeding is at most palliative, that nutrition education is of limited value because families frequently do not have either the facilities or resources to use the knowledge they have, and that amino acid supplementation is ineffective. The fundamental causes are social and economic in nature, and the need is to focus on the prevention of chronic malnutrition. [33]

No cases of kwashiorkor or marasmus were found in the three major surveys conducted in the United States. However, marasmus and kwashiorkor were both reported among Navajo children in Arizona in 1969; [34] this stimulated the establishment of infant and child feeding programs, and the incidence of both diseases had dropped markedly by 1976. [35]

NUTRITION, COGNITIVE DEVELOPMENT, AND BEHAVIOR

The effects of severe malnutrition on cognitive function and behavior, as observed in developing countries, become apparent in the post-infancy period. The most critical timing of brain development probably begins with the increase in neuronal multiplication at about the twelfth week of fetal life and extends to the third or fourth postnatal year when rapid myelination has passed its peak. [36] Severe malnutrition during rapid neuronal growth may result in reduced brain size, decreased brain cell number, and immature or incomplete biochemical organization of the brain. [37] Continued malnutrition during myelin formation has a cumulative effect. Several diverse areas of study have coalesced in the investigation of the relationship between nutrition and brain development or behavior. Research in cytology and embryology, both in animals and humans, has been amplified by extensive international work on protein-energy malnutrition and research on the social-cultural-economic etiology and consequences of malnutrition.

The complex interrelationships of the physiological and biochemical consequences of malnutrition and environmental influences make it difficult to delineate the effects of nutrition per se on learning ability. [37] Malnutrition severe enough to cause physical and mental retardation is usually associated with a deprived environment, which adds to the biological handicaps. The abnormalities of morphologic, biochemical, and physiological characteristics may alter brain function and reduce learning ability. The undernourished child is often apathetic, easily fatigued, lethargic, and immature, and therefore has less exposure to stimuli in the environment and is unresponsive at a critical period of development. Greater susceptibility to illness may increase social isolation. Adverse changes in personality, emotionality, and behavior may disrupt normal learning processes even more. Inactivity and unresponsiveness of the child further limit interaction with other family members, compounded by their own malnutrition. The lack of physical activity and external stimulation limits opportunity to learn and develop skills. In such an environment the fetus and infant are particularly susceptible to retardation in brain growth, and the infant and preschool child are subject to the complex of physiological and environmental factors that depress cognitive function.

It is not yet clear whether learning difficulties can be modified or reversed, and what degrees of nutritional rehabilitation and changes in environment are required. In most of the early studies, children who had recovered from protein-energy malnutrition returned to the same deprived environments, and when tested at school ages did more poorly than well-nourished controls. However, more recent studies have shown that reversibility of deficits in physical growth, head circumference, and psychological function may occur when nutritional rehabilitation is accompanied by enrichment of the environment and increased stimulation of the child.[38-40] Brožek[41] has published a chronology of the conferences on malnutrition and behavior between 1964 and 1974, along with an extensive bibliography.

The effects of less severe malnutrition on mental ability and function have not been intensively studied. A follow-up study[42] of children born in Holland during World War II whose mothers had been well-nourished except for a period of food shortage during pregnancy found no significant differences in adult performance. In the United States, the lesser degree of malnutrition observed is most likely to affect the ability to concentrate for learning rather than cause structural damage to the brain or cental nervous system.[43]

NUTRIENT REQUIREMENTS AND RECOMMENDED DIETARY ALLOWANCES

Fewer studies have been done on the nutrient intake or requirement of preschool children than of any other age group. Routine well-child care usually decreases by the end of the first year, and children between one and six years are seen by physicians only for illnesses. Except for longitudinal growth studies and occasional university-based studies, there have been few places where children in this age group congregated and could be available for study. The initiation of the Head Start Program in 1964 and the inclusion of children up to five years of age in the Special Supplemental Food Program for Women, Infants, and Children (WIC Program) authorized in 1972 were the first extensive federal programs for children of preschool age.

The three national nutrition surveys beginning in 1968 provided data on the dietary intakes of children over one year of age.

Experimental studies of nutrient requirements, however, have been concentrated on adults. Infants in the newborn period, usually under the age of four months, and preadolescents above 10 years of age have participated in some balance studies. The interim ages have been largely neglected except for a few mineral balance studies in the 1940s.

As a result, the physiological requirements of preschool children are not known, and the recommended allowances for these ages have been estimated. As discussed in Chapter 5, allowances for infants have been based to a large extent on the known composition of breast milk and the available data on the amount consumed at various stages of infancy. Using these allowances as the framework for one year of age, and adult requirements at the other end of the scale, the RDAs for intervening ages have been interpolated, supplemented where possible by data on preadolescents and adolescents. Growth rate and changes in body composition have been factored into the allowances.

ENERGY

The energy requirements of children are more closely related to body size than to age. Because of wide individual differences in physical activity, some children may require twice as many calories as others at the same age. The best indices of caloric balance of any child are the rate of growth in height and the weight gain in relation to deposition of subcutaneous fat. Since the preschool years are a period of slenderizing for most children, the maintenance of infant fat padding or an increase in fat thickness should be checked for possible obesity.

The mean RDA for energy at 1 to 3 years is 1300 kcal (5.5 MJ) and at 4 to 6 years it is 1700 kcal (7.1 MJ). The increase at these ages is curvilinear and the values apply to the midpoints of the age ranges. The mean RDA levels are slightly below the FAO/WHO[45] levels for these age groups because of the assumption that children in the United States tend to be less active.

Observed intakes of children in the United States tend to be somewhat lower than the mean RDA levels. Data from the PNS,[8] the 1971–1974 Health and Nutrition Examination Survey (HANES)[46] and the longitudinal studies of the Child Research Council (CRC)[47] show that median intakes ranged from 900 to 1200 kcal at one year of age and increased to 1600 to 1800 kcal by six years. All of the studies showed wide individual variation.

The Canadian Dietary Standard[48] for children was expressed as total energy, energy per kilogram, and energy per centimeter. Although the relationship between body weight and energy needs is high, height might be a better index because it is less dependent on energy balance and rules out the risk of everestimating the requirements of overweight children. Recommended allowances at 1 to 3 years were 1400 kcal, 107 kcal/kg, and 15.5 kcal/cm; at 4 to 6 years the allowances were 1800 kcal, 95 kcal/kg, and 16.0 kcal/cm. Recommended intakes per kg were higher than those observed in PNS and the CRC series, in which median levels of 97 to 100 kcal/kg at the beginning of the age span decreased to 83 to 88 kcal/kg at the end. In the CRC data, median intakes of boys rose from 12.5 to 15.1 kcal/cm and of girls from 12.0 to 13.7 kcal/cm between one and six years and therefore were also lower than the recommended intake.

LIPIDS

No allowances have been established for either lipids or carbohydrates. Nevertheless, the intake of essential fatty acids should be assured. The RDA text [44] suggests that the required intake of essential fatty acids lies within the range of 1 to 2 percent of calories, but in the discussion of vitamin E for children suggests a vitamin E allowance compatible with 4 to 7 percent of calories as linoleic acid. The Canadian Dietary Standard text [48] states that "no EFA requirement has been established for any class of humans other than infants" and suggests that 1 to 2 percent of calories as linoleate appears adequate after infancy.

PROTEIN

The RDA [44] for protein during this age span has been factorially determined by assuming that maintenance requirements of the adult (0.8 g/kg) apply also to the child, adding an arbitrary amount for growth, and adjusting for the efficiency of utilization of proteins of various quality. The efficiency of conversion of dietary protein to tissue protein during growth is unknown. However, protein content of the body, which rose from 11 percent to nearly 15 percent in the first year, increases still further between one and four years to 18 to 19 percent, which is similar to adult values. [49]

Until 1958 the RDA for protein was 40 g at 1 to 3 years and 50 g at 4 to 6 years. Since that time the allowance has been progressively lowered to 23 g at 1 to 3 years and 30 g at 4 to 6 years. The recommended allowance for energy has increased somewhat during this same time period, with the net result being that the protein recommendation decreased from approximately 13 percent of calories to its present level of 7.1 and 6.7 percent of calories in the two age groups. These are lower than usually considered adequate during growth.

The RDA is higher than the "safe" FAO/WHO[45] levels of 16 g and 20 g, but those figures are accompanied by a statement that they are based on protein of the biological value of egg and milk. They represent levels of less than 5 percent of calories supplied by protein. The Canadian Dietary Standard[48] allowed for a Net Protein Utilization (NPU) of 67 as the average quality of the Canadian diet and arrived at levels of 22 g at 1 to 3 years and 27 g at 4 to 6 years, equivalent to 6.3 and 6.0 percent of the recommended energy intake.

In contrast to the recommended allowances, observed intakes of preschool children tend to be much higher. Medians reported in the PNS,[8] HANES,[46] and the CRC series[47] ranged from 41 to 48 g/day at one year or shortly thereafter, increasing to 59 to 63 g at 6 years. Mean intakes in a California series were within the same ranges.[50] In the North Central region study,[51] median intakes were higher, rising from 52-53 g to levels of 67-73 g by the sixth year. Even in the low income ratio states of the Ten-State Nutrition Survey,[52] median protein intakes of children between 1 and 3 years of age were 47 to 48 g/day.

Whereas the RDA figure at 1 to 3 years allows 1.77 g protein/kg and 1.50 g/kg at 4 to 6 years, median intakes in HANES and the CRC series were 4.0 to 4.5 g/kg at one year and 2.9 to 3.2 g/kg at 6 years. Even higher intakes were found in the North Central region study, with mean intakes of 4.9 and 5.4 g/kg for the two sexes at 1-1½ years and 3.5 and 3.8 g/kg at 5 to 6 years. Therefore, on whatever basis they are calculated, observed intakes of children in several studies in the United States average at least twice the recommended allowances. These observed intakes are close to 15 percent of calorie intakes.

Eight metabolic studies on 44 preschool children published since 1917 showed conflicting results.[53] Protein requirements estimated for growth varied from 1 g/kg to 4 g/kg. The difference may be explained partly by daily fluctuations in nitrogen retention of individuals, suggesting that balance periods of 12 to 18 days are required to cover the range of fluctuations and partly by the dependence of protein requirement on caloric intake. Neither the minimal nor the optimal protein intake of children at this age has been determined.[7]

MINERALS

The Recommended Dietary Allowances for minerals are shown in Appendix 1. Calcium and iron deserve special consideration in this age group.

Calcium

The requirement for calcium during the preschool years in unknown, and neither minimal nor optimal dietary intakes can be specified with any degree of assurance. Balance studies and theoretical calculations of requirements have produced conflicting results and therefore conflicting interpretations.

In a review of balance studies reported since 1918, Irwin and Kienholz[54] found that retention of calcium varied from 2 to 18 mg/kg/day. Variations in estimations of dietary calcium needed between 1 and 6 years ranged from 250 to 1000 mg/day. Per unit of weight, children need two to four times as much calcium as adults for mineralization of growing bone and for maintenance.

Calcium retention is less during the preschool years than during infancy, and less than it will be during adolescence. Figure 6.4 shows a theoretical calcium retention curve formulated by Stearns[55] from estimations of the amounts of calcium needed at various stages of growth. Superimposed on the curve are the results of balance studies of children on two levels of milk and vitamin D intakes. This pattern of retention follows closely the curves of voluntary calcium intakes reported for preschool children (Figure 6.3).

The major difficulties in estimating calcium requirements are the ability of the body to adapt to varying levels of intake and the influence of other dietary factors on calcium metabolism. The adaptation of the rate of ab-

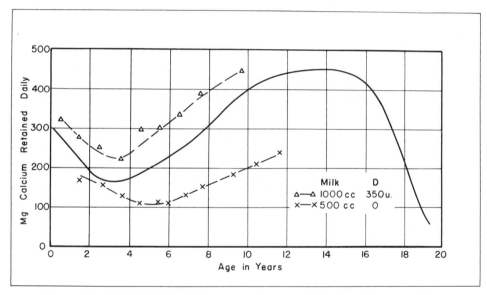

Figure 6.4   Theoretical calcium retention curve during growth, with observed retention of subjects on two levels of intake of milk and vitamin D. (Source: Stearns, G. Nutritional health of infants, children, and adolescents. In: Proceedings of the Food and Nutrition Institute, Agricultural Handbook No. 56, U.S. Department of Agriculture, Washington, D.C., 1952.)

sorption and utilization of calcium when habitual intakes are either low or high has long been recognized. In addition, the daily fluctuations in retention observed in balance studies were so great that it has been estimated that 15 to 21 days of continuous observation are necessary to get a true picture of actual retention. Absorption rates have been reported to vary from 30 to 60 percent of dietary intake,[54] influenced by the concomitant intake of vitamin D, phosphorus, lipid, phytate, oxalate, and other dietary components. Increased protein intake has been associated with increased urinary excretion of calcium.

As a result of the conflicting data on calcium metabolism and the difficulty of defining symptoms of calcium deficiency as a guide to dietary requirements, intakes recommended for the preschool child vary from one standard to another. The FAO/WHO recommendation[45] is 400 to 500 mg/day. The Canadian Dietary Standard[48] is 500 mg/day, and the RDA[44] is 800 mg/day.

Iron

There is equal uncertainty about the iron requirements of the preschool child. Historically, the RDA for iron during the early part of the preschool period has changed in parallel with the changes in allowances for the infant. Until 1958 the RDA for the child from 1 to 3 years was 7 mg/day, and for the child from 4 to 6 years 8 mg. In 1963 the values were increased to 8 mg and 10 mg respectively. In the 1968, 1974, and 1979 revisions, the allowance was raised to 15 mg/day for the child between 1 and 3 years, while the 10 mg figure was retained for the older preschool child.

The RDA is higher at the 1- to 3-year age level than other standards. The FAO/WHO recommendation[45] is 5 to 10 mg/day from 1 to 6 years, and the Canadian Dietary Standard[48] is 8 mg/day at 1 to 3 years and 9 mg/day at 4 to 6 years. Fomon[56] estimated a dietary requirement of 8 mg/day between 1 and 3 years, but suggested that the true requirement might be somewhat less.

It may be speculated that the iron requirement during the early preschool period depends on the iron status of the child at the end of the first year. If the child has had an adequate iron intake during the first year of life and therefore enters the preschool period with good iron storage and satisfactory blood levels, the risk of iron-deficiency anemia during the critical period from one to two years of age is relatively small and an intake lower than the present RDA level of 15 mg will continue to support hematopoiesis. If, on the other hand, iron nutriture is questionable or unsatisfactory toward the end of the first year, a higher intake will be protective, and a level approaching 15 mg may be indicated. This speculation is supported by the studies of Swedish children by Moe,[57] who concluded that if children received at least 10 mg/day during the first year, and especially between 8 and 12 months, they did not need more than 10 mg/day after the first year. In view of the relationship of family economic level to the risk of anemia, special attention should be given to the young preschooler from a low income family, preferably by evaluation of hemoglobin or hematocrit status and by estimation of iron storage as reflected in the saturation of transferrin.

VITAMINS

Recommended allowances for the vitamins during the preschool years have been determined primarily by interpolation from infant values to those of the adult, with estimations of growth needs. As a result, the allowances can be considered tentative pending further study.

Vitamin A

Despite findings in many United States surveys that dietary intakes of young children may be below the RDA and that serum vitamin A levels are often below the standard of 20 μg/100 ml, there was little or no supporting clinical evidence of vitamin A deficiency. In both the Ten-State Nutrition Survey[58] and the HANES survey,[59] serum vitamin A levels increased with age. The use of a single standard for all age groups may have overestimated the frequency of low serum levels in young children and underestimated the frequency in adults and the elderly.

In some developing countries vitamin A deficiency is widespread. The peak incidence of xerophthalmia occurs at 3 to 4 years of age, indicative of the greater vulnerability of the young child to nutritional deficiencies. Pure vitamin A deficiency is rarely encountered, however. Almost invariably the children with deficiency symptoms also lack other essential nutrients, and both protein-energy malnutrition and infections are commonly associated with xerophthalmia.[60] The general inadequacy of the diet as well as the interrelatedness of the absorption, transport, and metabolism of vitamin A and several other nutrients may in part account for the multiple findings.

The estimation of vitamin A requirements in various literature reports has varied with the criteria used. Optimal growth, maintenance of plasma levels, and addition of a margin for storage have been factored into some calculations. The RDA and Canadian Standard have both been based on body weight, with an arbitrary addition for growth. However, there is no fixed relationship between body size and the allowances as given. Both allowances provide for 400 RE (2000 I.U.) at 1 to 3 years, and 500 RE (2500 I.U.) at 4 to 6 years.

Hypervitaminosis A has been reported in both children and adults, but the acute form is most likely to occur in children under 3 years of age. Intakes of 20,000 I.U. or more taken daily for more than one or two months have produced symptoms of anorexia, slow growth, drying and cracking of the skin, enlargement of the liver and spleen, edema, pain in the long bones, bone fragility, and increased intracranial pressure.[7,61] Such high intakes are the result of vitamin supplementation rather than diet. The Food and Nutrition Board[44] has recommended that regular ingestion of more than 2000 RE (6700 I.U.) of preformed vitamin A above that in the diet should be carefully monitored by a physician.

Vitamin D
A recommended allowance of 10 μg (400 I.U.) is established by both the Food and Nutrition Board and FAO/WHO for children between 1 and 6 years of age. Allowing for exposure to sunlight, the Canadian Standard is lowered to 5 μg (200 I.U.)/day for children between 4 and 6 years.

Toxicity is possible at any age with large doses of vitamin D, but there is less evidence of risk for children beyond one year of age than for infants.

Vitamin E Activity
The requirement of vitamin E is related to the level of polyunsaturated fatty acids in the diet. In a diet with 4 to 7 percent of calories as linoleic acid, an allowance of 5 mg at 1 to 3 years and 6 mg at 4 to 6 years is believed to be adequate.

Vitamin K
Dietary levels and intestinal synthesis of vitamin K seem to be adequate after the period of early infancy. The estimated safe range of intake is 15 to 30 μg at 1 to 3 years and 20 to 40 μg at 4 to 6 years (Appendix 1).

Ascorbic Acid
It has been well established that 10 mg/day will prevent or cure scurvy. There is debate about the optimal intake of ascorbic acid, since there is little definite information on the requirements of preschool children. The FAO/WHO recommendation is 20 mg/day; the Canadian Dietary Standard recommends at least 20 mg/day; the RDA is 45 mg/day for the child between 1 and 6 years of age.

Some studies have found low intakes of ascorbic acid by preschool children when compared to the RDA. In the PNS[8] the intake of this vitamin was related to income. Median intakes of the lowest of four income groups increased from 24 mg in the second year to 39 mg in the sixth year by children who did not receive vitamin supplements, and in the highest income group median intakes rose from 45 mg to 67 mg. Median intakes, including supplements, ranged from 86 to 134 mg/day. The use of supplementary vitamins was also related to income; in the lowest income group 36 percent of the children were given supplements in the second year, and the number decreased to 22 percent in the sixth year. In the highest income group, the use of supplementary vitamins decreased from 84 percent to 56 percent. The correlation coefficient between vitamin C intake and plasma ascorbic acid was 0.60. Analysis of the data showed that intakes in excess of 125 mg resulted in little increase in plasma levels and the excess was probably excreted. In the 1971–1974 HANES data,[46] median ascorbic acid intakes of preschool children ranged from 40 to 54 mg/day, with the higher intakes observed among upper income families.

B Complex

Except for some studies of the thiamin and riboflavin requirements of preschool children, there are few data on which to base recommended allowances. The RDA values are shown in Appendix 1. FAO/WHO and Canadian Standards are similar to the RDA values for thiamin, riboflavin, niacin, and vitamin B_6. The 1979 RDA values are higher for folacin and vitamin B_{12}. However, these allowances are based on interpolation between infant and adult allowances.

MEETING NUTRIENT NEEDS

With the limited appetite of the preschool child, the major concern is that foods of high nutrient density should receive priority. Nutrient requirements for this age group can be met if attention is given to foods eaten between meals to ensure that they are high in nutritive value rather than primarily carbohydrate. Parents need to work out a balance between guidance of the child into good food choices and allowing the expression of independence which is essential to development. They must adopt an attitude toward the child's eating that is neither rigidly insistent on conformity nor totally permissive. There is no standard rule to follow, since the personality and standards of the parents as well as the characteristics of the child are different for each combination of parents and child. Even within a family, techniques that are effective with one child may not apply to another. However, some basic guidelines may be given.

MILK

The calcium content of milk is higher than in any other food, and it is difficult to supply adequate calcium for bone mineralization without milk in the diet. A total vegetarian (vegan) diet is not suitable for the young child unless great care is taken to ensure the quantity and balance of nutrients. Fortified soy milks are available as a substitute for cow's milk, but the inclusion of cow's milk in the child's diet offers protection for several nutrients. Yogurt, cheese, or buttermilk may be substituted if the child does not accept or tolerate whole cow's milk. Skim milk is not recommended for the child under two years of age;[56] there is little evidence to support the limitation of lipids in the diet of the young child in relation to later development of atherosclerosis, and there are more sensible ways to control weight gain.

The RDA of 800 mg of calcium can be met by the inclusion of 16 ounces of milk plus the small amounts of calcium from other foods. The additional contributions of milk to meet requirements of protein, phosphorus, riboflavin, and vitamins A and B_{12} are especially important. Milk may be consumed as a beverage, at or between meals, added to cereal and other foods, or included in the preparation of foods.

MEAT, FISH, AND POULTRY

Most children will take 1 to 3 ounces of meat, fish, or poultry per day. They prefer those that can be easily chewed, but meat cut into small pieces is a good finger food, either at or between meals. Although it is customary to serve these foods at the noon or evening meal, hamburger as a breakfast food will often be accepted by the child who resists conventional breakfast foods.

EGGS

One egg daily is usually recommended for the preschool child. Some children will eat only the yolk or only the white, but eggs may be included in foods. Baked custard, for example, is a highly nutritious dessert and usually well liked.

FRUITS AND VEGETABLES

At least four servings should be included in the daily diet. The size of servings will vary with the type and how well it is liked. Fruit is usually well accepted and a wide variety can be offered, cut into pieces for finger feeding or eaten by spoon. Citrus fruit or tomato is advisable daily for the vitamin C content. Green leafy or yellow vegetables, as high sources of carotene, should be included frequently. Potato is usually well accepted in any of a variety of forms.

Cooked vegetables may not be enthusiastically received, although most children have favorite vegetables which they will eat. However, raw vegetables are much more likely to be eaten, including carrots, peas, turnip, potato, and cauliflower. The child who may object to eating salad when it is served on a plate will probably accept the same raw vegetables when fed while the salad is being prepared. Small pieces of raw vegetables are often taken as willingly as fruit at between-meal snacks.

BREAD, CEREAL, AND PASTA

These foods are usually well accepted, although the servings may be small. Three or four servings a day may be typical, but they should be whole grain or enriched to supply a maximum of nutrients.

Within the past few years there has been concern about the use of sugar-coated cereals in the diet of the young child. When eaten with milk, there seems to be a minimum of increased risk of caries, and often the amount of sugar on the cereals is less than the child might add from the sugar bowl to a nonsugared cereal. Since sugar provides only calories and carbohydrate, its consumption by the preschool child should be limited; the substitution of honey provides little additional nutrient value, despite the mistaken belief of many mothers. However, the major hazard of sugar-coated cereals is the retention of sugar in the mouth when they are eaten dry as a snack between meals.

BUTTER, MARGARINE, AND OTHER FATS AND OILS

The increased palatability and flavor of foods to which fat is added may make the foods more acceptable to the young child. Daily intake of one to two tablespoons is recommended, with special emphasis on those containing vitamin A.

DESSERTS AND SWEETS

These foods have a place in the diet, but with the small appetite of the young preschool child they should receive little emphasis. Desserts of fruit, pudding, custard, or ice cream provide more essential nutrients than cake, pie, and other rich foods.

Too often the parents use sweets as a reward or withhold them as punishment, which places greater psychological value on them and makes them more desirable in the child's eyes. Desserts and sweets should be given no greater emphasis than other foods that are a usual part of the family diet.

CLARA M. DAVIS STUDIES

The statement is often made that if a young child is allowed to eat whatever foods he wants, he will, over time, eat a balanced diet. The person who makes that statement may refer to the work of Clara M. Davis, or may just have heard it so often that it has the stamp of truth. Any worker in the field of child nutrition should be familiar with the research as Davis conducted it; there were definite qualifications that are often ignored.

Dr. Davis[62,63] started her studies in the pediatric service of Mt. Sinai Hospital in Cleveland in 1926 and continued them at the Children's Memorial Hospital in Chicago. In all, she enrolled 15 infants between 7 and 10 months of age. For periods ranging from 6 months to 4½ years the children lived in a special nursery, with no visiting at home and no interruptions in the study. All but two of the infants had been breast fed, although some had been in institutions. None had been given solid foods prior to enrollment. Therefore they had not been conditioned by any method of feeding except by sucking.

The children were started on four meals a day, later changed to three, at specified times, with nothing but water between meals. At each meal a tray was placed on a table in front of the child; the tray contained 11 to 14 foods, each in a separate dish or glass. Each child sat at a separate table, so that one child could not influence another. A nurse sat beside the child, not speaking, not interfering, and not offering either approval or disapproval. She waited until the child indicated which food he wanted, then used a spoon to feed it to him if he opened his mouth. The children were allowed to feed themselves, either by hand or by spoon, when they were capable of it, usually by 15 to 16 months. When a dish was emptied, it was promptly refilled, and the child ate as much or as little of each food as he wanted. The position of foods was changed two to three times during the meal, so that each food was within reach.

The only foods offered were the following (an asterisk indicates foods that were served both raw and cooked):

Muscle meats (beef*, lamb, chicken)
Glandular organs (liver, kidney, brains, sweetbreads)
Fish (haddock)
Cereal (unprocessed whole wheat*, oatmeal*, barley, yellow corn meal)
Ry-Krisp
Bone marrow* and bone jelly
Eggs*
Milk, whole (raw sweet or lactic sour)
Fruits (apple*, orange, banana, tomato, peach, pineapple)
Vegetables (lettuce*, cabbage*, spinach, cauliflower, peas*, beets, carrots,
    turnips)
Sea salt
Water

Foods were cooked by low pressure steam without added water (except cereals) or salt. There were no "made" dishes, such as custard, bread, or soup, no "derived" foods, such as butter, sugar, or cheese, and no canned foods. Dishes were refilled as often as they were emptied; at a single meal one child ate 10 eggs. No limits were placed on the children, either for minimal or for maximal intake. Two infants drank no milk, one for 5 months and the other for 10 months, then resumed ordinary quantities. Salt was not put on foods, but some children ate salt plain. During the first week or two, each baby tried every food offered, but after that time most made a meal out of 3 to 4 foods and did not touch the others. Often the meals were odd; Dr. Davis used the examples of apples and liver for breakfast, raw beef and lactic milk for lunch, and orange juice, bananas, and milk for supper.

The children showed no fixed likes or dislikes, although they had waves of large amounts of a few foods, followed by normal amounts. One infant "lived for months" on orange juice, kidney, liver, egg yolk, and bone marrow. Favorite foods were meats, potato, carrots, peas, eggs, milk, apples, orange juice, and bananas. During the first six months after weaning, bone marrow was often a favorite food, but the children ate less of it as they grew older. For many, fruit constituted 50 percent of the food eaten. The most unpopular foods were spinach, lettuce, turnips, and barley. Cereals, even cooked, were often neglected and were rarely more than 8 percent of intake, even though two varieties were served at each meal.

The children had no digestive upsets and no anorexia during the study. There were no behavior problems connected with eating, and they approached each meal with enthusiasm. They were monitored for health and growth, with blood and urine analyses and X rays at intervals. Although some had infections during the study, all were "plump, solid, and looked well-nourished."

Nutrient intakes of some children during the first six months of study were published, and showed that the average protein intake was 4.6 g/kg/day, with a range of 3.5 to 7.8 g/kg in each of the monthly calculations. Caloric intake during the first six months ranged from 95 to 175 kcal/kg/day. The highest consumption was of animal proteins and fruit.

One measurement published from this study is rarely found in literature but is of interest. Loss of food and liquid averaged 39 g (range 20 to 50 g) on the bib and 17 g (range 10 to 25 g) on the sheet that was placed under the table and chair during the first six months, and 4 g and 5 g respectively (range for each 0 to 15 g) in the second six-month period.

In essence, then, the Davis studies show that children on self-selected diets may eat large amounts of some foods for a period of time, but that likes and dislikes change. However, these children had never been fed solids before the study, had not eaten in a family environment, and were fed—

with neither encouragement nor criticism—a diet that contained no sweet foods or highly processed foods of any kind. The conditions of this study are hardly applicable to children growing up in most households in the United States.

REFERENCES

1. Hamill, P.V. V., T. A. Drizd, C. L. Johnson, R. B. Reed, and A. F. Roche. *NCHS Growth Curves for Children Birth–18 Years.* DHEW Publ. No. (PHS) 78-1650. Supt. of Documents, U. S. Govt. Printing Office, Washington, D.C., 1977.
2. Hansman, C. Anthropometry and Related Data. In: McCammon, R. W. (Ed.) *Human Growth and Development.* Charles C. Thomas Co., Springfield, Ill., 1970.
3. Maresh, M. M. Linear body proportions: A roentgenographic study. *AMA J. Dis. Child. 98*:27-49, 1959.
4. Smith, D. W., W. Truog, J. E. Rogers, L. J. Greitzer, A. L. Skinner, J. J. MCann, and M. A. S. Harvey. Shifting linear growth during infancy: Illustration of genetic factors in growth from fetal life through infancy. *J. Pediat. 89*:225-230, 1976.
5. Tanner, J. M., M. J. R. Healy, R. D. Lockhart, J. D. McKenzie, and R. H. Whitehouse. Aberdeen Growth Study. I. The prediction of adult body measurements from measurements taken each year from birth to 5 years. *Arch. Dis. Child. 31*:372-381, 1956.
6. Maresh, M. M. Measurements from Roentgenograms. In: McCammon, R. W. (Ed.) *Human Growth and Development.* Charles C Thomas Co., Springfield, Ill., 1970.
7. Vaughan, V. C. III. Developmental Pediatrics. In: Vaughan, V. C. III., R. J. McKay, and W. E. Nelson. *Nelson Textbook of Pediatrics,* Tenth Edition. W. B. Saunders, Philadelphia, 1975.
8. Owen, G. M., K. M. Kram, P. J. Garry, J. E. Lowe, and A. H. Lubin. A study of nutritional status of preschool children in the United States, 1968–1970. *Pediat. 53* (Suppl. Part II):597-646, 1974.
9. Owen, G. M., and A. H. Lubin. Anthropometric differences between black and white preschool children. *Am. J. Dis. Child. 126*:168-169, 1973.
10. Garn, S. M., and D. C. Clark. Nutrition, growth, development, and maturation: Findings from the Ten-State Nutrition Survey of 1968–1970. *Pediat. 56*:306-319, 1975.
11. Habicht, J.-P., R. Martorell, C. Yarbrough, R. M. Malina, and R. E. Klein. Height and weight standards for preschool children. How rele-

vant are ethnic differences in growth potential? *Lancet 1*:611-615, 1974.

12. Robson, J. R. K., F. A. Larkin, J. H. Bursick, and K. P. Perri. Growth standards for infants and children: A cross-sectional study. *Pediat. 56*:1014-1020, 1975.

13. Owen, G. M., C. E. Nelson, and P.J. Garry. Nutritional status of preschool children: Hemoglobin, hematocrit, and plasma iron values. *J. Pediat. 76*:761-763, 1970.

14. Haughton, J. G. Nutritional anemia of infancy and childhood. *Am. J. Pub. Health 53*:1121-1126, 1963.

15. Gutelius, M. F. The problem of iron deficiency anemia in preschool Negro children. *Am. J. Pub. Health 59*:290-295, 1969.

16. Committee on Iron Nutritional Deficiencies. *Extent and Meanings of Iron Deficiency in the U.S.: Summary Proceedings of a Workshop, March 8–9, 1971.* National Academy of Sciences, Washington, D. C.

17. Garn, S. M., N. J. Smith, and D. C. Clark. Lifelong differences in hemoglobin levels between blacks and whites. *J. Nat. Med. Assoc. 67*:91-96, 1975.

18. Dallman, P. R., G. D. Barr, C. M. Allen, and H. R. Shinefield. Hemoglobin concentration in white, black, and Oriental children: Is there a need for separate criteria in screening for anemia? *Am. J. Clin. Nutr. 31*:377-380, 1978.

19. Beal, V. A. On the acceptance of solid foods, and other food patterns of infants and children. *Pediat. 20*:448-457, 1957.

20. Beal, V. A. Nutritional intake of children. II. Calcium, phosphorus, and iron. *J. Nutrition 53*:499-510, 1954.

21. Fox, H. M., B. A. Fryer, G. Lamkin, V. M. Vivian, and E. S. Eppright. Diets of preschool children in the North Central region. Calcium, phosphorus, and iron. *J. Am. Dietet. Assoc. 59*:233-237, 1971.

22. Sims, L. S., and P. M. Morris. Nutritional status of preschoolers. An ecological perspective. *J. Am. Dietet. Assoc. 64*:492-499, 1974.

23. Fomon, S. J., and T. A. Anderson (Eds.) *Practices of low-income families in feeding infants and small children, with particular attention to cultural subgroups.* Proceedings of a National Workshop. Maternal and Child Health Service, U.S. Dept. of Health, Education and Welfare, Rockville, Md., 1972.

24. Lowenberg, M. E. The development of food patterns in young children. In: Pipes, P. L. *Nutrition in Infancy and Childhood.* C. V. Mosby, St. Louis, 1977.

25. Lourie, R. S., E. M. Layman, and F. K. Millican. Why children eat things that are not food. *Children 10*:143-146, 1963.

26. Gutelius, M. F., F. K. Millican, E. M. Layman, G. J. Cohen, and C. C.

Dublin. Nutritional studies of children with pica. *Pediat. 29*:1012-1023, 1963.

27. Gutelius, M. F., F. K. Millican, E. M. Layman, G. J. Cohen, and C. C. Dublin. The treatment of pica with a vitamin and mineral supplement. *Am. J. Clin. Nutr. 12*:388-393, 1963.

28. Guinee, V. F. Pica and lead poisoning. *Nutr. Rev. 29*:267-269, 1971.

29. Hansen, J. D. L., N. Buchanon, and J. M. Pettifor. Protein Energy Malnutrition (PEM). In: McLaren, D. S., and D. Burman (Eds.) *Textbook of Paediatric Nutrition.* Churchill Livingstone, Edinburgh, 1976.

30. Viteri, F. E., and G. Arroyave. Protein-Calorie Malnutrition. In: Goodhart, R. S., and M. E. Shils (Eds.) *Modern Nutrition in Health and Disease,* Fifth Edition. Lea and Febiger, Philadelphia, 1973.

31. McLaren, D. S. The great protein fiasco. *Lancet 2*:93-96, 1974.

32. Scrimshaw, N. S. Through a glass darkly: Discerning the practical implications of human dietary protein-energy relationships. *Nutr. Rev. 35*:321-337, 1977.

33. Behar, M. Protein-calorie deficits in developing countries. *Ann. N. Y. Acad. Sci. 300*:176-187, 1977.

34. Van Duzen, J., J. P. Carter, J. Secondi, and C. Federspiel. Protein and calorie malnutrition among preschool Navajo Indian children. *Am. J. Clin. Nutr. 22*:1362-1370, 1969.

35. Van Duzen, J., J. P. Carter, and R. Vander Zwagg. Protein and calorie malnutrition among preschool Navajo Indian children. A follow-up. *Am. J. Clin. Nutr. 29*:657-662, 1976.

36. Dobbing, J. Cellular growth of the brain: Infant vulnerability. *Pediat. 55*:2-6, 1975.

37. Subcommittee on Nutrition, Brain Development, and Behavior of the Committee on International Nutrition Programs. *The Relationship of Nutrition to Brain Development and Behavior.* National Academy of Sciences, Washington, D. C., 1973.

38. Graham, G. G. Environmental factors affecting the growth of children. *Am. J. Clin. Nutr. 25*:1184-1188, 1972.

39. Barnes, R. H. Dual role of environmental deprivation and malnutrition in retarding intellectual development. *Am. J. Clin. Nutr. 29*:912-917, 1976.

40. Kallen, D. J. (Ed.) *Nutrition, Development and Social Behavior.* DHEW Publ. No. (NIH) 73-242. Supt. of Documents, U. S. Government Printing Office, Washington, D.C., 1973.

41. Brožek, J. Malnutrition and behavior. A decade of conferences. *J. Am. Dietet. Assoc. 72*:17-23, 1978.

42. Stein, Z., M. Susser, G. Saenger, and F. Marolla. *Famine and Human*

Development: The Dutch Hunger Winter of 1944–1945. Oxford Univ. Press, London, 1975.

43. Read, M. S. Malnutrition, hunger and behavior. II. Hunger, school feeding programs and behavior. *J. Am. Dietet. Assoc. 63*:386-391, 1973.

44. *Recommended Dietary Allowances,* Eighth Edition. National Academy of Sciences, Washington, D. C., 1974.

45. FAO/WHO Handbook on Human Nutritional Requirements, 1974. *Nutr. Rev. 33*:147-157, 1975.

46. Abraham, S., M. D. Carroll, C. M. Dresser, and C. L. Johnson. *Dietary Intake Findings, United States, 1971–1974.* DHEW Publication No. (HRA) 77-1647. Supt. of Documents, U. S. Government Printing Office, Washington, D. C., 1977.

47. Beal, V. A. Nutritional Intake. In: McCammon, R. W. (Ed.) *Human Growth and Development.* Charles C Thomas Co., Springfield, Ill., 1970.

48. *Dietary Standard for Canada.* Bureau of Nutritional Sciences, Department of National Health and Welfare Canada, Ottawa, 1976.

49. Widdowson, E. M., and J. W. T. Dickerson. Chemical composition of the body. In: Comar, C. L., and F. Bronner (Eds.) *Mineral Metabolism,* Vol. II. Academic Press, New York, 1963.

50. Crawford, P. B., J. H. Hankin, and R. L. Huenemann. Environmental factors associated with preschool obesity. III. Dietary intakes, eating patterns, and anthropometric measurements. *J. Am. Dietet. Assoc. 72*:589-595, 1978.

51. Fryer, B. A., G. H. Lamkin, V. M. Vivian, E. S. Eppright, and H. M. Fox. Diets of preschool children in the North Central region. Calories, protein, fat, and carbohydrate. *J. Am. Dietet. Assoc. 59*:228-232, 1971.

52. Ten-State Nutrition Survey. V. *Dietary.* DHEW Publication No. (HSM) 72-8133. Center for Disease Control, U. S. Dept. of Health, Education, and Welfare, Atlanta, Ga., 1972.

53. Irwin, M. I., and D. M. Hegsted. A conspectus of research on protein requirements of man. *J. Nutr. 101*:385-430, 1971.

54. Irwin, M. I., and E. W. Kienholz. A conspectus of research on calcium requirements of man. *J. Nutr. 103*:1019-1095, 1973.

55. Stearns, G. Nutritional health of infants, children, and adolescents. In: *Proceedings of the Food and Nutrition Institute,* Agric. Handbook No. 56, U.S. Dept. of Agriculture, Washington, D. C., 1952.

56. Fomon, S. J. *Infant Nutrition,* Second Edition. W. B. Saunders, Philadelphia, 1974.

57. Moe, P. J. Iron requirements in infancy. II. The influence of iron-fortified cereals given during the first year of life on the red blood picture of children at 1½-3 years of age. *Acta Paediatr. Scand.* *53*:423-432, 1964.

58. Ten-State Nutrition Survey. IV. *Biochemical.* DHEW Publication No. (HSM) 72-8132. Center for Disease Control, U. S. Dept. of Health, Education, and Welfare, Atlanta, Ga., 1972.

59. Abraham, S., F. W. Lowenstein, and C. L. Johnson. *Preliminary Findings of the First Health and Nutrition Examination Survey, United States, 1971-1972: Dietary Intake and Biochemical Findings.* DHEW Publication No. (HRA) 74-1219-1. Supt. of Documents, U. S. Government Printing Office, Washington, D. C., 1974.

60. Rodriguez, M. S., and M. I. Irwin. A Conspectus of Research on Vitamin A Requirements of Man. *J. Nutr. 102*:909-968, 1972.

61. Committee on Nutrition, American Academy of Pediatrics. Nutritional aspects of vegetarianism, health foods, and fad diets. *Pediat. 59*:460-463, 1977.

62. Davis, C. M. Self-selection of diets by newly weaned infants. An experimental study. *Am. J. Dis. Child. 36*:651-679, 1928.

63. Davis, C. M. Self-selection of diets. An experiment with infants. *The Trained Nurse and Hosp. Rev.* Vol. 86, May, 1931.

7

MIDDLE CHILDHOOD

The life span is a continuum with relatively few clear dividing lines between one period and the next. We have thus far based chapters in this book on physiological states, such as pregnancy and lactation, or on chronological age, arbitrarily selecting the first year as infancy and ages one to six years for the preschool period. However, the divisions for the remainder of the life span are biological and cannot be clearly circumscribed by chronological age. "Middle childhood" is here defined as beginning at six years and ending at the onset of pubertal changes. Therefore the end of this period varies between sexes and between individuals. The early-maturing girl may have the onset of acceleration of growth between 7 and 8 years of age and the late-maturing girl between 11 and 12 years. The early-maturing boy may begin his growth spurt between 9 and 10 years, and the late-maturing boy close to 14 years.

The Health Examination Survey of the National Center for Health Statistics (NCHS)[1] included children between the ages of 6 and 11 years in Cycle II and subjects from 12 to 17 years in Cycle III, but recognized that these age groups did not clearly distinguish between preadolescent and adolescent subjects. The Recommended Dietary Allowances[2] have used age groupings of 7 to 10 years and 11 to 14 years. In this chapter sources of data to 10 and 11 years are used, with an attempt to limit the discussion to the biologically prepubertal period. However, since there is a gradual flowing from childhood to puberty and adolescence, some of the characteristics of children during the early part of "middle childhood" reflect a continuation of the patterns of the preschool child, and during the latter part a transition from childhood to adolescence.

This interim period tends to be quite stable in somatic growth rates, development of physiological processes, and behavior. It is sometimes called a latent period because it is relatively more serene and has fewer problems than either the preschool period or adolescence. Growth is usually steady and linear. The child's appetite improves and food acceptances expand. Intake increases with age. Physical ability becomes more skillful and sports competition may begin. The daily routine of school provides regularity for much of the year. Independence extends to greater decision making, and access to money introduces a new aspect to food selection. Therefore, although changes are seen in this period, they are usually gradual.

PHYSICAL GROWTH

Growth in both weight and height is relatively slow between 6 years and the onset of the adolescent spurt. Sex differences are small at first, but the slightly faster growth of girls allows them to overtake and then surpass boys in both height and weight. At 6 years, boys are both taller and heavier. By 9 years the median height of girls is equal to that of boys and their median weight slightly more than that of boys in the NCHS tables[3] that are reproduced in Appendix 2. By 10 years the median girl is nearly 1 cm taller and more than 1 kg heavier than the median boy. For each sex the distributions become wider with increasing age; larger standard deviations and coefficients of variation show the greater differences between individual children as they get older.

HEIGHT AND SKELETAL MATURATION

Between 6 and 10 years the median height of boys increases from 116.1 cm to 137.5 cm, a gain of 21.4 cm, with annual increments ranging from 5.2 to 5.8 cm. The median height of girls increases from 114.6 cm to 138.3 cm, a gain of 23.7 cm, with annual increments of 5.8 to 6.5 cm.[3] The earlier maturation of girls, which will be more pronounced during puberty, is already becoming evident during childhood.

Individuality in growth rates becomes increasingly obvious during this age span. At 6 years there is a difference of approximately 16 cm between the 5th and 95th percentiles for both boys and girls. By 10 years the difference has expanded, and the child at the 95th percentile is 20 to 22 cm taller than the child at the 5th percentile. The early onset of pubertal changes in

298

girls accounts for some of the dispersion, but a similarly wide distribution of heights is also seen in boys.

Racial differences in growth in stature were relatively small in the Cycle II findings of the Health Examination Survey (HES) of NCHS.[1,4] Throughout the span from 6 to 11 years there were only slight differences in the heights of black and white boys. Black girls tended to be taller than white girls and, on the average, even taller than black or white boys. The small differences in stature were not considered to be of significance in evaluation, but body proportions were different. Black children had longer legs and shorter trunks, with consequently lower sitting heights, than white children. This finding was consistent for both sexes throughout the age span.

Increment in leg length tends to be greater than increment in trunk length between 6 and 11 years. There is little growth in head size. As a result, sitting height relative to total height decreases. This was shown in Figure 1.13 from data of the Child Research Council.[5] In the HES findings,[4] sitting height decreased from a mean of nearly 53 percent of height to 50.8 percent of height in black children and from 54.7 percent to slightly more than 52 percent in white children between 6 and 10 years.

Skeletal maturation was evaluated in HES by hand–wrist X rays.[6] There was a slight positive relationship between the degree of maturation and socioeconomic status. Black boys and girls were more advanced in skeletal development than white children, but the differences were not large enough for the establishment of separate standards. As expected, girls were more advanced than boys. At 9 years, 1 percent of the girls had reached "adult" bone ossification, and by 11 years 12 percent were judged adult, but no boys fell into this classification at 11 years.

WEIGHT AND ANTHROPOMETRIC MEASUREMENTS

Median weight of males in the NCHS data[3] increased from 20.7 kg at 6 years to 31.4 kg at 10 years, with an annual increment that rose from 2.2 kg to 3.9 kg with increasing age. Girls had higher weight increments, rising from 2.3 kg in the 7th year to 4.4 kg in the 10th year, with median weight increasing from 19.5 kg at 6 years to 32.6 kg at 10 years. The dispersion of weights was even greater than for heights. The boy or girl at the 95th percentile was approximately 9.5 kg heavier than a child at the 5th percentile at 6 years, but by 10 years the difference was 21 to 23 kg between these two percentile levels.

The greater weight gain of girls during this age span is accompanied by wider skinfold measurements. The triceps, subscapular, and midaxillary skinfold measurements in the HES[7] showed a steady increase with age for both sexes, although there was little change in the 5th and 10th percentiles for boys. Girls generally have skinfolds about 25 percent thicker than those of boys at the same age for the same site. Even among boys and girls of the same weight, girls have a greater amount of fat, indicating a true difference in body composition. The Seltzer-Mayer standards[8] for evaluation of obesity from triceps measurements during this age span also are 25 percent higher for girls. The minimum triceps skinfold indicating obesity rises from 12 mm to 16 mm for boys, and from 15 mm to 20 mm for girls between 6 and 10 years.

Measurements of girth, breadth, and length of body segments in the HES[4] also reflected sex differences in growth. Boys tended to have larger measurements of the hand, foot, and torso. Girls were larger in the buttocks and thigh areas, related in part to their greater deposition of soft tissues.

Racial differences were found in the HES in weight[1] and skinfold thicknesses[7] as well as in body proportions. Black boys were leaner than white boys throughout the span from 6 to 11 years, based on weight–height ratios. Black girls were leaner than white girls at the beginning of the age span, but by 10 years there was little racial difference. The distribution of fat was different, however, since white children of both sexes had median triceps measurements 25 percent higher than black children. In fact, white boys had more upper arm fat than black girls, suggesting "that racial mechanisms predominate over sex mechanisms as determinants of limb fat."[7] There was less racial difference in measurements of subscapular and midaxillary fat thickness, suggesting greater effect of sex than race on trunk measurements.

The changes in widths of bone, muscle, and fat as measured from X rays of children enrolled in the longitudinal studies of the Child Research Council were shown in Figure 1.15. Dietary intakes of 22 boys from birth to 10 years of age were analyzed in relation to weight and fat widths.[9] For this group, correlation coefficients of total caloric intake or the excess of intake over basal calories with weight, weight increment between 1 and 10 years, weight–height ratio, or fat widths were positive, but not statistically significant. They ranged from 0.13 for average caloric intake during the 10 years and weight at 10 years to 0.30 for caloric intake and weight–height ratio at 10 years. However, when the data were analyzed on the basis of the change in fat widths of each individual child, the correlation with energy intake was 0.42, which was statistically significant.

The individuality of energy requirements and food utilization as well as weight changes and fat deposition may be seen in subjects selected from this series. Boy 653 (Figure 7.1) had a low caloric intake throughout the first 10 years that rarely reached the median for boys. His weight maintained a position close to the 25th percentile. Fat widths were consistently in the lower

300

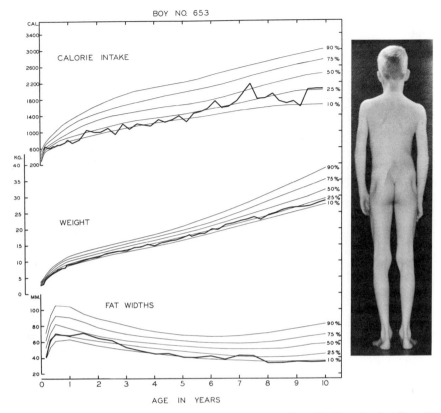

Figure 7.1   Calorie intake, weight, and fat widths of a boy in the first 10 years of life, plotted against the group percentiles for males, Child Research Council series.

half of the distribution, and remained close to the 10th percentile after 3 years of age. His photograph at 10 years shows a lean boy with little excess body fat. Boy 570 (Figure 7.2) is equally lean, but his energy intake after the first year was close to the median for males in the study. Boy 570 was athletically inclined and spent most of his free time in active sports. It can be assumed that much of his caloric intake was expended on physical activity.

Children may gain excessive weight at any age. Although there have been attempts to define ages when adiposity is most likely to develop, it can be observed in individuals at any age, either suddenly or gradually. This may be seen in the examples of boys whose fat widths increased during the first 10 years. Boy 659 (Figure 7.3) had a steady increase in caloric intake channel during the first 2 to 3 years, and thereafter maintained a position usually

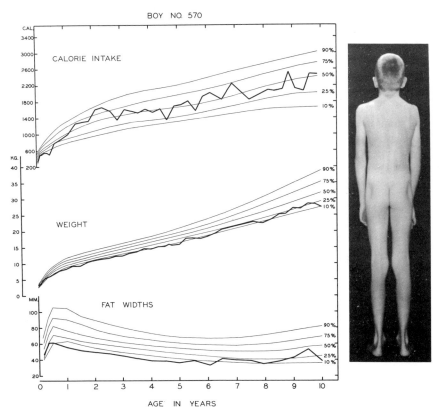

Figure 7.2 Calorie intake, weight, and fat widths of a boy in the first 10 years of life, plotted against the group percentiles for males, Child Research Council series.

above the 90th percentile, with occasional periods of dietary restriction that dropped his intake below the 75th percentile but were not maintained. His body weight was usually in the top 10 percent of the group, and fat measurements climbed to a level above the 90th percentile during the early school years. He became more obese during adolescence.

Concern about adiposity and attempts during childhood to control excessive fat are not often successful. This is shown by Boy 969 (Figure 7.4), who began to deposit excessive adipose tissue after 4 years of age and whose weight steadily increased. In his sixth year both his mother and his pediatrician became concerned about the change, and thereafter he was placed on dietary restrictions. The periods of severe restriction resulted in temporary

302   MIDDLE CHILDHOOD

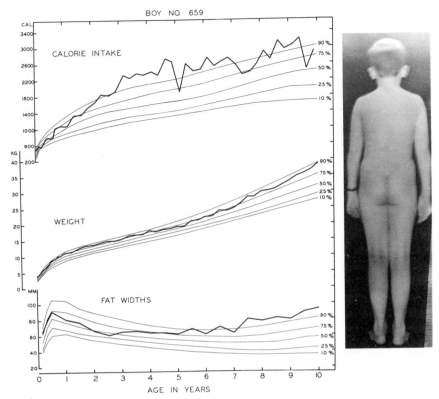

Figure 7.3 Calorie intake, weight, and fat widths of a boy in the first 10 years of life, plotted against the group percentiles for males, Child Research Council series.

decreases in measurements, but the overall trend was toward increasing weight and increasing fat widths. To ensure that he did not obtain food outside the home, he was driven to and from school and was brought home for lunch. As he became more obese, he withdrew from active sports and spent most of his free time reading or watching television. The decrease in physical energy expenditure obviously offset the value of the dietary limitation.

The patterns of weight increase in two brothers suggest the effects of heredity (Figure 7.5). Their mother was short and overweight, and their father very tall and thin. Both boys had low body weights until 8 years, then rose from the 10th to the 75th percentile of weight by 10 years. The younger brother (642) had slightly wider fat measurements after infancy than the

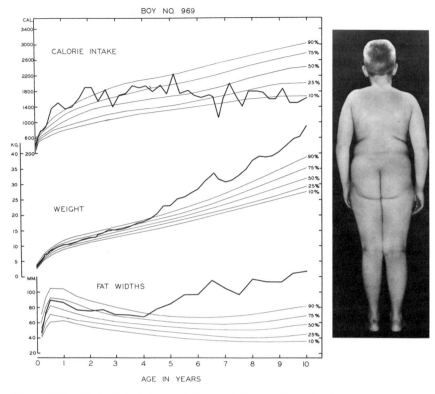

Figure 7.4   Calorie intake, weight, and fat widths of a boy in the first 10 years of life, plotted against the group percentiles for males, Child Research Council series.

older brother, but both had increased fat deposition between 8 and 10 years and were above the 90th percentile by 10 years. Neither boy had a remarkably high caloric intake when compared to the group standards, but the gain in weight and fat indicated that for them as individuals their intake exceeded expenditure. Both became more obese as adolescents, but the older boy increased greatly in stature and was tall and stocky but not obese as a young adult. The younger brother remained short and obese.

The individuality of caloric needs and expenditure is difficult to quantify. The caloric intake of Boy 570, who remained thin, was similar to those of the two brothers, who became obese. Even allowing for the measured differences in basal metabolic rates, there was obviously a different pattern of caloric utilization. The intake of a child in relation to his own needs is more significant than his intake in relation to a group distribution.

304

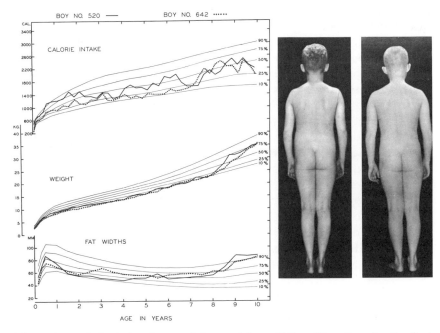

Figure 7.5 Calorie intakes, weight, and fat widths of brothers in the first 10 years of life, plotted against the group percentiles for males, Child Research Council series.

DENTAL DEVELOPMENT AND CARIES FORMATION

The eruption of the permanent dentition begins at about 6 years. In the 7th year, the first molars, central incisors, and probably the mandibular lateral incisors will have appeared in the mouth. By 10 years, four to six of the mandibular permanent teeth may have erupted, and three of the maxillary teeth. Calcification, which began within the first three to four postnatal months, continues in the teeth even after eruption.

Caries in the deciduous teeth reach a maximum prevalence at 6 to 8 years,[10] but of greater concern is the development of caries in the permanent dentition. The Ten-State Nutrition Survey found an average of 3 to 4 permanent teeth already carious at 10 years.[11] The three factors that have been identified as influencing the development of caries are the susceptibility of the tooth, the presence in the mouth of a fermentable carbohydrate, and bacteria capable of fermenting the carbohydrate. The bacteria in plaque on the tooth's surface ferment the carbohydrate, forming organic acids that act on the enamel, exposing the tooth to decay.[12]

Adequate nutrients during tooth formation are essential to the integrity of the tooth structure. The deposition of calcium and phosphorus as hydroxyapatite crystals in the protein matrix of the tooth is aided by vitamin D. Vitamin A is essential in the formation of enamel, and ascorbic acid in the formation of dentin. The incorporation of fluoroapatite increases the resistance of the tooth to decay. Since tooth formation occurs over a period of years, and is influenced by heredity, hormones, and other factors, the specific effect of nutrition is assumed but cannot be directly measured. After eruption of the teeth, the measurable effect of diet has been limited to fluorine, which may decrease caries prevalence by as much as 50 to 60 percent, and to the kind and timing of carbohydrate consumption, which may increase caries prevalence. Sucrose is a readily fermentable carbohydrate; its effect is greater if it is present in the mouth for an extended period of availability to the bacteria. Most conducive to tooth decay are candy and other sweet foods that adhere to the tooth surface or are slowly dissolved in the mouth. Honey, molasses, brown sugar, and dried fruits, as well as refined sugars, all seem to have significantly high cariogenic potential.[12]

PHYSIOLOGICAL DEVELOPMENT RELATED TO NUTRITION

The child between 6 and 10 years is still growing at a relatively slow but steady rate, and is considered a low risk insofar as most nutritional problems are concerned. Hemoglobin formation keeps pace with increased blood supply, and both hemoglobin and hematocrit rise somewhat during these years. Incidence of respiratory infections may be relatively high during the early school years, but resistance gradually increases. The child is not wholly free from nutrition-related problems, however.

LACTOSE INTOLERANCE

Lactase is a specific disaccharidase that hydrolyzes lactose to glucose and galactose in the brush border of mucosal cells in the small intestine. Milk and its derivatives are the only foods that contain lactose. Lactase activity is high in all mammals at birth, and remains high throughout the suckling period. In most mammals the activity of the enzyme declines when it is no longer needed after weaning. In the human, however, the decline of lactase activity is not universal, and is apparently governed by a combination of hereditary, dietary, and adaptive factors.

Among the populations that have been studied, high lactase levels are maintained consistently throughout life in 65 to 100 percent of adults in northern and western Europe and their descendants, and in some groups in Africa, India, and Pakistan, primarily herders or people who maintain milk-producing animals. In contrast, some degree of lactase deficiency has been reported in 60 to 100 percent of adults in many African blacks, Orientals, Latins, Eskimos, North and South American Indians, Australian aborigines, Southeast Asians, and some other population groups.[13] The age when lactase activity decreases in these people has not been extensively studied, but is believed to be in later childhood or in adolescence.

There are many different physiological kinds of intolerance to lactose. Lactase deficiency as an inborn error of metabolism is rare, and is identifiable with the first feedings of the neonate. Allergy to milk or its constituents has a different pattern of etiology. Lactose intolerance is recognized as part of the syndrome of protein–energy malnutrition, but may be related to atrophy of the mucosal cells. The intolerance with which we are concerned here occurs in otherwise healthy individuals. Lactose is well tolerated in infancy and early childhood, and then in some individuals the level of lactase activity gradually declines to the point of deficiency.

When mucosal lactase is deficient, lactose is not hydrolyzed and therefore is poorly absorbed. It passes unchanged into the large intestine. Its hyperosmolar effect results in drawing a large volume of water into the gut. Bacterial fermentation of the lactose causes formation of carbon dioxide, lactic acid, and other irritant volatile acids. Symptoms of distention, cramps, diarrhea, or general discomfort may appear within 1 to 24 hours after ingestion of lactose. The intensity of symptoms and their duration are related to the quantity of lactose consumed and the level of lactase activity in the individual.[14,15]

Lactose tolerance can be measured by administration of a load test of 50 to 100 g lactose in an aqueous suspension; sometimes the dose is set at 1 to 2 g/kg body weight. In malabsorption, fasting blood glucose levels do not increase above 20 mg/100 ml within two hours.[13,15] A biopsy of jejunal mucosa usually indicates that the cells are histologically normal but deficient in lactase activity.[13] The level of expired hydrogen after a test dose of lactose is another diagnostic tool. Since this defect is specific for lactase and does not involve other disaccharidases, it has been speculated that it is a dominant genetic defect with delayed manifestation or that it is an acquired trait due to the regression of enzyme activity as a result of a low-lactose diet. The malabsorption is related to race and to age.

Not all malabsorbers are milk-intolerant.[13-18] Many individuals with a flat glucose curve in a lactose tolerance test can consume milk in moderate amounts without symptoms. There has been criticism of the load test with a dose of 50 g lactose, which is equivalent to the lactose in a liter of milk, an amount greater than usual consumption at a time. Even a low dose, such as 1 g lactose/kg, is equivalent to 25 g lactose, or ½ liter of milk, for the average 8-year-old child. Milk consumed in smaller servings may cause no symptoms. There has also been some evidence that lactose is better tolerated in whole milk than in an aqueous suspension,[17] and that milk consumed with a meal is better tolerated than either aqueous lactose or milk consumed by itself.[13] In tests of malabsorbing children, only 50 to 55 percent have had symptoms of discomfort after consumption of milk; 70 to 90 percent of adult malabsorbers have been reported to have symptoms. However, in some studies in which adults or children with normal absorption have been used as controls, 20 to 30 percent of these normal controls have also had similar symptomatology after drinking milk,[18] so not all symptoms reported can be attributed to lactase deficiency.

The age when lactose malabsorption becomes prevalent has not been intensively studied. In a group of 69 black children, Garza and Scrimshaw[16] found a prevalence of 11 percent at 4 to 5 years, 50 percent at 6 to 7 years, and 72 percent at 8 to 9 years, although none of the children in this series had adverse symptoms after ingestion of 240 ml of milk. The prevalence of symptoms increased with higher intakes at a single serving.

The practical application of available data on the age and prevalence of lactase deficiency in some racial groups influences the recommendation of inclusion of milk in their diets. Although some extreme statements have been made that milk should not be recommended for black children or pregnant women and should not be used in international programs for the prevention or treatment of protein-energy malnutrition, a more widely accepted approach is that drinking moderate amounts of milk has no apparent adverse effects on most children and is nutritionally beneficial.[19] Since lactose malabsorption, as determined by load test, and milk intolerance are not synonymous terms, individual responses to milk ingestion are better guides than absorption tests. Most individuals who experience gastrointestinal symptoms learn to limit their consumption to levels that they tolerate without discomfort. In the HANES findings of 1971–1974, there was little difference between the races in milk consumption of persons 1 to 74 years of age.[20]

For those individuals who are intolerant of whole milk or who restrict intake to low levels, substitute products are available and should be recommended during any period of growth. Fermented milk, such as yogurt or buttermilk, is usually well tolerated, as are fermented or aged cheeses, including Swiss and cheddar. Low-lactose milks and milks in which the lactose has been enzymatically hydrolyzed by bacterial action have been commercially produced.

PSYCHOSOCIAL–BIOLOGICAL INTERACTIONS
HYPERACTIVITY

Hyperactivity is a poorly defined combination of symptoms, primarily behavioral, that has been estimated to have a prevalence between 3 and 20 percent of all schoolchildren in the United States. The lack of precise definition and the heterogeneity of classifications have led to confusion; terms such as hyperactivity, hyperkinesis, minimal brain dysfunction, and learning disabilities have all been used, and attempts by professional groups to narrow the definitions have been generally unsuccessful. Behavioral characteristics include short attention span, easy distractibility, impulsive behavior, overactivity, resistance to discipline, restlessness, emotional lability, and learning disabilities.[21]

Although hyperactivity has been reported in preschool children, it is difficult to diagnose until the child enters school, a situation that demands attention and sedentary behavior. The children are of normal intelligence but fail to learn at a normal rate and are often disruptive in the classroom. It may affect only one child in a family, often the oldest. The male-to-female ratio has been reported in various groups as 4:1 to 10:1. Symptomatology may diminish at puberty, but some workers have suggested that behavioral problems of adolescents and adults may sometimes be sequelae of earlier hyperactivity.

Therapy with central nervous stimulants, such as methylphenidate or amphetamines, or with other drugs has often been effective in amelioration of symptoms. More recently behavioral modification techniques have been used. The etiology is not clear, perhaps because of the diverse nature of the characteristics involved. When organic disease has been ruled out, factors that have been investigated or suggested in the causation of hyperactivity include genetics, perinatal hypoxia or other damage, and psychological and environmental conditions ranging from lead poisoning to family disruption, singly or in combination.

Food intake was proposed as a cause of hyperactivity by Feingold[22] in a popular book published in 1975; he stated that improvement in nearly 50 percent of his subjects could be accomplished by dietary changes. Feingold speculated that naturally occurring salicylates in foods and food additives of low molecular weight, specifically artificial flavors and colors, caused hyperactive behavior in children who have "genetic variations which predispose them to reaction." Since publication of the book, Feingold associations have been organized throughout the country and the diets of many children have been changed to the diet he recommended.

Since Feingold based his recommendation on subjective impressions and did no controlled studies, conferences were organized under two different sponsors[23,24] to review available data, and recommended carefully controlled double-blind crossover studies to test his hypothesis. The protocol included establishment of a definition of subjects, evaluation of the base diet, elimination of medication, alteration of the control and experimental diets, and repeated evaluations of the child by parents and teacher on a standardized questionnaire. Because of the placebo effect due to expectations and desire for success, this type of diet is difficult to devise without the parents and children being aware of its content. The studies with most scientific potential have supplied all food to the families in both experimental and control periods, comparable in appearance, taste, and palatability. Alternatively, or as a second study to test children who respond to the dietary restrictions with improved behavior, a specially prepared cookie or candy with or without the suspected additives has been given as a challenge and subsequent behavior observed.

To date the studies have not supported the degree of success reported by Feingold, and results have been inconclusive. The behavior ratings by parents and by teachers on either the control or the experimental diet have often not agreed; in some studies parents have reported improved behavior when teachers did not, and vice versa. However, two studies[25-27] noted that parents reported improvement on the Feingold diet only when it followed the ordinary diet, but not when the order was reversed. Even then the success rate did not reach the level reported by Feingold.

Relatively few preschool children have been studied, but there is some evidence that younger children may be more sensitive to food substances than older children. Further studies are in progress with both age groups to determine the conditions under which a child may respond to food additives. A consensus has emerged, however, that the studies thus far do not justify advocating sweeping changes in foods or in the diets of children.

NUTRIENT REQUIREMENTS AND RECOMMENDED DIETARY ALLOWANCES

Balance studies on children between 6 and 10 years of age have concentrated primarily on nitrogen and calcium, and the results have often not been in agreement. Most of the values for recommended allowances have been determined by interpolation, with arbitrary allowances for growth in the absence of more specific information.

ENERGY

The mean RDA for children 7 to 10 years of age is 2400 kcal (10.1 MJ) for both sexes, with an average weight of 28 kg. Both FAO/WHO[28] and the Canadian Dietary Standard[29] have used the age category 7 to 9 years. The FAO/WHO energy level is 2190 kcal (9.2 MJ) with an average weight of 28.1 kg. The Canadian Standard has provided separate figures for the sexes, with 2200 kcal (9.2 MJ) for boys and 2000 kcal (8.4 MJ) for girls, with average weights of 30 kg for both.

The RDA values are higher than most observed intakes in this age group. The HANES[30] data for 1971–1974 found that median intakes of boys rose from 1986 to 2051 kcal and of girls from 1774 to 1799 kcal between 6 and 9 years. In the Harvard growth study,[31] mean intakes between 6 and 10 years rose from 1970 to 2235 kcal for boys and from 1845 to 2125 kcal for girls. In the same age interval median intakes of boys in the Child Research Council[32] rose from 1780 to 2330 kcal and of girls from 1605 to 1900 kcal. Black children in the HANES data had generally lower average intakes than white children, but when income was taken into account, the differences were not always in the same direction.

Energy intakes per kilogram of body weight were similar in the HANES and in the Child Research Council series. During the age span from 6 to 10 years, median intakes of boys decreased from 87 to 71 kcal/kg and of girls from 78 to 61 kcal/kg in the latter series.

PROTEIN

The RDA for protein for both sexes in the 7 to 10 year age group is 34 g, which is equivalent to 1.2 g/kg or 5.7 percent of the caloric recommendation. The FAO/WHO recommendation is 25 g/day, equivalent to 0.9 g/kg or 4.6 percent of the energy recommended for the age group 7 to 9 years. The Canadian Dietary Standard is 33 g, or 1.22 g/kg, which is 6.0 to 6.7 percent of the energy allowances.

Irwin and Hegsted,[33] in summarizing 11 metabolic studies that have been done on 250 children since 1921, reported that estimates of protein requirement for the age group between 6 and 12 years ranged from 0.7 to 2.8 g/kg, with part of the difference attributed to variations in caloric intake. Nitrogen retention in one study was positive when protein comprised 15 percent of calories, although in another study previously malnourished children had positive nitrogen retention when 8 to 13 percent of calories were derived from protein.

The decrease in the RDA recommendation for protein since 1958, from 60 g/day to the current level of 34 g/day has resulted in lowering the protein from 2.2 g/kg to 1.2 g/kg and the percent of calories from 11.4 to 5.7. This change has reflected a trend away from using the early balance data and the usual intakes of well-nourished children as the major determinants of recommendations toward using a theoretical calculation of the requirements during growth as a factorial basis for setting the allowance levels.

Mean or median intakes of children in HANES,[30] the Harvard growth study[31] and the Child Research Council[32] have ranged from 57 to 72 g/day at the 6 to 7 year level to 66 to 84 g/day in the 9 to 10 year groups. These intakes are equivalent to a range of 13 to 15 percent of calories.

MINERALS

Calcium

Balance studies of calcium must be interpreted with caution because of the well-established ability of the body to adapt to varying levels of intake. As calcium intake is increased, retention increases, but retention is also influenced by age, rate of growth, and the presence of vitamin D. Negative balances in children have been reported on intakes of calcium lower than 23 mg/kg.[34] Estimated requirements for growth and maintenance have ranged from 0.69 to 0.85 g/day at 6 years, increasing to 1.00 to 1.53 g/day at 12 years, taking into account availability and utilization of dietary calcium.

In addition to the variable factors in calcium balance studies, the lack of identifiable symptomatology as a result of calcium deficiency has led to a difference of opinion on calcium allowances.[35] The RDA has continued to recommend an intake of 800 mg/day from 7 to 10 years of age. The FAO/WHO recommendation is 400 to 500 mg, and the Canadian Standard is intermediate at 700 mg.

Median intakes in the HANES survey during this age span ranged from 700 to 900 mg in black subjects to 960 to 1160 mg/day in white subjects, with intakes of boys higher than of girls. Median intakes in the Child Research Council series increased from 1.05 to 1.27 g/day for boys and from 0.92 to 1.06 g/day for girls between 6 and 10 years of age.

Iron

In a search of the literature, Bowering et al.[36] found only two balance studies of iron on children in this age group, although blood levels, especially hemoglobin concentration, have been determined on several thousand children. Mean hemoglobin concentrations have usually ranged between 11.2 and 13.7 g/100 ml. Although many studies have reported iron intakes of some children below the recommendations for this age group, iron-deficiency anemia is not a major problem.

Both the RDA and the Canadian Dietary Standard are established at a level of 10 mg/day. The FAO/WHO recommendation is 5 to 10 mg.

Other Minerals

The RDA for phosphorus is 800 mg, for iodine 120 μg, for magnesium 250 mg, and for zinc 10 mg for the age range of 7 to 10 years. The Canadian Standard is 150 mg for magnesium and 7 mg for zinc; other levels are similar to those of the United States. Estimated safe ranges of intake of other trace elements are shown in Appendix 1.

312

VITAMINS

The RDAs for vitamins are shown in Appendix I. Although several dietary surveys have found low intakes of vitamin A and ascorbic acid among some population groups within this age span, clinical symptoms of deficiency have rarely been observed.

There is difference of opinion on the recommendation for ascorbic acid at this age, as well as at other ages. The RDA has consistently been higher than the recommendations of other countries. For example, the RDA for ascorbic acid at 7 to 10 years is 45 mg. The FAO/WHO recommendation is 20 mg, and the Canadian Dietary Standard intermediate at 30 mg. The RDA values tend to be slightly higher than the other two standards for most vitamins of the B complex, and appreciably higher for folacin and vitamin B_{12}.

MEETING NUTRIENT NEEDS

During the early part of this age span there may be some residual of the poor appetite of the preschooler, but in general there is a gradual rise in intake and increasing acceptance of a variety of foods. Studies of plate waste in the school lunch program have shown that there is more waste in the early grades than in the upper grades. Food refusals are highest for vegetables and mixed casseroles, and lowest for milk, fruit, and desserts. As the child grows older, food refusals become fewer in number, but individual likes and dislikes of food may become more pronounced.

The healthy child who is moderately active will have an increasing appetite and a progressively larger intake of food that will meet nutrient requirements unless given too much access to foods high in carbohydrates. Emphasis should be placed on foods with high nutrient density, with attention to sources of vitamin A and ascorbic acid, which have often been reported low at this age.

Calcium needs can be met by the inclusion of at least 16 ounces of milk daily, although many school-age children willingly consume 24 ounces or more. Protein allowances can readily be achieved by 16 ounces of milk with the addition of meat (2 to 3 ounces), an egg, and additional plant sources. Peanut butter sandwiches often become a favorite of children and are good sources of protein, minerals, and vitamins of the B complex. Citrus fruit or another good source of ascorbic acid should be part of the daily routine, and green leafy or yellow vegetables served 3 to 4 times per week. The daily diet should include, in all, 3 to 4 servings of fruit or vegetables and 3 to 4 servings of whole grain or enriched bread or cereal. Fats on or in foods add to palatability and flavor, and usual intake is 1 to 2 tablespoons daily. Legumes and other protein-containing plant foods may be substituted for meat or eggs. If cow's milk is not served in the home, calcium-enriched soy milk should be provided for growing children rather than tea or soft drinks in order to provide the necessary calcium. Additional foods, including desserts, should be provided to satisfy caloric needs.

The importance of meeting energy needs during growth was shown in the study of Macy and Hunscher.[37] Even with a protein intake of 3 g/kg (14–16 percent of calories), as little as 10 kcal/kg difference in intake made a difference in the growth rate of healthy children between 4 and 9 years of age. Although there is a trend toward lowering the recommended allowances of protein, many early studies, including those of Macy and Hunscher, showed the importance of adequate protein to support a high level of nitrogen retention, and sufficient energy intake to protect the protein from deamination and conversion to energy.

The change in life-style of many families in the past few decades has led to more casual eating practices and fewer family gatherings for the traditional three meals a day. Many schoolchildren are left to prepare their own breakfasts, often without supervision. In a one-day survey of 80,000 children in Massachusetts,[38] nearly 20 percent of children in grades 1 to 3 had no breakfast or one that was rated poor; the number nearly doubled in grades 4 to 6. This report was appropriately entitled "You cannot teach a hungry child." When a child goes to school after having eaten no food since the previous evening, he is likely to be lethargic, hypoglycemic, and unable to concentrate on classwork, although few rigorous studies have been done to test school performance.[39] The Child Nutrition Act, passed by the U.S. Congress in 1966, provided a partial solution by the establishment of the School Breakfast Program. At the present time, more than one million breakfasts are served on each school day, primarily to children who live in low income areas or who travel long distances to school. However, not all school districts participate in the program. The problem of school attendance without breakfast may now be more common among children in middle and upper income families in districts without a school breakfast program.

Availability of food in the home does not ensure adequate nutrient intake for each family member, nor is the food shared equally even by children in the family. Individual choice of the type and amount of food consumed varies from one child to another. Three examples of the intakes of energy, protein, and calcium by like-sexed siblings are shown in Figures 7.6, 7.7, and 7.8, compared to the Child Research Council medians for the appropriate sex.[40]

314

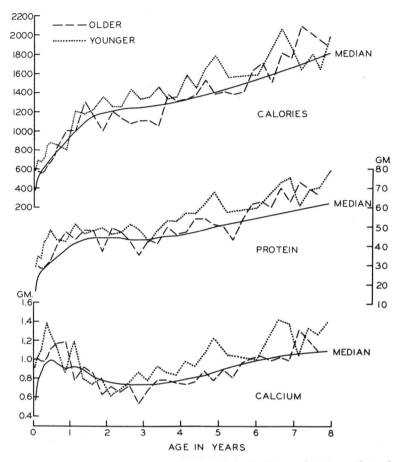

Figure 7.6   Calorie, protein, and calcium intakes of sisters, plotted against medians for girls, Child Research Council series. (Source: Beal, V. A. Dietary intake of individuals followed through infancy and childhood. Am. J. Public Health 51:1107–1117, 1961.)

The first pair are sisters, approximately two years apart in age. The younger sister consumed slightly more at comparable ages than the older sister, but the differences are small, and their intakes were close to the median for each nutrient.

The brothers in Figure 7.7 were also shown in Figure 7.5 as examples of siblings with similar gain in weight. Energy intake of the older boy was close

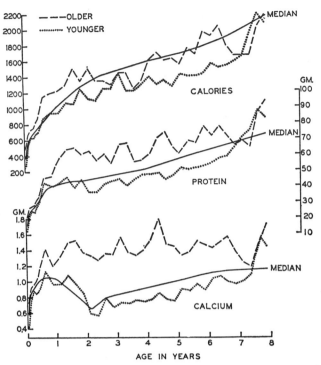

Figure 7.7 Calorie, protein, and calcium intakes of brothers, plotted against medians for boys, Child Research Council series. (Source: Beal, V. A. Dietary intake of individuals followed through infancy and childhood. Am. J. Public Health 51:1107–1117, 1961.)

to the group median, but his milk intake was consistently high, even during the preschool period, providing a calcium intake close to the maximum in this series and a relatively high protein intake. In contrast, his younger brother decreased milk intake during the preschool years in a pattern similar to the group median, resulting in lower intakes of calcium and protein. His increase in appetite and milk consumption after he reached school age led to intakes similar to those of his older brother after 7 years.

The brothers in Figure 7.8 ate very differently after infancy. The intake of the older brother was close to the group median for boys, with a rise after he entered school. In contrast, his younger brother had a large appetite. He usually had second servings and finished whatever food might be left at the end of the meal, and frequently prepared elaborate snacks for himself in the afternoon. His weight–height ratio and skinfold thicknesses were higher than his brother's.

MIDDLE CHILDHOOD

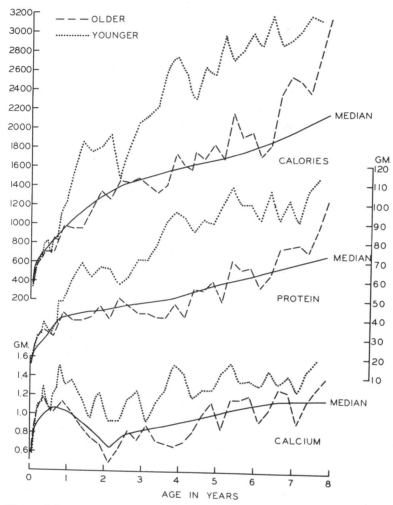

Figure 7.8   Calorie, protein, and calcium intakes of brothers, plotted against medians for boys, Child Research Council series. (Source: Beal, V. A. Dietary intake of individuals followed through infancy and childhood. Am. J. Public Health 51:1107–1117, 1961.)

The child of school age, although assuming greater independence in food, both at and between meals, needs guidance by parents or other caretakers in the selection of foods that are high in protein, minerals, and vitamins so that growth may not be compromised.Food patterns acquired at this age are likely to become life-long practices. The attitudes and standards of parents and older family members are often imitated, and should be good models for the child. Peer pressures become gradually more pronounced as the child grows older; for some children this leads to acceptance of foods that they formerly rejected, but for others it may lead to excessive intake of foods high in carbohydrate, such as candy and soft drinks.

As the child nears the end of this early school period and approaches the increased growth and nutrient demands of adolescence, he will be better able to cope with those stresses if he enters adolescence in good nutritional status and with food patterns that will contribute to optimal health.

REFERENCES

1. Hamill, P. V. V., F. E. Johnston, and W. Grams. *Height and Weight of Children, United States.* Public Health Service, Publ. No. 1000—Series 11—No. 104. Supt. of Documents, U. S. Government Printing Office, Washington, D. C., 1970.
2. *Recommended Dietary Allowances,* Eighth Edition. National Academy of Sciences, Washington, D. C., 1974.
3. Hamill, P. V. V., T. A. Drizd, C. L. Johnson, R. B. Reed, and A. F. Roche. *NCHS Growth Curves for Children Birth*-18 Years, United States. DHEW Publ. No. (PHS) 78-1650. Supt. of Documents, U. S. Government Printing Office, Washington, D. C., 1977.
4. Malina, R. M., P. V. V. Hamill, and S. Lemeshow. *Body Dimensions and Proportions, White and Negro Children 6-11 Years, United States.* DHEW Publ. No. (HRA) 75-1625. Supt. of Documents, U. S. Government Printing Office, Washington, D. C., 1974.
5. Hansman, C. Anthropometry and Related Data. In: McCammon, R. W. (Ed.) *Human Growth and Development.* Charles C Thomas Co., Springfield, Ill., 1970.
6. Roche, A. F., J. Roberts, and P. V. V. Hamill. *Skeletal Maturity of Children 6-11 Years, United States.* DHEW Publ. No. (HRA) 75-1622. Supt. of Documents, U. S. Government Printing Office, Washington, D. C., 1974.
7. Johnston, F. E., P. V. V. Hamill, and S. Lemeshow. *Skinfold Thickness of Children 6-11 Years, United States.* DHEW Publ. No. (HSM) 73-1602. Supt. of Documents, U. S. Government Printing Office, Washington, D. C., 1972.
8. Seltzer, C. C., and J. Mayer. A simple criterion of obesity. *Postgrad. Med. 38*:A101-107, 1965.
9. Beal, V. A., and M. M. Maresh. *Intake, weight, and body composition*

of boys to ten years of age. Presented at the International Congress of Dietetics, Stockholm, Sweden, 1965.

10. Valadian, I., and D. Porter. *Physical Growth and Development from Conception to Maturity.* Little, Brown, and Company. Boston, 1977.

11. Ten-State Nutrition Survey, 1968–1970. III. *Clinical, Anthropometry, Dental.* DHEW Publ. No. (HSM) 72-8131. Center for Disease Control, U.S. Department of Health, Education, and Welfare, Atlanta, Ga., 1972.

12. Nizel, A. E. Preventing dental caries: The nutritional factors. *Pediat. Clin. No. Amer. 24*:141–155, 1977.

13. Simoons, F. J., J. D. Johnson, and N. Kretchmer. Perspective on milk-drinking and malabsorption of lactose. *Pediat. 59*:98–109, 1977.

14. Stephenson, L. S., and M. C. Latham. Lactose tolerance tests as a predictor of milk tolerance. *Am. J. Clin. Nutr. 28*:86–88, 1975.

15. Garza, C., and N. S. Scrimshaw. Relationship of lactose intolerance to milk intolerance in young children. *Am. J. Clin. Nutr. 29*:192–196, 1976.

16. Stephenson, L. S., M. C. Latham, and D. V. Jones. Milk consumption by black and white pupils in two primary schools. *J. Am. Dietet. Assoc. 71*:258–262, 1977.

17. Leichter, J. Comparison of whole milk and skim milk with an aqueous solution in lactose tolerance testing. *Am. J. Clin. Nutr. 26*:393–396, 1973.

18. Paige, D. M., T. M. Bayless, and W. S. Dellinger, Jr. Relationship of milk consumption to blood glucose rise in lactose intolerant individuals. *Am. J. Clin. Nutr. 28*:677–680, 1975.

19. American Academy of Pediatrics Committee on Nutrition. Should milk drinking by children be discouraged? *Pediat. 53*:576–582, 1974.

20. Advance Data from Vital and Health Statistics, National Center for Health Statistics. *Selected findings: Food consumption profiles of white and black persons 1–74 years of age in the United States, 1971–74.* U. S. Dept. of Health, Education, and Welfare, Washington, D.C., June 26, 1978.

21. Ross, D. M., and S. A. Ross. *Hyperactivity: Research, Theory, Action.* John Wiley and Sons, New York, 1976.

22. Feingold, B. F. *Why Your Child is Hyperactive.* Random House, New York, 1975.

23. The National Advisory Committee on Hyperkinesis and Food Additives. *Report to the Nutrition Foundation June 1, 1975.* The Nutrition Foundation, New York.

24. *First Report of the Preliminary Findings and Recommendations of the Interagency Collaborative Group on Hyperkinesis.* Food and Drug Ad-

ministration, U.S. Department of Health, Education, and Welfare, Washington, D. C., 1976.

25. Conners, C. K., C. H. Goyette, D. A. Southwick, J. M. Lees, and P. A. Andrulonis. Food additives and hyperkinesis: A controlled double-blind experiment. *Pediat. 58*:154–166, 1976.

26. Harley, J. P., L. Tomasi, R. Ray, P. Eichman, C. Matthews, R. Chun, E. Traisman, and C. Cleeland. *An Experimental Evaluation of Hyperactivity and Food Additives, 1977—Phase I.* University of Wisconsin, Madison, 1977.

27. Harley, J. P., C. G. Matthews, and P. L. Eichman. *An Experimental Evaluation of Hyperactivity and Food Additives, 1977—Phase II.* University of Wisconsin, Madison, 1977.

28. FAO/WHO Handbook on Human Nutritional Requirements, 1974. *Nut. Rev. 33*:147–157, 1975.

29. *Dietary Standard for Canada.* Bureau of Nutritional Sciences, Department of National Health and Welfare. Ottawa, 1976.

30. Abraham, E., M. D. Carroll, C. M. Dresser, and C. L. Johnson. *Dietary Intake Findings, United States, 1971–1974.* DHEW Publ. No. (HRA) 77–1647. Supt. of Documents, U. S. Government Printing Office, 1977.

31. Burke, B. S., R. B. Reed, A. S. van den Berg, and H. C. Stuart. Caloric and protein intakes of children between 1 and 18 years of age. *Pediatrics 24* (Suppl. Part II):922–940, 1959.

32. Beal, V. A. Nutritional Intake. In: McCammon, R. W. (Ed.) *Human Growth and Development.* Charles C Thomas, Springfield, Ill., 1970.

33. Irwin, M. I., and D. M. Hegsted. A conspectus of research on protein requirements of man. *J. Nutr. 101*:385–430, 1971.

34. Irwin, M. I., and E. W. Kienholz. A conspectus of research on calcium requirements of man. *J. Nutr. 103*:1019–1095, 1973.

35. Walker, A. R. P. The human requirement of calcium: Should low intakes be supplemented? *Am. J. Clin. Nutr. 25*:518–530, 1972.

36. Bowering, J., A. M. Sanchez, and M. I. Irwin. A conspectus of research on iron requirements of man. *J. Nutr. 106*:985–1074, 1976.

37. Macy, I. G., and H. A. Hunscher. Calories—A limiting factor in the growth of children. *J. Nutr. 45*:189–199, 1951.

38. *Focus on Nutrition—You Cannot Teach a Hungry Child.* Mass. Dept. of Education, Boston, 1970.

39. Pollitt, E., M. Gersovitz, and M. Gargiulo. Educational benefits of the United States school feeding program: A critical review of the literature. *Am. J. Pub. Health 68*:477–481, 1978.

40. Beal, V. A. Dietary intake of individuals followed throughout infancy and childhood. *Am. J. Pub. Health 51*:1107–1117, 1961.

8

PUBESCENCE
AND
ADOLESCENCE

The transition from childhood to adulthood is accomplished by a series of physical, physiological, and psychological–social changes. Progress in the individual is usually characterized by an orderly sequence, but there is marked variation between sexes and between individuals in timing, intensity of change, and duration of the process. This period is usually called adolescence, but it really has two phases, pubescence and adolescence. Pubescence begins with the first increase in hormone secretion and appearance of secondary sex characteristics and ends when sexual reproduction becomes possible. Adolescence follows pubescence and terminates with the completion of physical growth at maturity.[1]

Only in the human and some primates is there a second acceleration of the growth curve before sexual maturity is attained. The first acceleration of the curve occurs during the fetal period and the peak velocity is reached during gestation, as was shown in Figure 1.6. Thereafter the rate of growth decelerates throughout childhood. In lower animals sexual maturity is attained during the deceleration, which continues until adult size is reached.[2] In the human, a relatively long period of childhood deceleration is followed by a second acceleration of the growth rate before sexual maturation occurs. This reacceleration of the growth curve is accompanied by gonadal maturation, appearance of secondary sex characteristics, modification of body contours and body composition, and alterations in metabolic functions. It is uniquely different from the pattern of childhood growth. It encompasses one-third of the entire period of growth and contributes nearly half of adult weight and 10 to 15 percent of adult stature.[3]

The majority of growth during this age period is attained during pubescence, which lasts an average of 2 to 3 years. The peak velocity of increase in stature and weight precedes menarche in girls and spermatogenesis in boys. Thereafter growth continues, but at a diminished rate. Increment in height during adolescence is much less than during pubescence, although the time span of adolescence is longer than the time span of pubescence. The adolescent phase may extend for an average of 5 to 7 years before final termination of growth. However, the term "adolescence" is commonly used to include both pubescence and adolescence and "adolescent growth spurt" to encompass the period from the start of the second acceleration to its cessation at maturity.

The factors that initiate the increase in hormonal secretions and lead to gonadal maturation and the second acceleration of physical growth are not well understood. It has been speculated that initiation may begin in the hypothalamus, but confirming evidence is lacking.[2] It is also difficult to establish the precise timing of the first pubescent changes in the individual. During the life span there is a gradual flowing from one developmental period to the next with few clearly identifiable points of demarcation. The earliest pubescent changes are relatively subtle. Although the stages of development of secondary sex characteristics (breasts, genital organs, and pubic and axillary hair) have been described,[4-6] subjective judgment is required in their evaluation. Menarche in girls is a landmark signaling a stage of hormonal and physical development sufficient to initiate the menstrual cycle, even though regularity of the cycle may not be accomplished for several months. No similar landmark is easily identifiable for males.

Rarely is the stature of individual children measured frequently enough to identify the precise age of departure from the childhood growth curve, and in some children the change is so gradual that it is difficult to determine an age when the slope changes. Most individual data on adolescent growth have been derived from longitudinal growth studies, in which measurements have usually been obtained at specified chronological ages, which identify only the age boundaries within which the acceleration began. These studies, however, provide identification of the timing of peak height velocity. Few data are available on the measurement of levels of hormones and metabolites in blood or urine that might be early indicators of the onset of pubescent changes.

It is equally difficult to establish the precise timing of the end of adolescence.[1] The cessation of growth in stature is commonly used as an index. In the longitudinal studies of the Fels Research Institute, growth in stature ceased at a median age of 17.3 years in females and 21.2 years in males, with a range from 10th to 90th percentiles of 15.8 to 21.1 years in females and 18.4 to 23.5 years in males.[7] In various other published studies median ages at the termination of growth have ranged from 16 to 18 years in females and from 18 to 22 years in males. Slow growth may continue for some time at a rate within the error of measurement or within the range of diurnal variation, which makes the point of termination difficult to establish. Garn and Wagner[8] reported a mean increment in stature between 17 and 28 years of 1.2 ± 0.8 cm in females and 2.3 ± 1.8 cm in males, stating also that late-maturing individuals may continue to grow until 30 years of age. Muscle mass may increase into the third decade and skeletal mass into the fourth decade of life. Chest circumference continues to increase in both sexes after stature measurements become stable.[9]

The fusion of epiphyses to the diaphyses of long bones is sometimes used as an index to the end of adolescent growth, since long bone length cannot increase after replacement of the cartilaginous plate by ossified tissue. However, fusion in different bones occurs at different ages, with reported median ages ranging from 12.3 to 15.9 years in females and from 15.2 to 18.2 years in males for various sites of the extremities.[1] Late growth in the vertebral column after fusion of the long bones results from apposition of bone at the upper and lower surfaces of the vertebral bodies. In the Fels subjects, a median increase of 1.4 cm height in males and 1.0 cm in females was observed after fusion of the femur was mature.[7] The concept of physiological age as an index to maturity is equally elusive, since different physiological functions reach maturity at different times.[10]

Growth is self-limiting, but the reason for the cessation of growth is no more clearly understood than the reason for the second acceleration in rate. Hypotheses have included an automatic passive deterioration of the growth potential or an active self-inhibitory system of negative feedback when a critical mass has been attained.[2] Therefore, while events during pubescence and adolescence may be described and evaluated, the mechanisms responsible for either the initiation or the termination of the processes have not been identified.

PHYSICAL GROWTH

Differences between the sexes and between individuals of the same sex become more pronounced during this age span. The patterns of change allow for some generalizations in the section that follows, but it must be kept in mind that there are overlapping distributions of weight, height, and other physical measurements of boys and girls.

In some respects the order of maximal growth in various segments of the body is the reverse of the order during fetal growth, which was characterized by a cephalo-caudal progression. During adolescence the peripheral parts of the extremities tend to be more advanced in maturation than the proximal. The peak growth of leg length is usually reached before hip width reaches its maximum increase. Trunk length and chest depth are usually the last of the skeletal measurements to reach their peak growth. Therefore, the ratio of trunk length to leg length rises during adolescence in both sexes. The peak velocity in muscle size and in strength usually follows the age of maximal increase in stature, and the peak velocity of weight gain occurs approximately 6 months after peak height velocity.[5]

SEX DIFFERENCES

From infancy boys tend to be slightly taller and heavier, with wider bones and less subcutaneous fat than girls, as discussed in Chapter 1, but the differences in total body size and in growth rates are relatively small during childhood. For example, median heights of boys and girls in the standards of the National Center for Health Statistics (NCHS)[11] differed by less than 1 cm and median weights by less than 1 kg at 8 years of age. Sex differences become marked with the onset of puberty, as shown by the NCHS median height curves in Figure 8.1. Girls become taller by 10 years, but after 13 years boys surpass girls and attain greater ultimate height. By 18 years males were 13 cm taller and 12 kg heavier than girls, on the average.

Despite the similarity in body size during childhood, there is a difference in skeletal maturation. Girls are 4 weeks more advanced than boys at birth, on the average, and continue to be 20 percent faster in skeletal development than boys.[12] In the longitudinal studies of the Child Research Council, 64 percent of girls but only 5 percent of boys had 7 ossified carpal centers at 5 years; all girls in the study had 8 ossified centers by 11 years, but it was not until 14 years that all boys in the series had reached that level.[13] The advanced skeletal maturation of girls is consistent with their earlier onset of pubescent growth.

Increased production of adrenal steroids is believed to be the first indication of approaching puberty and occurs in both sexes at approximately 7 years of age,[14] but progress toward puberty is then faster in girls, both in appearance of secondary sex characteristics and in acceleration of growth. The onset of the more rapid growth of puberty begins in girls at an average age of 10 years, and in boys about 2 years later. Therefore boys have a longer period of childhood growth, adding perhaps an additional 10 cm of height[13]; they enter puberty older, taller, and heavier than girls.

The intensity of growth is greater in males. The later and larger increments of boys as contrasted with girls are shown in Figure 8.2. Height incre-

Figure 8.1   NCHS mean heights of males and females 7 to 18 years of age.

PUBESCENCE AND ADOLESCENCE

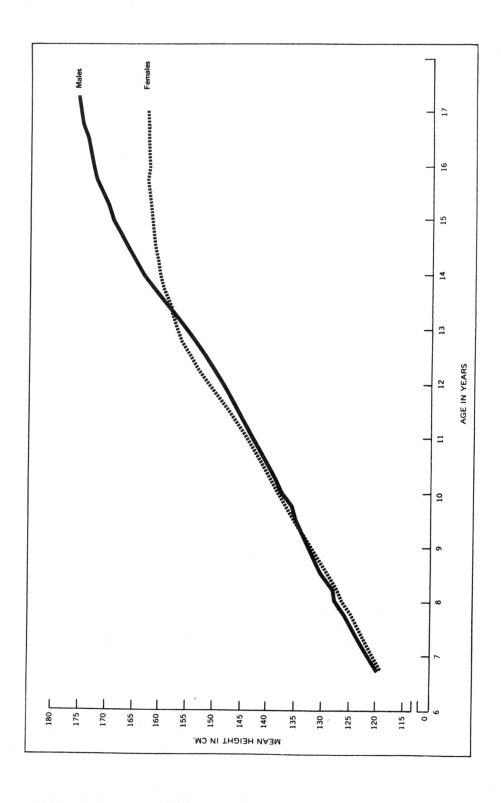

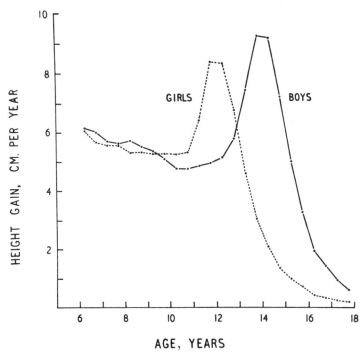

Figure 8.2   Adolescent spurt in height increments; peak velocity of girl at 12–13 years and of boy at 14–15 years. (Reprinted from Tanner, J.M. Growth at Adolescence. Blackwell Scientific Publishers, Oxford, England, 1962.)

ment during the year of peak velocity may be 10 cm in the male but only 8 cm in the female.[5] Between 10 and 18 years the median values of height and weight in the NCHS data[11] increased 40 cm and 37.5 kg for males but only 26 cm and 24 kg for females. Males also have a longer period of growth. The sex difference in the onset of pubertal growth is approximately two years, but the male is closer to four years older than the female at the termination of growth. As a cumulative result of a longer span of childhood growth, greater increments during the spurt, and a longer period of adolescent increase, males are, on the average, taller and heavier than females at maturity.

Sex differences in body contours, proportions, and composition become more pronounced during pubescence and adolescence. As a result of greater production of androgens, primarily testosterone, males develop wider shoulders and greater muscle mass. Females, with higher estrogen secretion,

326

develop wider hips and more adipose tissue. A longer forearm relative to the length of the upper arm or to total height is a characteristic of males that becomes increasingly evident during growth. Males have longer legs and shorter sitting height in relation to total height than do females, partially as a result of their longer childhood growth, since legs grow more rapidly than the trunk during prepubescent growth. These changes, in combination with the development of secondary sex characteristics, contribute to increasing differences in physical size and appearance between males and females.

INDIVIDUAL VARIATIONS

Variations within each sex become more pronounced during pubescence. During infancy and early childhood the range of variation in stature or skeletal age within each sex is relatively narrow at any given chronological age. However, the range of variance among individuals increases markedly during pubescence and adolescence with the differences in the timing, peak velocity, and total duration of growth. For example, the standard deviation of skeletal age is only 6 months in the third year, increases to 10 months in the seventh year, and is between 12 and 15 months at later ages.[14] In the Child Research Council series,[9] standard deviation was highest in relation to mean height at 11 to 12 years in girls and at 13 to 14 years in boys, ages that are close to the ages of fastest growth reported in several longitudinal studies.[15] Variance diminishes again as subjects approach maturity.

This wide variance during this age span reflects the inclusion within a single chronological age group of early-maturing children who are already in the decelerating phase of growth with late-maturing children who have not yet reached their peak velocity. This variation is shown in Figure 8.3, in which the height increments in each six-month interval of an early-maturing boy and a late-maturing boy are plotted against the median increments of boys in the Child Research Council study. The early-maturing boy reached peak height velocity at approximately 12 years and the late-maturing boy at 16 years. Therefore the distribution at the median age of peak velocity, between 14 and 15 years, included boys at different stages of growth from early pubescent to nearly mature.

Similar variations are observed among girls, as shown in Figure 8.4, drawn by Tanner[5] from data of Shuttleworth from the Harvard Growth Study of the 1930s. Individual patterns of timing of the growth spurt were evident when height increments of the girls were plotted by chronological age, and the mean velocity curve was smoothed and extended in time. However, when the same individual curves were plotted so that the focus was not on chronological age but on the age of maximum velocity, the similarity in

INCREMENTS IN HEIGHT

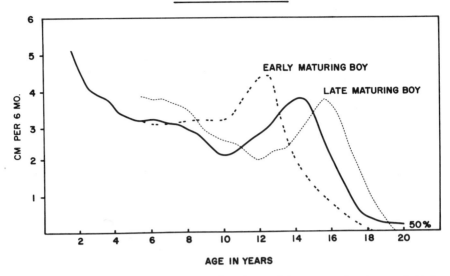

Figure 8.3 Increments in height of early- and late-maturing boys plotted against the median for boys in the Child Research Council series. (Reprinted with permission from Marion M. Maresh, M.D.)

growth patterns of individuals became evident, and the average curve more nearly reflected individual patterns. This illustrates both the distortion of the average and the underestimation of the velocity of growth during pubescence when the index is chronological age.

The wider individual variations during pubescence indicate that chronological age is an inadequate index of physical growth and, therefore, of nutritional requirements. Maturational age, based on growth rate, skeletal development, or some other index of biological stage, must be used in the evaluation of an individual. Although 10 years is the average age of acceleration of growth rate in girls, the range may be from 7 years to nearly 12 years. Maximum velocity of growth in stature follows the onset of pubescent growth by an average of 2 to 2.5 years, and maximum velocity of weight gain is usually about six months later than peak height velocity. Therefore, the age at maximum increment in growth, and in nutritional re-

Figure 8.4 Height curves of girls plotted against chronological age (left) and according to time of maximum velocity (right). (Reprinted from Tanner, J.M. Growth at Adolescence. Blackwell Scientific Publishers, Oxford, England, 1962.)

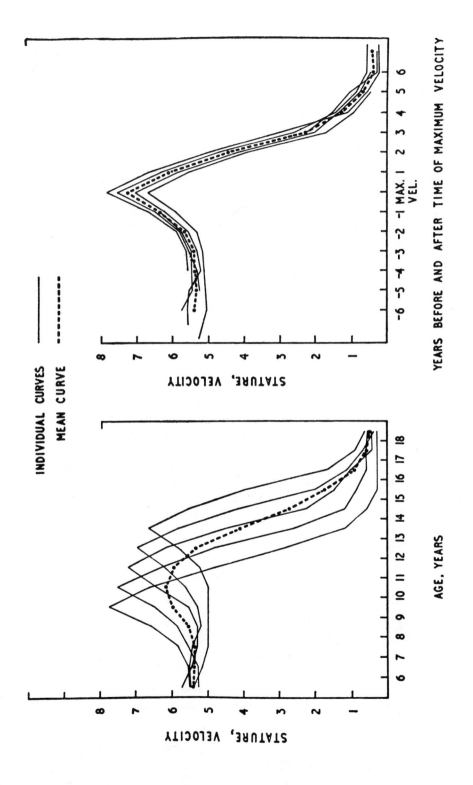

INDIVIDUAL CURVES ————
MEAN CURVE ▪▪▪▪▪

STATURE, VELOCITY

AGE, YEARS

STATURE, VELOCITY

YEARS BEFORE AND AFTER TIME OF MAXIMUM VELOCITY

-6 -5 -4 -3 -2 -1 MAX. 1 2 3 4 5 6
VEL.

quirements as well, may be as early as 10 years in some girls or as late as 14 years in others. Comparable ages of greatest growth and nutrient need in boys are two years later than in girls, with similar variations between individuals.

The total duration of growth also shows wide individual variations. The average duration of pubescent-adolescent growth spans an interval of 8 to 9 years, but for the individual the period of increased nutrient requirements may be shorter or longer. For some individuals the entire period from growth acceleration to mature size may be telescoped into as little as 5 years, and others extend the time span to as much as 13 to 14 years following onset of pubescent growth.[16]

The amount of growth is also variable from one individual to another. The average height gain of girls in the Child Research Council series[16] was 31 cm between the onset of acceleration and final cessation of growth in stature, but individual girls ranged from 18 to 39 cm. The average gain of boys was 33 cm, with a range from 21 to 45 cm. The individual with large gains in height and weight obviously has need of more nutrients to support that gain, in contrast to the individual with relatively small increase in body size.

With the wide variations in both the timing and the magnitude of growth, the use of a standard table of nutrient requirements based on chronological age is unsatisfactory when applied to the individual child during this age span. Early-maturing children tend to have a greater velocity of growth over a relatively short period of time. Their nutrient requirements to support this pattern of growth increase at an early chronological age, are high during rapid growth, and then decrease to adult maintenance needs relatively early. In contrast, the late-maturing individuals continue for a longer period of time to have requirements for slowly increasing prepubescent growth; the elevated requirements for increased rates of growth occur at a later age, and the decrease to adult maintenance is later. Although it is convenient to use average chronological ages or age spans in discussing growth and nutrient needs during pubescence and adolescence, within any given age span some children may be prepubertal, some at the peak of the growth process, and some postadolescent. Therefore, each child must be treated as an individual with evaluation of his or her unique maturational stage and biological age.

HORMONAL INFLUENCES ON GROWTH AND MATURATION

Physical growth, sexual maturation, and physiological development during pubescence and adolescence are under the control of a complex series of alterations in the rates of secretion of a number of hormones. The mechanisms by which they function are poorly understood, and much of our interpretation is either theoretical or indirect. However, there is evidence that the sequence of changes, including the appearance of secondary sex characteristics, the acceleration of growth, the modification of body composition and body contours, and the attainment of reproductive ability, are influenced by hormone secretions or by differences in the responsiveness of tissues to hormones.

The onset of puberty may result from a gradual and quantitative change rather than a qualitative change in hormone secretion.[2] For example, sex hormones (estrogen, progesterone, and androgens) are secreted in small amounts during childhood, but the rate of secretion increases during pubescence. It has been speculated that their secretion and effect may be altered by the removal of inhibiting factors that check gonadotropin secretion by the hypothalamus, or that there is a change in the sensitivity of the brain to sex steroids because of the maturation of central nervous system tissue.

Although the sex hormones exert a major controlling influence, many other hormones participate in adolescent development. No attempt will be made here to explore fully the endocrinological aspects of this age period, but a brief summary is essential to understand the physical and physiological changes that influence nutrient requirements.

GROWTH HORMONE

Somatotropin is a polypeptide produced by the pituitary. It is highly species-specific and is necessary for growth, but its role in adolescent growth is still unresolved. The blood concentrations of growth hormone are higher during both the prepubertal and pubertal periods than in the adult, and there is some evidence that levels are elevated in adolescent females. Growth hormone stimulates protein anabolism at the cellular level. Experimental data indicate that it increases nitrogen retention and plasma levels of phosphate, glucose, and free fatty acids and decreases the plasma levels of urea nitrogen and amino acids and the excretion of sodium and potassium.[2] There is some speculation that it interacts with the central nervous system, which may in part control the secretion of growth hormone; in turn growth hormone may contribute to the maturation of the central nervous system.

THYROID HORMONES

Triiodothyronine (T_3) and thyroxine (T_4) influence overall body growth and skeletal maturation, although the mechanisms are poorly understood. Their action may be permissive rather than controlling.[12] They contribute to the maturation of the central nervous system. Metabolic effects of the thyroid hormones include increases in oxygen consumption, heat production, nitrogen retention, protein synthesis, glucose absorption, glycolysis, and gluconeogenesis.[2] Their effects are both anabolic and catabolic. The mass of the thyroid gland increases more rapidly during adolescence than in earlier childhood, but there is no increase in thyroid hormones or in protein-bound iodine (PBI) during adolescence.[17] The increase in size of the thyroid, which is usually self-limited and subsides without treatment, is maximum in boys at 13 to 14 years and in girls at 17 to 18 years.[18]

Large deviations in thyroid function result in definite changes in the growth spurt. Hypothyroidism reduces the growth spurt and delays bony development and epiphyseal ossification; the ratio of the upper body to lower body segments remains in an infantile or early childhood range. Hyperthyroidism, if of sufficient duration, results in increased linear growth and advanced skeletal development. However, the significance of the role of thyroid hormones in the adolescent growth spurt in normal euthyroid individuals is not clear.[18]

INSULIN

The effect of insulin on growth is indirect, through its regulation of intermediary metabolism. Insulin increases the uptake and metabolism of glucose, glycogenesis, and the synthesis of fatty acids. It also stimulates the transport of amino acids into cells and catalyzes the incorporation of amino acids into protein. There may be some interdependence of the functions of insulin with gonadal and pituitary hormones. Cheek has speculated that insulin may play a major role in the increased fat deposition in the female.[19]

ADRENAL CORTICAL STEROIDS

The adrenal cortex, possibly due to stimulation by ACTH, secretes several steroid hormones that promote and regulate growth as well as sexual development and function. The adrenal cortex is the major, and possibly the sole, source of estrogens in the male and of androgens in the female.[5] The androgens (primarily androsterone), estrogens (especially estradiol and estrone), and progesteroids secreted by the adrenal cortex are anabolic in their action in both sexes. However, glucocorticoids (primarily cortisol) are catabolic, diverting amino acids of the metabolic pool from protein synthesis toward the synthesis of carbohydrate and fat.[2]

GONADOTROPINS

Gonadotropins, which are glycoproteins released by the pituitary under the influence of the hypothalamus and CNS centers, can be detected in urine prior to puberty but their secretion is markedly increased during puberty.[17] Follicle-stimulating hormone (FSH) in the male stimulates the growth of tubules in the testes, which then leads to testosterone production by the testes. In the female FSH stimulates follicle maturation in the ovaries, which then leads to ovarian production of estrogen. Luteinizing hormone (LH), or interstitial-cell-stimulating hormone (ICSH), in the male stimulates the Leydig cells of the testes,[14] thus also leading to testosterone production. In the female LH is responsible for ovulation and the initial formation of the corpus luteum. Secretion of gonadotropins is relatively steady in the male, but occurs in a cyclic pattern in the female.[2]

Gonadal Hormones

The accelerated growth of adolescence is probably due primarily to the sex hormones, but the interrelationships among many hormones are complex. The contributions of each to total body growth, to the development of specific organs and tissues, and to skeletal maturation have not yet been clarified. Androgens and estrogens are produced in both sexes, but the differences in amounts and target organs result in charactistics that are typically masculine or feminine.

Androgens

These steroids have potent anabolic action. They have been demonstrated to increase the retention of nitrogen, potassium, phosphorus, and calcium. They increase protein synthesis, probably through their stimulation of production of RNA and ribosomes,[20] thus influencing growth of the whole body and of specific tissues and organs. They accelerate skeletal maturation.

In the male, testosterone secreted by the testes combines with adrenal androgens to produce greater growth than in the female, including larger muscle and erythrocyte masses. Testosterone is a masculinizing compound, and secondary sex characteristics appear when the testes begin to function at adult levels. Testosterone levels rise rapidly between 12 and 14 years, and there is a twentyfold increase in levels between 10 and 17 years.[17] In the female, the ovaries secrete androgens in small amounts, but the growth acceleration in the female is probably due primarily to adrenal androgens.[12] It has been speculated that the lesser growth of females may be due to a controlling influence of estrogens.[17]

Estrogens

In the male, the testes secrete small amounts of estrogen, which may be responsible for the temporary rounding of hips and changes in the breast often seen early in puberty. In the female, the outer cortex of the ovaries contains follicles, which secrete estrogens, and corpora lutea, which secrete both estrogens and progesterone.

The ovarian estrogens are primarily estradiol and estrone. In influencing the development and maintenance of secondary sex characteristics and reproductive functions, they result in significant morphological, physiological, and behavioral changes. They regulate the secretion of FSH and LH by the pituitary, increase uterine weight, and induce vaginal cornification. Although they are anabolic with respect to specific tissues, such as the secondary sex organs, they do not appear to influence total body growth, although they may hasten epiphyseal closure. They have little, if any, effect on nitrogen retention, and may even inhibit it.[2] The steep rise in estrogen secretion in early puberty becomes cyclic about 18 months prior to menarche.[21]

Progesterone

Secreted by the corpora lutea of the ovarian cortex, progesterone causes changes in the uterine endometrium and is responsible also for cyclic changes in the vagina. It stimulates the development of lobules and alveoli in the breasts, resulting in the continuing maturation of breast function.

SEQUENCE OF DEVELOPMENTAL CHANGES

The timing of changes in the body varies between sexes and within each sex between individuals. However, once the process has begun in an individual, the sequence of changes follows a relatively consistent pattern. Under the influence of the gonadotropins, the first visible signs of puberty are development of secondary sex characteristics. As the ovaries and testes mature, estrogens and androgens result in major alterations in body size, composition, and function. The stages of maturation have been described in a number of publications,[4-6,21] and will only be summarized here.

DEVELOPMENT OF THE FEMALE

Girls have somewhat less variation than boys.[21] The total span of time from the onset of puberty to maturity is shorter and there is less difference between early- and late-maturing girls. The smaller increment in height is accomplished sooner and sexual maturity is attained more quickly after the initial pubertal changes begin.

The sequence of events in relation to the spurt in height[21] is shown in Figure 8.5, which is based on an average of published data and may be shifted in either direction of age to adjust for earlier or later maturation. The first visible change is breast bud formation, with elevation of papilla and enlargement of the areola, followed by initial elevation of the breast. Breast changes may become evident at any age between 7 and 12 years, and usually

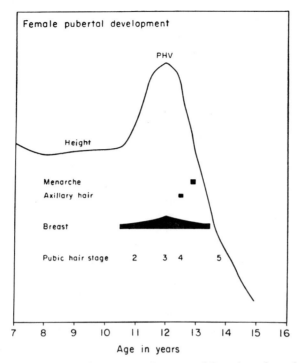

Figure 8.5   Sequence of events of female pubertal changes related to height spurt. (Reprinted from Hammar, S.L. Adolescence. In: Brennemann's Practice of Pediatrics, Vol. 1. Harper and Row, Hagerstown, Md., 1975.)

precede the appearance of the first pubic hair, although the timing may be simultaneous. This is soon followed by the acceleration of both the rate of linear growth and the deposition of body fat.

Breasts continue to enlarge. Pubic hair becomes progressively thicker, darker, curlier, and more extensive. As the ovaries mature, their secretion of estrogen results in thickening of the epithelium of the enlarging vagina. Maximum height velocity is attained relatively early in genital development and precedes menarche, which occurs during the decelerating phase of linear growth. Axillary hair may appear before or after menarche. The ovaries continue to increase in size following menarche; ovulation may begin shortly after the onset of the menstrual cycle but regularity in ovulation may not be attained for as long as two years. It has been estimated that the average female becomes fertile at 14 to 15 years, but that it may be as early as 11½ years in some females.

In attempts to identify better indices of maturation than chronological age, height age and skeletal age have sometimes been used. In addition, the measurement and description of the breasts and pubic hair have been rated, as indicated for pubic hair in Figure 8.5. Since menarche is a measurable landmark in girls, a great deal of atttention has been focused on the variations in age at menarche in various populations.

Age at Menarche

The age of a girl at the time of her first menstrual period is one of the few objective and precise measures of her stage of maturation. As a result, extensive data have been amassed on age at menarche. This has led to calculations and hypotheses related to physical measurements and predictions of adult height. It has also led to investigation of associated factors, including genetics, socioeconomic status, geographical location, ethnic background, season of birth, chronic disease, and nutritional status in efforts to determine their influence on maturation. The interrelationships among all of these factors are complex and the variety of hypotheses that have been proposed have been accepted or refuted with much controversy. Until the factor or factors that trigger pubescent growth and the sequence of hormonal and other physiological alterations that follow are more clearly defined, the influence of genetics and many environmental factors will continue to be controversial.

Data in the literature on age at menarche are subject to misinterpretation for several reasons. The only accurate way of determining precise menarcheal age is by repeated longitudinal follow-up of girls, beginning before the age of earliest menarche and continuing until the last girl in the series has reached that landmark. Many cross-sectional studies have included subjects who have not yet menstruated because the upper age limit of the group was set too low. The method of recording age has not been consistent. For example, "age 13 years" may mean in the thirteenth year, which is between 12 and 13 years, or following the thirteenth birthday, which is between 13 and 14 years. Retrospective data are inaccurate, and the inaccuracy increases as the women questioned become older[22,23]; a middle-aged woman is unlikely to remember with precision the date of an event several decades earlier. The statistical handling of data also introduces a difference in interpretation; the inclusion of subjects with markedly delayed menarche elevates the mean age but has less effect on median age, and many literature reports have presented mean age of a group of girls without showing the frequency distributions.

Menarche usually occurs between 10 and 16 years of age, although earlier or later ages have been reported without evident pathology. Mean or median ages reported from various parts of the world in the past 50 years have usually been between 12 and 14 years, with a clustering close to 13 years. In the data abstracted from Cycles II and III (ages 6 through 17 years) of the Health Examination Survey,[24] the median age at menarche was 12.8 years, with 0.2 percent before 10 years and 0.3 percent after the 17th year. In this survey, age was based on the last birthday, with 0.5 years added for the calculations. The observed cumulative percentage distribution and a fitted curve are shown in Figure 8.6. In a summary of 11 studies of girls in four countries, Johnston et al.[25] reported mean ages at menarche ranging from

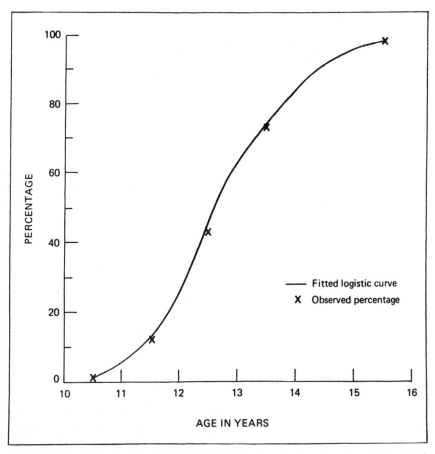

Figure 8.6 Cumulative percentage curve of age at menarche. (Reprinted from MacMahon, B. Age at Menarche. DHEW Publ. No. (HRA) 74-1615. Supt. of Documents, U.S. Government Printing Office, Washington, D.C., 1973.)

12.4 years to 13.1 years; in four longitudinal studies in the United States, mean ages ranged from 12.8 to 13.1 years, with standard deviations between 0.96 and 1.16.

Since menarche is one event in a series of sequential developments during puberty, it is closely related to changes in height, weight, skeletal development, and other body measurements. Early-maturing girls tend to be taller and heavier, with more advanced bone age, than their peers of the same chronological age. Late-maturing girls tend to be slower in all aspects of physical and physiological development. For example, the correlation between age at peak height velocity and age at menarche has been reported between 0.84 and 0.93 in longitudinal studies.[26] This relationship is shown in Figure 8.7, based on Shuttleworth's studies. In early-maturing girls, peak height velocity occurs at a younger age, followed by menarche about 6 months later. In late-maturing girls the longer time interval of more than 1½ years between peak height velocity and menarche suggests a general

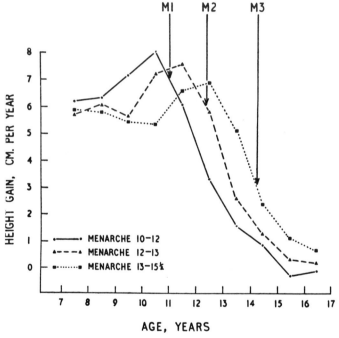

Figure 8.7   Relation of peak height velocity to age at menarche in early, average, and late maturing girls. (Reprinted from Tanner, J.M. Growth at Adolescence. Blackwell Scientific Publishers, Oxford, England, 1962.)

PUBESCENCE AND ADOLESCENCE

slowing of the entire pubescent sequence. Figure 8.8 shows the advancement in skeletal age over chronological age in the early-maturing girls when compared to those with later menarche.

The interrelationships of various measurements of physical development and age at menarche have led to attempts to define more precisely the correlations between events. When height is held constant, early menarche is associated with greater body weight. After analysis of data from longitudinal studies, Frisch and Revelle[27] hypothesized that a "critical" body weight of 47.8 kg must be attained before menarche could occur. They later refined the hypothesis to suggest that menarche was more closely related to body composition than to weight, and used weight and height to calculate body

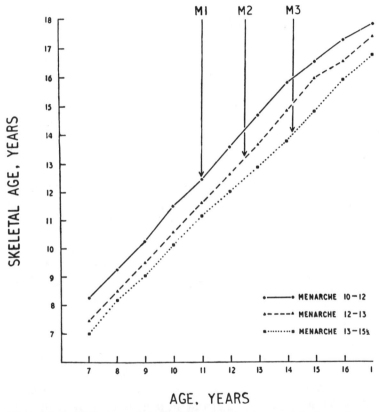

Figure 8.8 Relation of skeletal age to age at menarche in early, average, and late maturing girls. (Reprinted from Tanner, J.M. Growth at Adolescence. Blackwell Scientific Publishers, Oxford, England, 1962.)

water, according to the formula of Mellits and Cheek,[29] and thereby estimated body fat. They hypothesized that when total body water was 55.1 percent of body weight and fat comprised 23.5 percent of weight, this correlated with completion in the fall of metabolic rate from childhood to adult levels. This, in turn, triggered menarche through an impact on the hypothalamic sex steroid receptor, reducing its feedback sensitivity and accounting for a sufficient secretion of estrogen to support menstruation. Although this theory has since had some partially confirming evidence, as would be expected from the interrelationships of growth and menarche, it does not allow for the wide variations among individuals in all measurements. In an analysis of 11 studies, Johnston et al.[25] found that mean weights at menarche varied from 39.8 to 55.0 kg, with individual girls in those studies weighing as little as 25.9 kg or as much as 97.3 kg when their menses started. The coefficients of variation for weight in the 11 studies ranged from 13.4 percent to 24.9 percent, which were two to four times the coefficients of variation for stature at menarche for the same girls. In other words, the weight of individuals at menarche was one of the most variable measurements of their adolescent development. Billewicz et al.[26] stated that weight and body composition are factors in the process of maturation without having critical levels related to menarche. Johnston et al.[25] attributed the closer relationship of estimated total body water with menarcheal age found by Frisch and Revelle to statistical artifacts associated with regression analysis. It seems, therefore, that simplistic approaches to the complex interrelationships of events during puberty and adolescence have been relatively unproductive to date.

Secular changes in the age at menarche have been equally subject to differences in interpretation. As discussed in Chapter 1, a secular increase in height during childhood has been established in many populations, although no further increase among advantaged groups is now evident. Increased height of children, associated with earlier maturation but little change in adult stature, would be consistent with earlier menarche in girls. However, historical records indicate that menarche occurred at 13 years in ancient China, in the 12th year in Hindus, and at 14 years (12–16 years) in Greek girls; Romans and Jews set the age at 12 years.[30] The admixture of religious and cultural practices and beliefs may have influenced these records, and there are no scientific data to confirm or deny whether these were actual ages of physiological change. However, they suggest that age at menarche in early times was not very different from the present. Records dating from the early nineteenth century indicate older ages at menarche, at least in some segments of the population; an increase in average age about the time of the Industrial Revolution has been suggested but is impossible to verify.

After reviewing reports of ages at menarche from several northern European countries since the 1840s, Tanner[5] concluded that in the past century mean age at menarche has been reduced 3 to 4 months per decade, with the result that girls now begin to menstruate 2½ to 3½ years earlier than girls 100 years ago. These data as presented by Tanner are shown in Figure 8.9. Brown,[31] however, reported that the decline was not uniform and universally consistent, but that different patterns of change occurred in different countries. In addition to the retrospective errors in much of the earlier data, Brown's analysis showed no changes in age for girls who experienced menarche between 10 and 14 years, but a decrease in the number of girls with menarche after 16 years. The greater dispersion of ages, with larger numbers in the upper levels of the distribution, may have resulted in elevation of the mean age in the nineteenth century in Tanner's graph. Brundtland and Walløe,[32] in a review of the Norwegian data used by Tanner, found errors in the interpretation of ages in the original reports, in calculation of the means, and in the translation of the Norwegian reports into other languages. Some of the original reports were translated by a Swede from Norwegian to German. Brundtland and Walløe reevaluated the method of recording and interpreting ages and divided the subjects into socioeconomic classes. These recalculations are also shown in Figure 8.9 and differ from Tanner's. Brundtland and Walløe concluded that there was no change in age at menarche in either upper or lower classes in the nineteenth century but that menarche was two years later in the lower class. The decrease in age of menarche occurred between 1900 and 1940, primarily in the lower socioeconomic group, and the difference in age between the two groups has now disappeared.

Data from longitudinal studies in the United States and from a number of epidemiological studies throughout the world have shown little or no decrease in menarcheal age in the past 40 to 50 years, when most reported mean ages have been between 12 and 14 years. From the data now available, one may speculate that during the Industrial Revolution, for reasons not clear, many females, especially in the lower socioeconomic classes, did not reach menarche until 16 years or later and that the major secular change has been a lowering of menarcheal age among that group. As with stature, the secular change in age at menarche may now have ceased, at least among advantaged populations.

Investigation of factors that might be related to age at menarche and, therefore, to the maturational processes of adolescence has ranged from genetics to urbanization. Associated with late menarche in various studies have been the following: late adolescent development of parents, low socioeconomic status, poor nutritional status, low protein intake, large number

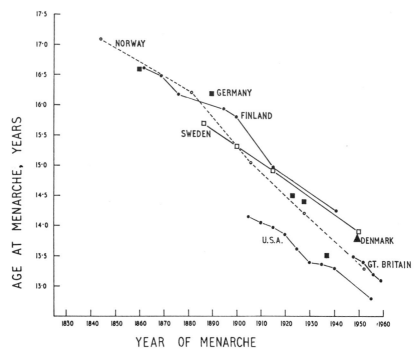

Figure 8.9 Left: Secular trend in age at menarche, 1830–1960, by Tanner. Right: Secular trend in age at menarche in Norway, 1820–1960, by Brundtland and Walløe. (Reprinted from Tanner, J.M. Growth at Adolescence. Blackwell Scientific Publishers, Oxford, England, 1962, and Brundtland, G.H., and L. Walloe. Menarcheal age in 18th century Norway. Ann. Human Biol. 3:363–373, 1976.)

of siblings, and rural residence. Studies have also investigated relationships with birth month, attendance at coeducational or girls' schools, race, breast or formula feeding in infancy, climate, and ambient temperature, but the findings from those studies have been unconfirmed or controversial. The most consistent relationships have been those which are related, whether as cause or concomitant development, with early maturation: taller and heavier girls with advanced skeletal development tend to have earlier ages at menarche than shorter, lighter girls with slower skeletal development.

DEVELOPMENT OF THE MALE

The first clinical sign of puberty in the male is usually an increase in size of the testes, with development of the seminiferous tubules and interstitial cells

342   PUBESCENCE AND ADOLESCENCE

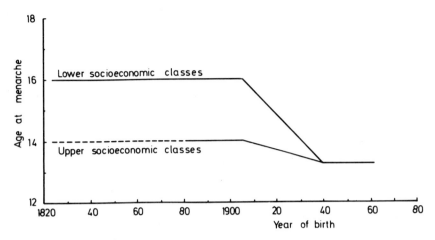

Figure 8.9   (Continued)

as a result of stimulation by gonadotropins. This occurs at an average age of 11 years, although the range may be from 9 to 15 years.[22] With maturation of the testes, secretion of testosterone accelerates growth. The penis increases first in length and then in breadth; genitalia are usually well developed by 14 to 15 years in the average male.[1,33] The outline of the usual sequence of changes in the male are shown in Figure 8.10. Stages of testicular size and growth of pubic hair may be evaluated as indices of maturation.

During early puberty, under the influence of estrogens or adrenal corticoids, the male may have increased deposition of body fat, and hips and breasts may show some signs of female configuration, but this is usually temporary. Subcutaneous fat thicknesses in the male decrease once puberty has become established. The secretion of testosterone results in marked increases in muscles and in shoulder width, as well as in linear growth. Peak height velocity occurs at an average of approximately 14 years, close to the age of attaining adult genitalia, but the timing may vary from 12 to 16 years. Adolescent increase in strength and endurance is more marked in the male than in the female.

Facial and axillary hair usually do not appear until after the peak velocity of increase in stature. Voice changes are gradual and usually late in the sequence of adolescent development; as a result, alterations in voice tone or depth are not clearly indicative of any particular stage of development.

PHYSIOLOGICAL MATURATION

Physical growth, hormonal secretion, body composition, and other aspects of physiological development are so closely interwoven during pubescence

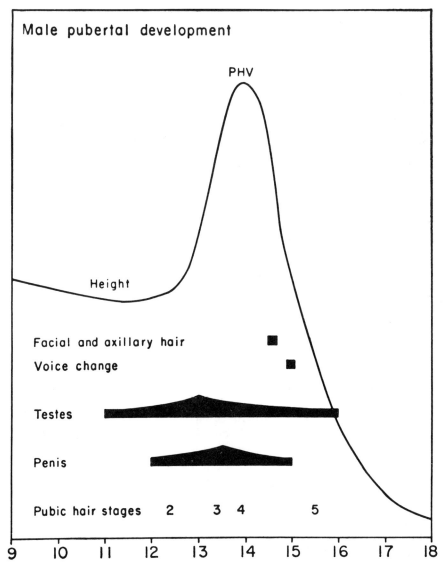

Figure 8.10 Sequence of events in male pubertal changes related to height spurt. (Reprinted from Hammar, S. L. Adolescence. In: Brennemann's Practice of Pediatrics, Vol. 1. Harper and Row, Hagerstown, Md., 1975.)

and adolescence that it is difficult to compartmentalize them. The increment in weight during this period is approximately equivalent to the total weight attained between conception and the onset of puberty. The sex differences in major components of weight result in physiological and metabolic separation of males and females. The male doubles his muscle mass, while the major soft tissue change in the female is the increase in body fat. Sex differences become pronounced in body water and its distribution, electrolyte levels, body temperature, respiratory rate, blood pressure, metabolic rate, blood components, and other physiological functions.

Throughout the life span different physiological functions reach maturity at different periods. Therefore a concept of physiological age is not valid. For example, glomerular filtration rate reaches adult values by 2 to 3 years of age, but blood pressure continues to rise throughout the life span. However, many physiological functions reach maturity during the pubescent-adolescent period concurrent with physical maturation.

BASAL METABOLIC RATE

Approximately 80 percent of the BMR is derived from the metabolic activity of the internal organs, including the brain, liver, lungs, heart, and kidneys.[19] Most of the remainder is derived from muscles at rest. In the adult, the brain and viscera comprise less than 10 percent of body weight and less than 20 percent of cell mass.[34] However, in the child, these organs comprise a larger proportion of cell mass, so BMR per unit of size is higher in the child. Since internal organs grow at a slower rate than other body constituents, BMR per unit size decreases throughout childhood as body weight increases. There are inconsistent reports of whether there is a temporary increase in resting metabolism per unit size at the onset of puberty[5,19]; at best the rise is small, more often observed in the male than the female. The BMR of males is higher than of females because of their higher muscle and lower fat content.

BODY WATER

Total body water increases from birth to 20 years as tissues grow, and is higher in males than in females.[19] In young adult males, 60 to 62 percent of body weight is composed of water, and in females 51 to 55 percent. The ratio of body water to weight decreases very rapidly in the first year of life, from 0.80 liters/kg to 0.60 liters/kg, but through the rest of childhood and adolescence the change is small and gradual, to 0.50 liters/kg by 20 years.[5,10]

The compartmentalization of body water reflects the changes in body composition. Intracellular water per unit of weight rises during growth. It has been estimated that approximately 72 percent of lean body mass is water between infancy and adulthood. Therefore lean body mass is related to body water as well as to total electrolytes, especially potassium. Muscle accounts for 30 percent of intracellular water at 4 years, but this rises to 70 percent in adolescence. The greater muscle development of males results in a higher ratio of intracellular to extracellular water, as indicated by the increased ratio of potassium to chloride. Since fat is almost completely anhydrous, the greater accumulation of body fat in the female results in a ratio of intracellular to extracellular water lower than that in males. Extracellular water maintains a relatively constant relationship to body weight after the first year, with a mean of 0.175 liter/kg.[19]

BLOOD AND ITS COMPONENTS

The volume of blood is linearly related to weight, and is more highly correlated with weight than with stature, age, or surface area.[10] The increase in blood volume during pubescence and adolescence is greater than the proportional increase in either height or age, especially in males. Blood volume per unit of weight shows little sex difference in childhood, but beginning in the adolescent period it is higher in males than in females.

Plasma volume per kilogram remains relatively constant. Red blood cell volume, however, increases from an average of 25.4 ml/kg at 1 year to 28.2 ml/kg in the adult male but decreases to 24.2 ml/kg in the adult female.[35] The relationship between red blood cell volume and lean body mass, however, is similar in both sexes, indicating that the higher level of males is consistent with their greater muscle mass. Nevertheless, there is some evidence that even when the muscle-to-fat ratio is equivalent, the red cell volume per unit of weight is still higher in males than in females.[2]

During the childhood years, the gradual rise in hemoglobin concentration is similar in both sexes, but after 12 years there is a significant sex difference. In the male androgens stimulate erythrocyte production in the bone marrow. The role of female sex hormones has not been extensively studied, but it has been speculated that progesterone stimulates erythropoiesis while estrogen has a depressing effect.[2] The increase in hemoglobin concentration in the male accelerates, attaining an average of 15.5 to 16.5 g/100 ml at 18 to 20 years. In the female the childhood increase stabilizes earlier and remains at an average of 13.5 to 14.5 g/100 ml.[10,36] The erythrocyte count of the male averages more than 5 million cells/mm³ during adolescence while the female maintains an average close to 4.7 million/mm³. The greater blood volume of the male, then, is associated with a higher concentration of hemoglobin and a higher volume of erythrocytes than the female. As is true at other ages, the levels of blacks tend to be lower than the levels of whites.

Total cholesterol in the blood changes little with age during childhood, but there is a tendency toward higher levels in females and in blacks. In two cross-sectional studies[37,38] a peak in the mean or median of girls was observed at 8 years, followed by a decrease to approximately 13 years, and then a plateau or rise throughout the rest of adolescence. The peak in males was maintained until 14 years and was followed by a greater decrease to 17 years. After 13 years the average plasma cholesterol level of females was higher than that of males.

The individuality of patterns of change in total serum cholesterol during adolescence was shown in a longitudinal study.[39] In the period of most rapid growth between onset of the acceleration of growth and fusion of the capitellum to the shaft of the humerus, 12 boys had a decrease in blood level, averaging 9 percent; 2 boys had no consistent pattern of change. Of 16 girls, 12 had a decrease in serum cholesterol, 2 showed no change, and 2 girls had increases in levels.

In contrast to the usual pattern of decrease in total cholesterol in adolescence, triglyceride levels rise. In a cross-sectional study,[37] the rise in girls between 10 and 13 years was followed by a decline. In boys a rise between 11 and 15 years was maintained to 17 years.

PULSE AND RESPIRATION

The heart rate of the individual is highly variable, but under basal conditions it falls during childhood in both sexes. There is no sex difference to 10 years, but beginning in pubescence the heart rate of the male tends to be lower than that of the female.

Blood pressure, however, tends to be higher in the male. Systolic pressure rises gradually in both sexes during growth, but after 14 years remains relatively constant in the female but continues to rise in the male, stabilizing at adult values when growth is complete.[5,10] The total rise in the male during adolescence is greater than in the female. Hypertension during this age period was found in less than 1 percent of subjects in the Health Examination Survey.[40]

Vital capacity increases during adolescence and is highly correlated with height. The male has a marked increase in respiratory rate, basal tidal volume, maximum breathing capacity, and alveolar CO_2 tension.[10] These measurements change little, if at all, in females during adolescence.[5]

The physiological response to exercise changes markedly during adolescence, and performance improves, especially in males. In addition to the increase in body size and strength, there is maturation of several functions that are essential to physical performance and more rapid recovery from exercise; all of these factors combine to increase proficiency. Alterations in circulation include heart rate and blood pressure; respiratory changes include increase in ventilation and rate; metabolic maturation involves differences in oxygen consumption and in blood levels of lactate, pyruvate, and bicarbonate.[2]

There is no significant difference in work performance between boys and girls prior to puberty, but during the adolescent period males become more efficient. The sex difference may be related to greater muscle growth in males and the increased fat deposition in females, or to lower motivation in females, but physiological changes that affect work capacity are also sex-related. Maximal oxygen uptakes, expressed as liters per minute, increase with age in both sexes, but if expressed as uptake per kilogram per minute, values are unchanged in males after 9 years but decrease in females to a level 17 percent lower than in males.[41] In addition to his more efficient respiration, the male's higher hemoglobin concentration increases the availability of oxygen for cell function and his greater muscle mass allows for higher glycogen storage. Strength and endurance increase in the male throughout the second decade of life, but reach their peak in girls about the time of menarche and then decline.

Since the physiological responses to exercise are based on functions that mature in relation to physical growth, wide individual variations in physical ability may be observed at each chronological age. In evaluating the individual's ability, his or her stage of maturation must be considered.

The interrelationships of the menstrual cycle and athletic performance in women have been extensively studied.[42] No consistent alterations related to phases of the menstrual cycle have been found in strength, heart rate, blood pressure, pulmonary capacity, or general athletic performance except in women with dysmenorrhea. Menstrual discomfort tends to lower performance. Reductions in basal metabolic rate or red blood cell count during or immediately following menstruation tend to be less among women who are physically active than those who are physically inactive.

NUTRITIONAL ASPECTS OF HEALTH

Despite the concern that is often expressed about the dietary patterns of teenagers in the United States, their nutritional health is generally good. The major cause of death in this age group is accidents, and the most frequent infections are infectious mononucleosis, serum hepatitis, and venereal diseases.[33] Most adolescents tend to resist infectious diseases, and the prevalence of respiratory infections is lower than during early childhood. In the Ten-State Nutrition Survey "there was no evidence of widespread, severe, clinically evident malnutrition in the population examined."[43]

348

In the Health Examination survey[44] of youths between 12 and 17 years of age, only 4 percent of whites and 10 percent of blacks rated their own health as fair or poor. The large majority of ratings ranged from good to excellent, and parents rated their children's health somewhat higher than did the children themselves. Youths in the lowest income group were more concerned with underweight and those in the upper income group with overweight.

OBESITY

Obesity in the adolescent is more complex than at other ages in the life span. The healthy individual approximately doubles body weight during pubescence and adolescence, but not necessarily at a constant rate. The boy tends to have a temporary increase in body fat measurements early in puberty and then becomes leaner. The girl, on the other hand, tends to have a persistent increase in adipose tissue throughout adolescence; the peak in weight velocity usually follows the peak in height velocity, so that increase in fatness is greater during the deceleration phase of increment in stature. It is important to separate a temporary tendency toward fatness, which is transient, from a permanent acquisition of excess fat, which may not be recognized until after it has occurred. It must also be recognized that the increments of muscle and bone during this period add to body weight, so that some individuals may be overweight without being overfat.

The definition of obesity, if based on weight or weight-to-height ratio, is further confused by individual differences in the timing of the growth spurt. The early-maturing child may reach a position in the upper quartile of weight distribution for age merely because of a growth spurt earlier than average. For adults the standard of a weight 20 percent or more above "ideal" weight for age is often used to identify the obese, but this frame of reference is less satisfactory for the adolescent, and the stage of maturation must be considered. The timing of the growth spurt must also be considered if, for example, the top 15 percent of a weight distribution for age are to be considered obese. As a result of the use of different standards, published figures on the incidence of obesity during this age span show wide variations, and the true incidence of excessive adiposity in this country is unknown.

The multiple etiology of obesity further confuses its identification in the adolescent. Forbes[45] identified two different patterns. One pattern is of the child who has not only increased fat but also increased lean body mass; this child tends to be tall, with advanced skeletal development. This pattern, which may be recognized well before puberty, was described by Bayley,[46] as shown in Figure 1.10. It is also consistent with the observations of Garn and Clark[47] in their analysis of patterns of obesity found in the Ten-State Nutrition Survey. The second pattern is of the adolescent whose height and skeletal growth are within the expected range but who has excessive deposition of fat. Forbes speculated that this type of obesity developed during childhood years. On the other hand, a child may become obese during adolescence and fit neither of these patterns.

Social and cultural attitudes toward obesity in any given era affect not only the definition and recognition of the obese state, but also the self-image and personality problems of the obese child and acceptance by family and peers. With the current emphasis on leanness, fostered both by television and movie personalities and by health specialists, many teenagers who are not obese consider themselves so,[48] and there is an exaggerated interest in weight reduction, especially among girls,[49] often leading to inadequate and sometimes bizarre dietary intakes.

If obesity is persistent and excessive, it may be associated with alterations in metabolic function in the adolescent as in the adult, with elevation of blood pressure and of blood levels of triglycerides, glucose, and insulin.[50] This may lead to increased health risk in adulthood. Obesity also affects the psychological and social maturation of the adolescent. It may interfere with the normal progression from dependence to independence, with participation in athletics and other activities, with the development of social relationships with both sexes, with the ability to obtain employment or college acceptance and, therefore, with the choice of a career. As a result, the sequelae of obesity in adolescence are far-reaching.

Therapy for the obese adolescent is more complicated than for the adult. Drugs that depress appetite by stimulation of the central nervous system or by altering the appetite control center of the hypothalamus have limited success at any age, may interfere with normal metabolic function in this critical period of growth, or may create dependence and be subject to abuse.[51] Hormone therapy should be restricted to unusual cases; it has little long-range benefit and may be harmful in its effect on metabolic processes and skeletal growth.[51,52] With our present state of knowledge, treatment of the obese adolescent depends on dietary restriction, either directly through control of intake or indirectly through behavior alteration, and on the increase in caloric expenditure of physical activity.

Dietary control in the growing child must be considered differently from that in the adult. There must be adequate provision of calories, protein, and other nutrients to permit growth and development of lean body mass while controlling or decreasing body fat. When caloric intake is reduced sufficiently to cause loss of weight, protein anabolism is altered. A loss of more than 1 percent of body mass results in a marked depression of growth.[53] If adult stature is limited, the problem of obesity during adulthood is accentuated. As Knittle[54] has so aptly stated, "No one diet can be devised that will deny calories and protein to the fat depot while providing the necessary nu-

350

trients to other tissues." If the degree of overweight is moderate, dietary restriction that is sufficient to maintain body weight at a stationary level while stature increases is safer than restriction that results in weight loss. If the degree of obesity is so great that weight loss is essential, growth in stature and skeletal maturation should be carefully monitored. If treatment is initiated when growth is complete or nearly complete, techniques applicable to adults may be used without concern about possible interference with the growth processes.

Motivation is a major factor in successful weight control or reduction at any age, and it presents a special problem to the young. Dietary restriction requires forgoing immediate pleasure for long-term benefit; it means being different from others within one's family circle or social milieu. Adoption of a change in life-style and behavior is more difficult during a period when peer acceptance is important. Effective therapy, then, depends on support and encouragement of family and friends. Since obesity may also be found in parents or siblings, involvement of the entire family may be indicated and may be helpful to the adolescent in adherence to a dietary regime.

Many studies have reported a higher degree of inactivity and slower motions in obese adolescents than in those of average weight,[48,55,56] but it is not clear whether the inactivity contributed to the development of obesity or was a result of the added exertion due to greater body mass or of the embarrassment of the obese child on the playing field and in the dressing room. In either case dietary restriction of foods high in carbohydrate or fat while maintaining adequate intake of protein and other nutrients is more effective when combined with a program of increased physical activity. Not only does the ativity raise energy output, but it provides diversion and limits the time available for contact with food. The increased muscle tone and sense of well-being that accompany exercise are both physically and psychologically beneficial.

With study of the internal and external cues that alter hunger-satiety signals and of the environmental factors that may override satiety signals in obese individuals in contrast to people of normal weight, the concept of emphasis on eating behavior rather than on caloric intake has given a new dimension to therapy. The purpose is to identify activity patterns, psychological and emotional states, social factors, and physical environments that affect eating behavior and then to alter factors that lead to excessive consumption.[51,57] The initial results of behavior modification have been promising. Since it stresses awareness of situations that affect food consumption and rewards for control over their effects, this therapeutic technique may prove to be effective in long-term alteration of eating behavior.

Most methods of weight control or reduction have been successful with some individuals for short periods of time but disappointing in long-term results. Since the obese adolescent may have a poor self-image, temporary success followed by relapse at the end of treatment may increase the sense of failure.[58] Continued contact with the therapist and support of family members after initial success is important in maintaining weight control and creating a feeling of accomplishment, which contributes to psychological development. Learning a pattern of moderate eating and of regular exercise that can be followed for life is the most effective way of preventing the continuation of obesity into adulthood.

ANOREXIA NERVOSA

In contrast to obesity, anorexia nervosa is willful self-starvation. Once considered rare, the prevalence of this illness is believed to have increased during the past half century. It has been repeated more often in the upper and middle classes of affluent societies and has its origin usually during puberty, although a few cases have been diagnosed just before puberty or after 20 years of age. Primary anorexia nervosa combines distortions of normal physiological, psychological, and social developments in adolescence. Its prevalence is not known and the disease may not be recognized until it is well advanced. The etiology is not clear and there is controversy about whether the psychological disturbance[59] or immature hypothalamic function[60] is the basic cause. Organic disease is usually absent at onset.

Anorexia nervosa has been diagnosed in adolescent girls 10 times more frequently than in boys.[61] The eating history usually reveals no previous problems, and prior excessive body weight has been reported in only 15 to 20 percent of patients. The child has usually shown conforming behavior. The family of the anorexic girl is likely to be socially ambitious and financially successful. Although the family relationships may appear happy, Bruch[59] suggests that marital discord results in parental demands on the child for conformity and loyalty at a time when the child is trying to establish independence. It is also possible that early feeding methods have distorted normal hunger-satiety signals.

The first clinical sign is weight loss. While many adolescent girls diet, they usually dislike the program. The anorexic girl, on the other hand, delights in it, and carries it to the stage of emaciation. Although there are individual differences, a common pattern has been observed. There is compulsive control over food intake with obsession about food. Hunger pains are persistently denied, but in approximately 25 percent of girls the periods of minimal intake may be interspersed with periods of compulsive eating, often followed by self-induced vomiting or use of laxatives or diuretics.[62] The girl develops a distorted self-image, takes pride in her weight loss, and denies its abnormality, even when it is extreme. Hyperactivity and a drive for intellectual excellence are typical.

352

Amenorrhea is characteristic of the disease, usually following weight loss, but there have been some reports of cessation of menses prior to clinical recognition of anorexia nervosa. As weight loss continues, the chronic semistarvation state has many of the biochemical characteristics of protein-energy malnutrition.[62] There is a loss of body fat and of muscle, a decrease in blood pressure and basal metabolic rate, and alteration in the levels of circulating hormones. Hemoglobin and trace mineral concentrations are usually within normal limits. Vitamin deficiency symptoms are rarely seen; it has been speculated that the general lowering of metabolic processes lowers their requirement and that nutrients from lean tissue catabolism may be reutilized. As the emaciation progresses, apathy and lethargy replace hyperactivity, and the mortality rate in severe cases may be as high as 10 percent.

Treatment is more effective in the early stages, and becomes progressively more difficult as the condition progresses. Willful control by the patient is a deterrent to therapy. Behavior modification techniques have shown some initial effects in reversing weight loss, but it is generally accepted that effective therapy should include removal of the patient from the home environment by hospitalization, treatment of the entire family to alter basic attitudes and problems, and extensive psychotherapy for the anorexic patient in addition to nutritional therapy.

IRON-DEFICIENCY ANEMIA

The risk of iron-deficiency anemia is higher during adolescence than during midchildhood. In addition to body maintenance, iron is needed for growth of body tissues and its concomitant increase in blood volume and, for the female, replacement of iron losses in menstrual blood. Anemia during the adolescent period was considered in Chapter 2.

The proportions of lean body mass and fat that comprise every level of growth vary with age and with sex. The need for iron as a component of growth is closely related to the deposition of lean body mass. Hepner[63] has calculated a need of 46 mg iron/kg lean body mass. This suggests an average need during infancy of 35 mg iron for each kilogram of body weight gained; between 10 and 16 years the female requires utilization of 31 mg iron/kg weight gain and the male 42 mg/kg because of his higher muscle increment.

Individual variations in the amount of menstrual blood loss in normal women were shown by Hallberg[64] to range from 1.6 to 199.7 ml/period. Using these data, Beaton[65] constructed a graph (Figure 8.11) in which menstrual losses of iron were added to basal maintenance losses. The median amount of iron that must be utilized to maintain homeostasis was calculated

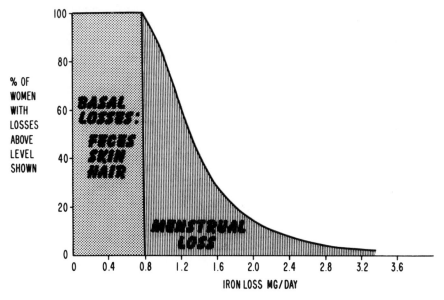

Figure 8.11 Cumulative distribution of iron losses of women for maintenance and to replace menstrual losses. (Adapted from Beaton, G.H. The use of nutritional requirements and allowances. In: White, P.L. (Ed.) Proc. Western Hemisphere Nutr. Congress III, Futura Publishing Company, Mt. Kisco, New York, 1972.)

as approximately 1.4 mg/day, with a range from less than 1 mg to more than 3 mg. In the adolescent female, iron needed for the decreasing rate of growth in lean body mass after menarche is less than during the pubescent phase.

The risk of anemia in the male adolescent, then, is closely related to the growth of lean body mass and is highest when growth is most rapid. In the female the majority of increase in lean body mass occurs before menarche, after which the risk is highest in those with large menstrual losses.

GOITER

In the Ten-State Nutrition Survey,[43] goiter was found in 2.1 to 8.1 percent of individuals between 10 and 16 years of age, but was unrelated to iodine excretion. It was concluded, therefore, that the goiter observed was not associated with iodine deficiency.

In a later study in four states, Trowbridge[66] reported goiter prevalence ranging from 4.5 to 9.8 percent of subjects between 9 and 16 years of age.

The highest iodine excretion was found in the area with the highest goiter prevalence. Measurements of thyroxine and protein-bound iodine and clinical examinations did not identify any abnormalities in most of these children. He concluded that some of the goiter may be pathological and some may be an artifact of the examination criteria, but suggested that "the thyroid enlargement which is called goiter may be part of a normal variation in thyroid size in adolescence which is not accompanied by physiologic or health consequence."

ACNE VULGARIS

Complexion problems are often a source of embarrassment for the teenager. Acne occurs primarily on the face, chest, and back, due to inflammation of the sebaceous glands. Its cause is believed to be related to changes in hormonal secretion. The most effective treatment is skin care, involving cleanliness and the use of topical preparations or antibiotics.

Popular belief is that dietary restrictions are effective in the treatment of acne, most commonly the limitation of chocolate, soft drinks, peanut butter, and other foods high in sucrose or fats. However, these recommendations are largely empirical and several controlled studies have failed to demonstrate their consistent effectiveness. More logical is the maintenance of healthy skin and overall good metabolic function by the consumption of a diet high in fruits, vegetables, protein foods, and other dietary components that will assure adequate intakes of nutrients.

Supplementation with daily doses of vitamin A ranging from 25,000 to 200,000 I.U. has sometimes been recommended, despite lack of evidence of benefit in the treatment of acne. This practice is hazardous, since large intakes of vitamin A can produce toxic effects, including increased intracranial pressure mimicking brain tumors.[67]

ORAL CONTRACEPTIVES

Since their introduction in 1960, the use of oral contraceptives (OC) has increased. It has been estimated that more than 10 million women in the United States, including many adolescent girls, have taken OC at some time. The most commonly used products are a combination or sequence of synthetic estrogen (usually ethinyl estradiol or its 3-methyl derivative, mestranol) and one of several synthetic progestogens. They prevent conception by interfering with the release, movement, or implantation of ova or by inhibiting passage of spermatozoa.[68]

Although these steroids are structurally similar to hormones naturally formed by the woman, they do not replicate the effects of natural steroids, nor do they represent pseudopregnancy.[69] They have been reported to influence the metabolism of almost all nutrients, as identified primarily by biochemical studies of blood and urine, although the alterations in most nutrients are small, controversial, and of minor health significance.[68-72] Few clinical findings have been related to the use of OC, and these have been found usually when prior nutritional status was marginal or poor. The effects of OC have been reported to vary with the components and dosage of the product, length of time used, prior nutritional status, present nutrient intake, unknown factors of individual susceptibility and response, and socioeconomic status as represented by income and education. Many of the effects have been related to the level of estrogen, which was 80 or 100 μg/day in early products but has been lowered to 30 μg in many current products.[68]

Total serum protein is usually unchanged, although serum albumin may be somewhat lower in OC users. Serum triglycerides, free fatty acids, and cholesterol have been reported to increase. These steroids tend to have a hyperglycemic effect in some women, but without clinical evidence of diabetes, and it has been suggested that this may be related to the impairment of tryptophan metabolism and alterations in pyridoxine nutrition.

The estrogen component has been reported to increase the absorption of calcium. Serum copper and ceruloplasmin are elevated by estrogen, without change in urinary copper excretion, suggesting increased absorption and decreased requirement. Plasma zinc concentrations may be decreased, but the level of erythrocyte zinc is increased, perhaps because of the increased binding of zinc in red blood cells to the apoenzyme of carbonic anhydrase; this suggests a redistribution rather than a change in total body zinc. The combination of estrogenic effect and decrease in menstrual blood loss of up to 50 percent results in an increase of serum iron and iron-binding capacity; the iron requirements of a woman on OC may be somewhat lowered.

Blood levels of vitamin A are increased, apparently because of the estrogen-induced greater concentration of the lipoprotein that binds the vitamin. Lower concentrations of carotene suggest enhancement of its conversion to vitamin A. Vitamin K has been investigated in relation to the thromboembolisms observed in some women on OC, and it is possible that the need for vitamin K may be reduced in OC users.

The water-soluble vitamins have been extensively studied in relation to alterations in metabolism by steroids. Ascorbic acid levels in plasma, leukocytes, and platelets tend to be lower, probaby as an effect of estrogen. Changes in thiamin status have been suggested by biochemical tests, including erythrocyte transketolase activity. Red cell riboflavin may be lowered, but evidence of glossitis has been found only in women in India with poor or marginal intakes of many nutrients. Lower serum B_{12} has been reported in some women, but tissue levels do not appear to be affected. The changes in these vitamins are relatively small, and the lack of clinical symptoms implies that supplementation is not necessary.

Major interest and concern about the effects of OC on nutrients have centered on folacin and pyridoxine. A decrease in serum and erythrocyte levels of folacin has been well documented, occurring in a minority of women. The women at risk of folate depletion are those with marginal folate intakes, excessive alcohol consumption, malabsorption, or other diseases increasing folate requirements or requiring treatment with anticonvulsant drugs. The low folate levels may enhance the possibility of folate deficiencies in women who become pregnant soon after discontinuing the use of OC. Megaloblastic anemia has been reported in a small number of women using OC, but usually a malabsorption syndrome has been found in these cases. There is conflicting evidence on whether OC interferes with the absorption of the polyglutamate form of folic acid. Roe[69] has suggested that if the erythrocyte folate level is decreased 50 ng/ml, an increased intake of 35 μg folic acid/day would compensate for the difference, but that a daily supplement of 100 μg/day would be required to overcome depletion in women who had been using OC for a long period of time.

A majority of the users of OC excrete increased amounts of xanthurenic acid and other tryptophan metabolites after an oral load of tryptophan, which is reversible with the administration of pyridoxine.[73] Pyridoxal phosphate is a coenzyme essential for the conversion of tryptophan to niacin. However, only 15 to 20 percent of users have low plasma levels of pyridoxal phosphate. Therefore, most users do not become B_6-deficient but may have abnormal tryptophan metabolism. However, the higher frequency of mental depression among women on OC has stimulated investigation of its possible relationship to pyridoxine. Depression has been associated with a decrease in amines in certain parts of the brain, particularly norepinephrine, derived from tyrosine, and 5-hydroxytryptamine, derived from tryptophan. Since OC may alter the metabolism of both amino acids, and the alteration may be related to pyridoxine deficiency, pharmacological doses of pyridoxine may be effective in treatment.

There is little consensus on the need for vitamin supplementation during use of oral contraceptives. Biochemical changes are relatively small for most nutrients, and some blood levels revert spontaneously to normal even though use of OC is continued. However, many believe that pyridoxine and/or folacin should be given as supplements.

The effects of use of these contraceptive steroids on adolescent girls have not been intensively studied. Biochemical changes have been investigated primarily in women whose adolescent growth has been completed. The increased risk of embolism and other vascular problems, hypertension, migraine, and depression have been documented, but there is a dearth of information on the effects of these steroids on growth and skeletal maturation in the adolescent girls who use them.

PREGNANCY

The increasing prevalence of pregnancies among adolescent girls in the past few decades has focused attention on the special problems associated with reproduction during or soon after a period of rapid growth. Pregnancy was considered in detail in Chapter 3, including nutrient requirements of adolescent girls during pregnancy (Table 3.4), but a brief discussion is essential here in the context of physiological maturation and physical growth during this age period.

Many early studies of the effects of "teenage" pregnancy on mothers and their infants included within a single group all mothers under 20 years of age without regard to biological maturation. In addition, until recent years most adolescent pregnancies studied were those of nonwhite girls in low income groups. Therefore the risks associated with specific age groups were not delineated, and the obstetric complications associated with race, income, and their attendant educational and environmental variables were not differentiated from risks related to age. Grant and Heald[74] warned that erroneous conclusions may be drawn from studies in large medical centers, which tend to attract a large number of abnormal cases with racial and socioeconomic bias, and that demographic characteristics may be more important determinants of obstetric complications than age.

Recent trends toward earlier sexual freedom and societal acceptance of maternity without marriage have influenced the prevalence of pregnancy in very young teenagers and in white adolescents in higher income and educational levels, providing a wider range of subjects for the study and clarification of the influence of variables. It is estimated that approximately one million teenage girls in the United States become pregnant each year, the majority unmarried. Of this total number, 400,000 are less than 18 years of age and 30,000 are under 15 years. Approximately 60 percent of the pregnancies continue to delivery. One-fourth of the teenagers who give birth become pregnant again within a year, so there is a strong likelihood of subsequent pregnancies at short time intervals while these girls are still in their teens.

Many factors interfere with adequate preconceptional and prenatal care, in addition to the limiting influences of income and race. Girls who are unwed must depend on family or community services for support. Those who are married face the instability that is common in young marriages. The emotional stress of pregnancy is superimposed on the uneven psychological development of the adolescent. Denial of pregnancy in its early stages and unwillingness to apply for early prenatal care or a tendency to consider early care unimportant often lead to inadequate medical care until adverse symptoms occur or the pregnancy is well advanced.

The most consistent and well-documented risk in the young adolescent is the delivery of an infant weighing less than 2500 g.[74,75] This is accompanied by increased frequency of malformations and higher infant mortality. The risks are greater for the nonwhite adolescent with low income. Further studies with populations diverse in demographic characteristics as well as age are essential to clarify the relative influence of these variables on other complications for which reports have been inconsistent. These include increased prevalence of toxemia, anemia, contracted pelvis, and prolonged labor.[74-76]

It is becoming clear that the very young adolescent, 14 years of age or less, has the greatest risk of delivering an infant with low birth weight. Grant and Heald[74] concluded from a study of published data that age–demographic characteristics are more important determinants of obstetric complications than age alone. Erkan et al.[75] found that the relationship between age at menarche and age at pregnancy was critical. Girls who conceived within 24 months after menarche were nearly twice as likely to deliver infants weighing less than 2500 g than those who conceived more than two years after menarche. The shorter time interval was also associated with a higher incidence of preeclampsia, but this relationship was not statistically significant. Physiological maturity is related to greater control of hormonal production, stability of ovarian function, and size of the uterus and the pelvis.

The sequence of maximum increments in growth in height and weight in relation to menarche and possible pregnancy are shown schematically in Figure 8.12, with the rates of pregnancy from British data of 1970.[76] Since menarche occurs after the peak velocity of increase in height and weight, fertility becomes possible only after the girl has already experienced her most rapid growth. Few studies have been done on age at the start of fertility, but irregular menses are common during the first one or two years following menarche, and it is believed that many of the early menstrual periods are anovulatory.[76] The potential for conception is more closely related to maturational age than to chronological age, and occurs earlier in the early-maturing girl. Ideally, then, analysis of the risks associated with pregnancy should be based on menarcheal age rather than on chronological age.

Individual variation in the amount of linear growth attained after menarche may also be a factor in the degree of risk of superimposing prenancy on a period of continuing growth of the mother. Roche and Davila[77] reported a median increment of 7.4 cm of stature following menarche, with a range of 4.3 cm at the tenth percentile to 10.6 cm at the ninetieth. Dreizen et al.[78]

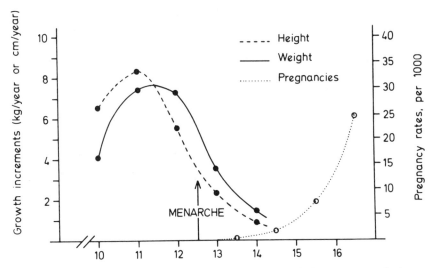

Figure 8.12 Schematic presentation of age in relation to growth increments, menarche, and incidence of pregnancies in adolescent girls. (Reprinted from Thomson, A.M. Pregnancy in Adolescence. In: McKigney, J.I., and H.N. Munro (Eds.) Nutrient Requirements in Adolescence. MIT Press, Cambridge, Mass., 1976.)

found a mean difference of 8.4 cm between menarche and completion of skeletal maturation in well-nourished girls and 5.6 cm in girls who had been poorly nourished and who had delayed menarche. The amount of potential growth remaining at conception may influence the degree of limitation of fetal development when the mother is very young. In addition, little is known about possible effects of pregnancy on the growth potential of the adolescent mother herself.

The weight gain of the adolescent during pregnancy should allow for gain to her own body as well as for the fetus and products of conception. A gain of 5 to 10 kg may be expected between menarche and maturity, on the average, with a rapid gain in the first year following menarche tapering off gradually to approximately 18 years. As with adult women, preconceptional weight and gain during pregnancy may be expected to affect fetal weight, but the allowance for gain of the adolescent should be higher than for the adult.

The nutritional status of the adolescent at the start of pregnancy may be compromised as a result of the recent demands of rapid growth, and further diminished if she has consumed a marginal or poor intake or if she has restricted her intake for weight control. Most of the studies of pregnant adolescents[79] have shown low intakes of calcium, iron, vitamin A, and sometimes vitamin C when judged by the Recommended Dietary Allowances. When vitamin–mineral supplements are prescribed, many girls do not take them regularly. Dietary improvement is not always accomplished, even with intensive counseling.

Programs for the adolescent during and following pregnancy should not be restricted to medical or nutritional care alone but should address the multiple problems of continued education, family planning, home management, consumer education, and other aspects of social and economic management.

ATHEROSCLEROSIS

The relationship of nutrition to atherosclerosis will be considered in more detail in Chapter 9, but some aspects of change in blood vessels during growth should be considered here. The relationship of fatty streaks during childhood to fibrous plaques in the adult has been the subject of controversy, and this had led to diverging opinions about the effects and wisdom of altering the diets of children with the aim of preventing later coronary artery disease.

Fatty streaks are abnormal lipid accumulations in the intima of the large arteries and are believed by some to be the first recognizable stage of atherosclerosis. In the aorta, fatty streaks have been identified within a few months after birth and are thought to be present in almost all children after 3 years. In the second decade of life the extent of the aortic intimal surface involved by fatty streaks increases. However, there is wide individual variation, with greater involvement observed in blacks than in whites, and in females than in males. No consistent relationship has been found between aortic fatty streaks and the factors commonly associated with severe adult atherosclerosis, including diet, obesity, geographic residence, or other illnesses. In the coronary artery, fatty streaks are usually not observed until about 15 years of age, and have been found in all populations regardless of their propensity to develop fibrous plaques or clinical atherosclerotic disease.[80]

Epidemiological studies have shown a strong statistical correlation between high total serum cholesterol concentrations and premature coronary artery disease. There is, however, no conclusive evidence that in humans a reduction of the intake of cholesterol or saturated fat prevents, decreases the development of, or reverses the atherosclerotic process or its attendant morbidity or mortality. Nevertheless, since these dietary factors have been implicated in the etiology of some forms of coronary artery disease, one school of thought recommends limitation of saturated fats and of foods high in cholesterol, either for their direct effect during childhood or as aiding in the establishment of eating patterns that may be beneficial to the adult. A more moderate recommendation is for the identification of children with specific risk factors, including family history, obesity, diabetes, hypertension, hyperlipidemia, and hypercholesterolemia; education about a change in eating patterns is more likely to be acceptable to this group of children.

Recent studies indicate that the risk of atherosclerosis is greater when the highest concentration of total plasma cholesterol is found in the low density lipoprotein (LDL) cholesterol. In cord blood and in the neonate, more than 50 percent of cholesterol consists of high density lipoprotein (HDL) cholesterol, but by one year the HDL concentration is similar to that of older children and adults.[81] One group of children who can be identified early are those with Type II familial hyperlipidemia; during the first year of life a decrease in plasma cholesterol can be accomplished by a diet low in cholesterol and high in polyunsaturated fats, but older children have a less sensitive response to such dietary manipulation. The long-term effects of this diet have not yet been explored.[82]

NUTRIENT REQUIREMENTS AND RECOMMENDED DIETARY ALLOWANCES

Nutrient needs during puberty and adolescence are dictated primarily by the rate of growth. Requirements increase from childhood levels at the onset of the growth spurt, reach their maximum at the time of peak growth, and gradually approach adult levels as growth subsides. The convenience of using chronological age categories in establishing standards limits the confusion of attempting to adapt standards to individual requirements and they are generally satisfactory when applied to population data. However, they are misleading when applied to individuals, especially those with early maturation. The girl whose menarche occurs at 10½ years has already passed through the period of her highest requirement for somatic growth before 10 years and is in the decelerating phase of growth when standards devised for the average girl recommend increases in nutrient intake.

Physical activity also has considerable influence on nutrient requirements and is extremely variable. The adolescent who participates in athletics and has periods of high exertion is likely to have an increase in appetite commensurate with energy output; higher caloric intake is accompanied by increased intake of all nutrients if the diet is varied. However, the sedentary individual has lower needs for calories but little decrease in other nutrient needs and, therefore, requires foods of higher nutrient density.

362

Sex differences in nutrient requirements become pronounced during puberty and continue throughout the rest of life. These differences begin with the onset of pubertal growth; the rise in needs for somatic growth is earlier in girls. The peak requirement of girls is lower than the peak for boys because of their lesser total increment in size and because of the differences in body composition. A larger proportion of male growth consists of lean body mass, which has more active metabolic function than adipose tissue and therefore requires more nutrients both for its growth and for its maintenance. As a result of different patterns of growth, metabolism, and physical activity, the total requirements of the male for calories and nutrients are higher, but the differential is greater for calories than for protein, minerals, and vitamins. Therefore the male has a higher allowance for calories within which to meet the requirements of other nutrients. The female, on the other hand, must have a higher ratio of nutrients to calories in her diet in order to meet all of her requirements.

There is some evidence that the efficiency of absorption and utilization of nutrients may increase during puberty and adolescence. This would be consistent with other observations of adaptation of digestive and metabolic processes of the body during periods of increased requirement or inadequate intake. However, physical or psychological stress may decrease absorption, and the teenager is subject to emotional lability, vulnerable to pressures of school or family or peers, and sometimes stressed in competitive athletics.

Few balance studies have been done on adolescents, and there is little experimental data on which to base requirements.[83,84] Therefore most estimations of requirements and dietary standards have been established from studies of intakes of presumably healthy subjects, interpolation, and factorial calculations. All of these methods are subject to varying interpretations by different individuals and committees, and each includes large factors of error and judgment. Some of the final values are difficult to support scientifically.[83]

During this age span maturational age is a better basis than chronological age for establishing requirements or evaluating intakes. Attempts to improve the delineation of age categories is evident from the fact that five different divisions for age groups between 9 years and adulthood have been used in the nine editions of the Recommended Dietary Allowances. Decisions have also differed on the age of maximum allowances, especially for girls. For example, in all editions through 1968 the allowances for energy intakes of girls increased to a peak between 13 and 16 years before dropping to adult levels, even though this age is later than the average peak growth velocity and is characterized by decelerating growth in most girls (see Figure 8.12). In the 1974 revision the maximum energy allowance for girls was between 7 and 14 years, and in 1979 between 7 and 10 years, ages more consistent with average maximum growth.

Historical changes in allowances have been much greater for the adolescent that for the child. A comparison of the first edition with the ninth edition shows the following decreases in maximum allowances for males and females, respectively: ascorbic acid 40 and 25 percent, protein 44 and 42 percent, riboflavin 43 and 35 percent, and energy 24 and 21 percent. Decreases of 25 percent or less have occurred in maximum allowances for vitamin A, thiamin, niacin and calcium. During the same time span, the only allowances which have increased have been for iron, which is now 20 percent higher for both sexes.

Despite repeated warnings against such use,[84-86] the RDA levels have commonly been used in dietary studies to determine the prevalence of low or marginal intakes and to estimate the risk of deficiency. However, the progressive changes in the RDA levels, particularly for the age groups between 10 and 20 years, complicate comparisons of such prevalence data over time. For example, fewer diets are given low ratings for ascorbic acid, protein, or riboflavin, but more diets are given low iron scores when compared to the present RDA levels.

ENERGY

The requirements of adolescents for energy vary widely from one individual to another, not only because of the different timing and magnitude of somatic growth but also because of great variations in physical activity. It is not uncommon to observe a twofold or greater difference in caloric intake of boys at a given age or of girls at a given age. In males the difference is often related to the amount of exercise. The requirements of girls are more difficult to estimate from studies of habitual intake because they are more prone to restrict voluntary food consumption for weight control.

The most recent recommended intakes of males are similar in the standards established by the United States,[87] Canada,[88] the Caribbean Food and Nutrition Institute,[89] and FAO/WHO.[90] There is a gradual increase during puberty from the childhood recommendations, to a peak of 2900 to 3200 kcal (12.2 to 13.4 MJ) in the age groups that center around 17 to 22 years, followed by a decrease to adult levels.

There is somewhat more variation in the recommendations for females, both in level and in maximum age. The RDA reaches a maximum of 2400 kcal (10.1 MJ) between 7 and 10 years, and the Canadian standard a maximum of 2300 kcal (9.6 MJ) at 10 to 12 years. The FAO/WHO and Caribbean standards are alike, reaching a maximum of 2490 kcal (10.4 MJ) at 13 to 15 years before declining to adult levels. Although the RDA committee stated that their allowances for children were lower than FAO/WHO standards "because American children are, on the whole, less active than those in other countries," the only significant deviation is for adolescent girls.

Studies of intakes of adolescents show some differences in the ages and levels of calories when average or median intakes of groups reach their maximum. In a review of data published between 1931 and 1955, Heald et al.[91] found that average intakes increased in males to a maximum of 3470 kcal/day at 16 years, followed by a decline of approximately 200 kcal/day by 18 years. In a collaborative study by 39 State Agricultural Experiment stations[92] between 1947 and 1958, mean intakes of males reached a peak of 3100 kcal/day at 16 to 17 years. In the Health and Nutrition Examination Survey (HANES),[93] white males had a peak median intake of approximately 2900 kcal/day between 15 and 19 years, while the peak in black males was 2475 kcal at 18 to 19 years. In two longitudinal studies at the Harvard School of Public Health (HSPH)[94] and the Child Research Council (CRC),[95] observations were discontinued at 18 and 17 years, respectively, but in both studies the intake of males at these ages had reached a plateau or was still increasing. The mean intake in the HSPH study at 17 to 18 years was 3535 kcal/day and in the CRC study a median close to 2800 kcal/day was maintained from 15 to 17 years. In the CRC study, the range in intake between 15 and 17 years was from 1900 kcal at the 10th percentile to 4000 kcal at the 90th percentile.

The females in the studies reviewed by Heald et al. reached their highest mean intake of 2550 kcal/day at "12 years," which presumably means between 12 and 13 years. In the collaborative study, the highest mean intake of 2300 kcal was observed at 11½ years. In the HANES survey, the highest median intakes of both black and white girls was 1850 to 1900 kcal/day at 10 to 11 years. In the Ten-State Nutrition Survey,[96] highest means were observed in girls 12 to 14 years of age, with levels ranging from 1750 to 2100 kcal in the low income ratio states and from 2100 to 2350 in high income ratio states for various ethnic groups. In the HSPH study, mean intakes reached a maximum of 2600 kcal/day at 14 to 15 years. The highest median in the CRC study was 2100 kcal/day at 13.5 years, with a range from 1450 at the 10th percentile to 2950 at the 90th percentile.

In summary, the mean or median maximum energy intake of females in these studies was between 1750 and 2600 kcal, attained at some age between 10 and 15 years. Maximum intakes of males were between 2475 and 3535 kcal at some age between 15 and 19 years. Differences may be due to study methodology, demographic characteristics of the populations, and other factors, but both the caloric level and the age at maximum intake showed distinct sex differences.

The requirements for calories, as well as for other nutrients, vary with the rate of growth and therefore with maturational stage of the child. In the HSPH study, early-maturing girls tended to have higher intakes of calories and protein between 8 and 12 years and early-maturing boys between 10 and 14 years than children who matured later. Since it is difficult to estimate maturational age without more complex examination facilities than are commonly available, an index of body size may be more meaningful than chronological age. Weight is altered by caloric intake and is a poor index; most studies show lower caloric intake per kilogram of body weight in obese than in normal weight individuals merely because the denominator is larger. The CRC study reported percentile levels of energy intake per centimeter of height. In males the highest level of the median was reached at 11 to 12 years, when the intake was approximately 18 kcal/cm, followed by a decline to 15 to 15.5 kcal/cm by 17 years. In females the highest median was observed at 9.5 years, when intake was 14 kcal/cm, and the median declined to 11 to 11.5 kcal/cm at 18 years.

CARBOHYDRATE

Since carbohydrate can be made in the body from some amino acids and from the glycerol of fats, no recommended allowances have been established. In the usual American diet 45 to 50 percent of calories are derived from carbohydrate; this level is observed in adolescence as well as at other ages. In the CRC study,[95] carbohydrate intakes increased during childhood but showed less change with age within the adolescent period than did energy. For example, the median intakes of males ranged between 300 and 325 g/day from 10 to 17 years of age, with 10th percentile levels close to 200 g and 90th percentile levels approximately 400 g/day.

Carbohydrate assumes particular importance to the adolescent who participates in athletic competition.[97] Carbohydrate is the most efficient source of energy at the high levels of oxygen demand that occur in maximal muscular effort. During physical training and competition, the primary increased dietary needs are for calories, water, salt, and carbohydrate. In prolonged exercise or in repeated intense bursts of exercise of short duration, muscle and liver glycogen may be depleted. Studies of carbohydrate metabolism in competitive athletics have focused on techniques for prolonging endurance and delaying muscle fatigue resulting from glycogen depletion. These have led to methods for increasing glycogen storage at the start of competition by "glycogen loading." Several days in advance of the competition glycogen stores are lowered by a low carbohydrate intake; during this period fatigue and inefficiency may be common. In the 3 to 4 days preceding competition the diet is changed to a carbohydrate intake that comprises 75 percent or more of the total calories consumed. This has been shown to double the glycogen storage in muscles.[98] This technique significantly increases endurance and has been shown effective in sports requiring endurance.

366

LIPIDS

No allowances have been established for fat intakes. The usual U.S. diet contains 35 to 45 percent of calories from fat. It has been suggested that a decrease to 35 percent or less should be recommended for adults, and some have recommended that the lower fat intake should begin during adolescence. In the CRC series,[95] the median fat intakes of children and adolescents after the first six months of life ranged between 37.5 and 39 percent of calories. The range from minimum to maximum intakes during adolescence was 27 to 47 percent for males and 24 to 51 percent for females.

Median intakes of fat of the CRC males rose from 100 g/day at 10 years to 126 g at 17 years. The median daily intakes of girls, on the other hand, rose from 80 g at 9 years to 93 g at 13.5 years and then gradually decreased to less than 80 g by 18 years.

PROTEIN

The RDA values for protein were progressively lowered between 1958 and 1974, as was discussed in Chapter 2 (Figure 2.1). In 1943 the RDA provided 10 to 11 percent of calories as protein. At the present time, the recommendations represent 6.7 to 8.7 percent of calories during adolescence. However, in a series of balance studies on adolescents, Johnston[99] found that the protein requirement could be met only when protein contributed at least 15 percent of calories on a diet adequate in calories. In balance studies of weight reduction in adolescents, Heald and Hunt[100] concluded that even 15 percent of calories from protein may be inadequate for optimal nitrogen retention when caloric intake is restricted. Protein anabolism is essential during the accelerative phase of growth and therefore a positive nitrogen balance must be maintained. Limitation of either protein or calories during rapid growth has repeatedly been shown to inhibit growth. There may be increased absorption of nitrogen during rapid growth.[99]

The RDA levels for males increase from 45 g (1.0 g/kg) at 11 to 14 years to 56 g (0.85 g/kg at 15 to 18 years and 0.8 g/kg at 19 to 22 years). For females the allowance is 46 g at 11 to 18 years and then decreases to 44 g at 19 to 22 years. The allowance per kilogram is the same for both sexes at comparable ages. The recommended allowances for both Canada[85] and the Caribbean area[89] are similar to the U.S. allowances during adolescence for males, but the highest allowance for females is 43 g in the Canadian standard and 45 g in the Caribbean allowances. The FAO/WHO figures[90] are lower at all ages, reaching a maximum of 38 g for the 16 to 19 year-old male and 31 g for the 13 to 15 to year-old female; however if the dietary protein score is 70, the levels would reach a maximum of 57 g for the male and 46 g for the female.[101] Both TSNS and HANES used a standard of 1.2 g/kg for both sexes between 10 and 16 years of age in evaluating intakes.

Intakes reported from both cross-sectional and longitudinal studies of adolescents are appreciably higher than the RDA levels. In most reports protein has contributed 12 to 16 percent of calories. Mean or median values for males in TSNS, HANES, and the HSPH and CRC growth studies fell within ranges of 78 to 84 g/day at 10 to 11 years, 86 to 98 g at 12 to 14 years, and 106 to 111 g at 16 to 17 years. Comparable intakes for females at the same ages were 69 to 74 g, 69 to 81 g, and 64 to 78 g. In all four studies the intakes of males rose throughout that age span, but intakes of females rose to a peak at some age between 12 and 16 years and then declined somewhat.

MINERALS

The data base for minerals is somewhat more extensive than for vitamins, but there are areas of controversy in the interpretation of balance studies as well as in factorial calculations and interpolation of recommended allowances during adolescence.

Calcium

Standards for calcium intake differ markedly during adolescence. The U.S. allowance increases to 1.2 g between 11 and 18 years, with allowances of 0.8 g prior to 10 years and after 19 years, with no sex difference. The FAO/WHO standard, in contrast, allows for 0.6 to 0.7 g between 10 and 15 years, and 0.5 to 0.6 g from 16 to 19 years, and the Caribbean allowance is set at the upper value of the FAO/WHO range. The Canadian recommended dietary intake is usually lower than the RDA, but closer to the RDA than to the FAO/WHO standard. The Canadian standard, however, provides for a sex difference, with the female level rising to a peak of 1.0 g at 10 to 12 years and the male level rising to a peak of 1.2 g at 13 to 15 years.

Since bone grows in volume and density as well as length, calculations of calcium requirement based on height increments alone underestimate calcium needs. It has been estimated that the female must retain 200 mg calcium/day for bone growth alone during the peak increment in stature between 10 and 14 years, and that the male must retain nearly 300 mg/day for bone growth at his peak between 12 and 14 years. However, individuals of the same stature may differ by at least 30 percent in bone volume and, therefore, differ in calcium requirement.[102] Calcium retention increases during adolescence, with the increase at an earlier age in females than in males.[103]

Many dietary studies in the United States have reported that some adolescents, especially girls, have calcium intakes that do not meet the RDA; however, few consume less than the FAO/WHO standard for that age

368

group. Mean or median intakes of males tended to increase steadily through the second decade of life, reaching a peak at 19 to 20 years.[103] Females, on the other hand, reached a peak between 12 and 16 years in various studies and then lowered their milk consumption and calcium intake toward the end of adolescence.

In the TSNS findings, mean intakes of males 10 to 16 years of age ranged from 0.7 to 1.5 g calcium/day and of females from 0.5 to 1.1 g; lowest mean intakes were reported in ethnic minority groups in low income ratio states. In the HANES data of 1971–1974, median intakes of males between 10 and 16 years rose from 1.1 to 1.25 g/day, but decreased in females from 0.96 to 0.72 g/day. In the CRC study of middle income children, median intakes of males 10 to 17 years of age ranged from 1.3 to 1.6 g; median intakes of females were 1.1 to 1.2 g/day between 10 and 16 years, then decreased to 0.7 to 1.0 g between 16 and 18 years.

Phosphorus

This mineral is included in both the United States and Canadian standards, with a Ca/P ratio of 1:1. Dietary studies show that the ratio is above 1:1 only during the first two years of life and drops slowly through childhood. The Ca/P ratio in the CRC study[95] was 0.80 to 0.85 in males between 10 and 17 years and in females between 10 and 14 years, but fell to 0.71 in females by 18 years when their milk consumption decreased.

Although a wide variation in Ca/P ratio can be tolerated so long as the vitamin D intake is adequate,[87] large intakes of phosphorus from soft drinks by adolescents with low milk intakes have raised some concern about low Ca/P ratios.

Iron

Perhaps the most controversial allowances are for iron during adolescence. The RDA recommends an intake of 18 mg/day by both males and females from 11 to 18 years, after which the female allowance continues at that level until menopause, but the male level drops to 10 mg at 19 years when most of his growth has been completed. In contrast, the Canadian Dietary Standard is 14 mg/day for the female after 13 years, and the male allowance reaches 14 mg only at 16 to 18 years. The FAO/WHO standard provides a range at all ages dependent on bioavailability of the food iron. The ranges for the male are 9 to 18 mg at 13 to 15 years and 5 to 9 mg after 16 years; the ranges for the female are 12 to 24 mg/day at 13 to 15 years, and 14 to 28 mg from 16 years into adulthood.

Most diets in the United States provide approximately 6 mg of iron per 1000 kcal. An allowance of 18 mg is unlikely to be reached except by athletes or occasionally by other adolescents with high intakes, and will rarely be reached by females. Most dietary studies have reported average intakes of adolescent females at levels close to 9 to 10 mg and of males 12 to 16 mg. The prevalence of "low" ratings for dietary iron is therefore very high and is inconsistent with the much lower prevalence of iron-deficiency anemia. This discrepancy has led to controversy about level of the allowance and about recommendations for iron supplementation.

VITAMINS

The RDA levels for vitamins have not been firmly established, but are dependent primarily on the judgment of the committee. Concern has been expressed about the prevalence of low intakes of vitamin A and ascorbic acid by some adolescents. The RDA values have decreased for both of these vitamins, although the allowances for ascorbic acid were increased again in 1979. Prevalence studies based on earlier editions of the RDA need to be reevaluated in the light of present standards. Since little clinical evidence of deficiency has been found in national surveys even when low dietary intakes were reported, one may question either the methodology of dietary surveys or the appropriateness of standards for rating as possible explanations for the discrepancy. The RDA table is in Appendix 1.

MEETING NUTRIENT NEEDS

Dietary recommendations during adolescence must take into account the social and attitudinal characteristics of the individual as well as the timing and rate of growth. Greater independence from family supervision and guidance is associated with increased peer conformity and influences of mass media. Rapid changes in body size create alterations in body image and individual reactions to those changes. Emotional instability may cause intermittent stress. Physical activity may be high among individuals who participate in competitive sports but very low in those with sedentary pursuits. Time schedules may lead to the omission of some meals or to greater frequency of eating. Meals may be consumed more often away from home and may commonly be bought in franchised food outlets. Interest in vegetarianism and nontraditional eating patterns may increase. In short, adolescence is a period of alteration in life-style and self-concept as well as of alteration in physical size.

Intermittently over the years concern has been expressed about the "poor diets" of adolescents. However, there are few data to substantiate these concerns. Although some teenagers do not make wise food selections, intakes below contemporary standards are most often observed among members of minority ethnic groups who are economically disadvantaged. Earlier studies that compared intakes to the former RDA standards showed a higher prevalence of "inadequate" diets than would be true using the present RDA levels. At the present time, iron and calcium intakes are of greatest concern. The RDA level of 18 mg iron is difficult to reach by dietary means. The tendency of some adolescents, especially girls, to decrease their milk consumption results in a lower calcium intake. However, concern about the nutrient contribution of between-meal snacks is not justified by recent studies.[104]

Analysis of the 24-hour intake records of 10 to 16 year-old subjects in TSNS[96] revealed that 7 to 30 percent of the day's intake of calories, protein, calcium, iron, thiamin, and riboflavin and up to 55 percent of vitamin A and ascorbic acid intake was supplied by between-meal snacks. The nutrient density of between-meal foods met or exceeded the RDA ratio for several nutrients, belying the common assumption that such foods are low in nutritive value. Huenemann et al.[48] found that frequent snacking was associated with higher total nutrient intake. Since the traditional pattern of three meals daily, usually eaten at home, is rapidly being replaced by fewer conventional meals but greater access to food at frequent intervals, nutrition education must accept this fact and place greater emphasis on selection of foods at any time of day to meet total nutrient needs.

Unless there is conscious control, the higher energy needs of the healthy adolescent will usually be met by increased appetite. Limitation of caloric intake is sometimes recommended by coaches for males in training for competitive sports, especially for wrestling. If caloric intake is limited enough to result in weight loss, the diversion of protein for energy may interfere with somatic growth. Reduction of caloric intake may be undertaken by adolescents, especially girls, for weight control. In the Berkeley study of high school students,[48] the number of girls who described themselves as too fat increased from 43 percent in the ninth grade to 56 percent in the twelfth grade, and 70 percent of the girls desired a weight loss, although only 11 to 17 percent were actually rated as mildly or markedly obese by measurements of body composition. The restriction of calories during adolescence is often done without professional advice and may lead to inadequate or even bizarre diets. Because so many adolescents are concerned about weight, this can provide the basis for effective nutrition education.

The inclusion of milk, cheese, or yogurt in the diet is essential to meet the RDA for calcium. Other foods in the U.S. diet rarely provide more than a total of 300 mg Ca/day. The daily consumption of 24 ounces of milk or its equivalent will ensure an intake close to the RDA. Although a deficiency of calcium has not been recognized clinically, there is ample evidence of its need for the mineralization of bone. A generous body storage of calcium provides extra protection for the adolescent who becomes pregnant soon after the peak of height velocity. Dairy products are also good sources of protein of high quality, other minerals, and several vitamins. They provide more protection in meeting nutrient allowances than any other single food.

Meat is an excellent source of protein, as well as of several minerals and vitamins. One advantage of inclusion of meat in the diet, which is often overlooked, is of special significance during adolescence. Meat contains heme iron, which is more readily absorbed than other forms of iron and which also enhances the absorption of iron from other foods in the small intestine.[105] The high requirements of iron for both sexes during adolescence can more readily be met if meat is eaten. Moreover, the risk of anemia is greater at this age if a vegetarian diet excluding meat is consumed.

Ascorbic acid also enhances the absorption of iron. Since it is customary to serve citrus fruit at breakfast, special attention to its inclusion in the diet should be given to anyone who chooses not to eat breakfast.

Vitamin A has sometimes been found to be low in the diets of teenagers. The frequent inclusion of yellow fruits, which are usually popular, and of green leafy and yellow vegetables, which may be less well liked and sometimes omitted at fast-food service establishments, should be encouraged. If low-fat milks are consumed, care should be taken to ensure that they are fortified with vitamin A.

Meeting nutrients needs can better be achieved when the diet contains a wide variety of foods than when variety is limited. With appetite as a guide to amounts for individuals, the allowances of all nutrients (with the possible exception of iron) can be met if the following protective foods are consumed daily:

24 ounces or more of milk or its nutritional equivalent
Two servings of meat, fish, poultry, or legumes
One egg (subject to limitation if plasma lipids are high)
Two or more servings of fruit, including citrus
Two or more servings of vegetables, including green leafy or yellow three or
    four times a week
Potato or a substitute
Two to six servings of bread or cereal, whole wheat or enriched
One to two tablespoons of butter or fortified margarine
Additional foods to meet energy needs

If, for any reason, the diet is restricted either in total quantity or in specific food groups, an evaluation of customary intake of the individual should be done to identify deficiencies and to provide a basis for nutrition counseling. The development of good food patterns in the adolescent should be encouraged because they may become the more stable food habits of the adult.

REFERENCES

1. Roche, A. F. Some aspects of adolescent growth and maturation. In: McKigney, J. I., and H. N. Munro (Eds.) *Nutrient Requirements in Adolescence.* MIT Press, Cambridge, Mass., 1976.
2. Timiras, P. S. *Developmental Physiology and Aging.* Macmillan, New York, 1972.
3. Heald, F. P. New reference points for defining adolescent nutrient requirements. In: McKigney, J. I., and H. N. Munro. *Nutrient Requirements in Adolescence.* MIT Press, Cambridge, Mass. 1976.
4. Reynolds, E. L., and J. V. Wines. Physical changes associated with adolescence in boys. *Am. J. Dis. Child. 82*:529–547, 1951.
5. Tanner, J. M. *Growth at Adolescence,* Second Edition. Blackwell Scientific Publishers, Oxford, 1962.
6. Young, H. B., W. W. Greulich, J. R. Gallagher, T. Cone, and F. Heald. Evaluation of physical maturity at adolescence. *Develop. Med. Child. Neurol. 10*:338–348, 1968.
7. Roche, A. F., and G. H. Davila. Prepubertal and postpubertal growth. In: Cheek, D. (Ed.) *Fetal and Postnatal Cellular Growth.* John Wiley and Sons, New York, 1975.
8. Garn, S. M., and B. Wagner. The adolescent growth of the skeletal mass and its implications to mineral requirements. In: Heald, F. P. (Ed.) *Adolescent Nutrition and Growth.* Appleton-Century-Crofts, New York, 1969.
9. Hansman, C. Anthropometry and related data. In: McCammon, R. W. (Ed.) *Human Growth and Development.* Charles C Thomas, Springfield, Ill., 1970.
10. Shock, N. W. Physiological growth. In: Falkner, F. (Ed.) *Human Development.* W. B. Saunders, Philadelphia, 1966.
11. Hamill, P. V. V., T. A. Drizd, C. L. Johnson, R. B. Reed, and A. F. Roche. *NCHS Growth Curves for Children Birth–18 Years.* DHEW Publ. No. (PHS) 78-1650. Supt. of Documents, U.S. Government Printing Office, Washington, D.C., 1977.
12. Tanner, J. M. Human growth and constitution. In: Harrison, G. A., J. S. Weiner, J. M. Tanner, and N. A. Barnicot (Eds.) *Human Biology. An Introduction to Human Evolution, Variation and Growth.* Oxford University Press, New York, 1964.
13. Hansman, C. F., and M. M. Maresh. A longitudinal study of skeletal maturation. *Am. J. Dis. Child. 101*:305–321, 1961.
14. Vaughn, V. C., III. Developmental pediatrics. In: Vaughn, V. C., III, R. J. McKay, and W. E. Nelson (Eds.) *Nelson Textbook of Pediatrics,* Tenth Edition. W. B. Saunders, Philadelphia, 1975.

15. Thissen, D., R. D. Bock, H. Wainer, and A. F. Roche. Individual growth in stature: A comparison of four growth studies in the U.S.A. *Ann. Human Biol. 3:*529–542, 1976.

16. Maresh, M. M. Variations in patterns of linear growth and skeletal maturation. *J. Am. Phys. Therapy Assoc. 44:*881–890, 1964.

17. Brasel, J. A. Hormonal changes during adolescence: A selected review of the literature. In: McKigney, J. I., and H. N. Munro (Eds.) *Nutrient Requirements in Adolescence.* MIT Press, Cambridge, Mass. 1976.

18. Rivlin, R. S. Thyroid hormone and the adolescent growth spurt: Clinical and fundamental considerations. In: Heald, F. P. (Ed.) *Adolescent Nutrition and Growth.* Appleton-Century-Crofts, New York, 1969.

19. Cheek, D. B. Growth and body composition. In: Cheek, D. B. (Ed.) *Fetal and Postnatal Cellular Growth.* John Wiley and Sons, New York, 1975.

20. Kochakian, C. D. Effect of androgens on cellular growth and metabolism. In: Heald, F. P. (Ed.) *Adolescent Nutrition and Growth.* Appleton-Century-Crofts, New York, 1969.

21. Hammar, S. L. Adolescence. In: Kelley, V. K. (Ed.) *Brennemann's Practice of Pediatrics,* Vol. I. Harper and Row, Hagerstown, Md., 1975.

22. Damon, A., and C. J. Bajema. Age at menarche. Accuracy of recall after thirty-nine years. *Human Biol. 46:*381–384, 1974.

23. Livson, N., and D. McNeill. The accuracy of recalled age of menarche. *Human Biol. 34:*218–221, 1962.

24. McMahon, B. *Age at Menarche.* DHEW Publ. No. (HRA) 74-1615. Supt. of Documents, U.S. Government Printing Office, Washington, D.C., 1973.

25. Johnston, F. E., A. F. Roche, L. M. Schell, and H. N. B. Wettenhall. Critical weight at menarche. Critique of a hypothesis. *Am. J. Dis. Child. 129:*19–23, 1975.

26. Billewicz, W. Z., H. M. Fellowes, and C. A. Hytten. Comments on the critical metabolic mass and the age of menarche. *Ann. Human Biol. 3:*51–59, 1976.

27. Frisch, R. E., and R. Revelle. Height and weight at menarche and a hypothesis of menarche. *Arch. Dis. Child. 46:*695–701, 1971.

28. Frisch, R. E., R. Revelle, and S. Cook. Components of weight at menarche and the initiation of the adolescent growth spurt in girls. Estimated total water, lean body weight and fat. *Human Biol. 46:* 469–483, 1973.

29. Mellits, E. D., and D. B. Cheek. The assessment of body water and

fatness from infancy to adulthood. *Monogr. Soc. Res. Child Dev. 35* (7):12–27, 1970.

30. McCammon, R. W. Are boys and girls maturing physically at earlier ages? *Am. J. Pub. Health 55*:103–106, 1965.
31. Brown, P. E. The age at menarche. *Brit. J. Prev. Soc. Med. 20*:9–14, 1966.
32. Brundtland, G. H., and L. Walløe. Menarcheal age in 19th century Norway. *Ann. Human Biol. 3*:363–373, 1976.
33. Millar, H. E. C. *Approaches to Adolescent Health Care in the 1970s.* DHEW Publ. No. (HSA) 75-5014. Supt. of Documents, U.S. Government Printing Office, Washington, D.C., 1975.
34. Holliday, M. A. Discussion. In: McKigney, J. I., and H. N. Munro (Eds.) *Nutrient Requirements in Adolescence.* MIT Press, Cambridge, Mass. 1976.
35. Hepner, R. Discussion. In: McKigney, J. I., and H. N. Munro (Eds.) *Nutrient Requirements in Adolescence.* MIT Press, Cambridge, Mass. 1976.
36. Meyers, A.J. Hematology. In: McCammon, R. W. (Ed.) *Human Growth and Development.* Charles C Thomas, Springfield, Ill., 1970.
37. deGroot, I., J. A. Morrison, K. A. Kelly, J. L. Rauh, M. J. Mellies, B. K. Edwards, and C. J. Glueck. Lipids in school children 6 to 17 years of age: Upper normal limits. *Pediat. 60*:437–443, 1977.
38. Abraham, S., C. L. Johnson, and M. D. Carroll. *Total Serum Cholesterol Levels of Children 4-17 Years. United States, 1971–74.* DHEW Publ. No. (PHS) 78-1655. Supt. of Documents, U.S. Government Printing Office, Washington, D.C., 1978.
39. Lee, V. A. Individual trends in the total serum cholesterol of children and adolescents over a ten-year period. *Am. J. Clin. Nutr. 20*:5-12, 1967.
40. Roberts, J. *Cardiovascular Conditions of Children 6–11 Years and Youths 12–17 Years, United States, 1963–1965 and 1966–1970.* DHEW Publ. No. (PHS) 78-1653. Supt. of Documents, U.S. Government Printing Office, Washington, D.C., 1978.
41. Consolazio, C. F. Physical activity and performance of the adolescent. In: McKigney, J. I., and H. N. Munroe (Eds.) *Nutrient Requirements in Adolescence.* MIT Press, Cambridge, Mass., 1976.
42. *Physical Activity during Menstruation and Pregnancy.* Physical Fitness Research Digest, Series 8, No. 3. President's Council on Physical Fitness and Sports, Washington, D.C., July, 1978.
43. Ten-State Nutrition Survey, 1968–1970. *III. Clinical, Anthropometry, Dental.* DHEW Pub. No. (HSM) 72-8131. Supt. of Documents, U.S. Government Printing Office, Washington, D.C., 1972.

44. Roberts, J. *Examination and Health History Findings among Children and Youths, 6–17 Years, United States.* DHEW Publ. No. (HRA) 74-1611. Supt. of Documents, U.S. Government Printing Office, Washington, D.C., 1974.

45. Forbes, G. Lean body mass and fat in obese children. *Pediat. 34*:308–314, 1964.

46. Bayley, N. Growth curves of height and weight by age for boys and girls, scaled according to physical maturity. *J. Pediat. 48*:187-194, 1956.

47. Garn, S. M., and D. C. Clark. Nutrition, growth, development, and maturation: Findings from the Ten-State Nutrition Survey of 1968–1970. *Pediat. 56*:306–319, 1975.

48. Huenemann, R. L., M. C. Hampton, A. R. Behnke, L. R. Shapiro, and B. W. Mitchell. *Teenage Nutrition and Physique.* Charles C Thomas, Springfield, Ill., 1974.

49. Dwyer, J. T., J. J. Feldman, and J. Mayer. Adolescent dieters: Who are they? Physical characteristics, attitudes, and dieting practices of adolescent girls. *Am. J. Clin. Nutr. 20*: 1045–1056, 1967.

50. Bray, G. A. *The Obese Patient.* W. B. Saunders, Philadelphia, 1976.

51. Coates, T. J., and C. E. Thoreson. Treating obesity in children and adolescents: A review. *Am. J. Pub. Health 68*:143–151, 1978.

52. Rivlin, R. S. The use of hormones in the treatment of obesity. In: Winick, M. (Ed.) *Childhood Obesity.* John Wiley and Sons, New York, 1975.

53. Heald, F. P. Juvenile Obesity. In: Winick, M. (Ed.) *Childhood Obesity.* John Wiley and Sons, New York, 1975.

54. Knittle, J. L. Obesity in childhood: A problem in adipose tissue cellular development. *J. Pediat. 81*:1048–1059, 1972.

55. Johnson, M. L., B. S. Burke, and J. Mayer. Relative importance of inactivity and overeating in the energy balance of obese high school girls. *Am. J. Clin. Nutr. 4*:37–44, 1956.

56. Spargo, J. A., F. Heald, and P. S. Peckos. Adolescent obesity. *Nutr. Today 1*:2–9, 1966.

57. Barlow, D. H., and J. L. Tillotson. Behavioral science and nutrition. *J. Am. Dietet. Assoc. 72*:368–371, 1978.

58. Hammar, S. L. Obesity and the pediatrician. *Am. J. Dis. Child. 125*:787-788, 1973.

59. Bruch, H. *Eating Disorders. Obesity, Anorexia Nervosa, and the Person Within.* Basic Books, New York, 1973.

60. Katz, J. L., and H. Weiner. A functional anterior hypothalamic defect in primary anorexia nervosa? *Psychosom. Med. 37*:103–105, 1975.

61. Hurd, H. P. II, P. J. Palumbo, and H. Gharib. Hypothalmic-endocrine dysfunction in anorexia nervosa. *Mayo Clinic Proc.* *52*:711–716, 1977.

62. Bruch, H. Anorexia nervosa. *Nutr. Today 13*:14–18, 1978.

63. Hepner, R. Discussion. In: McKigney, J. I., and H. N. Munro (Eds.) *Nutrient Requirements in Adolescence.* MIT Press, Cambridge, Mass. 1976.

64. Hallberg, L., A. Hogdahl, L. Nilsson, and G. Rybo. Menstrual blood loss: A population study. *Acta Obstet. Gynecol. Scand. 45*:320–351, 1966.

65. Beaton, G. H. The use of nutritional requirements and allowances. In: White, P. L. (Ed.) *Proc. West. Hemisphere Nutrition Congress III.* Futura Publ. Co., 1971.

66. Trowbridge, F. L. Discussion. In: McKigney, J. I., and H. N. Munro (Ed.) *Nutrient Requirements in Adolescence.* MIT Press, Cambridge, Mass., 1976.

67. Am. Acad. Pediat. Committees on Drugs and on Nutrition. The use and abuse of vitamin A. *Pediat. 48*:655–656, 1971.

68. Rose, D. P. The pill and nutrition: A most intricate relationship. *The Professional Nutritionist* (Foremost Foods Co.). *9*:1–5, 1977.

69. Roe, D. A. Nutrition and the contraceptive pill. In: Winick, M. (Ed.) *Nutritional Disorders of American Women.* John Wiley and Sons, New York, 1977.

70. Symposium. Effects of oral contraceptive hormones on nutrient metabolism. *Am. J. Clin. Nutr. 28*:329–412 and 515–560, 1975.

71. Committee on Nutrition of the Mother and Preschool Child. *Oral Contraceptives and Nutrition.* National Academy of Sciences, Washington, D.C., 1975.

72. Theurer, R. C. Effect of oral contraceptive agents on vitamin and mineral needs: A review. *J. Reprod. Med. 8*:13–19, 1972.

73. Luhby, A. L., M. Brin, M. Gordon, P. Davis, M. Murphy, and H. Spiegel. Vitamin B_6 metabolism in users of contraceptive agents. Abnormal urinary xanthurenic acid excretion and its correction by pyridoxine. *Am. J. Clin. Nutr. 24*:684–693, 1971.

74. Grant, J. A., and F. P. Heald. Complications of adolescent pregnancy. Survey of the literature on fetal outcome in adolescence. *Clin. Pediat. 11*:567–570, 1972.

75. Erkan, K. A., B. A. Rimer, and O. C. Stine. Juvenile pregnancy: Role of physiological maturity. *Maryland Med. J. 20*:50–52, 1971.

76. Thomson, A. M. Pregnancy in adolescence. In: McKigney, J. I., and H. N. Munro (Eds.) *Nutrient Requirements in Adolescence.* MIT Press, Cambridge, Mass. 1976.

77. Roche, A. F., and G. H. Davila. Late adolescent growth in stature. *Pediat. 50*:874–880, 1972.

78. Dreizen, S., C. N. Spirakis, and R. E. Stone. A comparison of skeletal growth and maturation in undernourished and well-nourished girls before and after menarche. *J. Pediat. 70*:256–263, 1967.

79. Weigley, E. The pregnant adolescent: A review of nutritional research and programs. *J. Am. Dietet. Assoc. 66*:588–592, 1975.

80. McGill, H. C., S. C. Mitchell, and R. M. Lauer. *Development Nutrition: Atherosclerosis.* Ross Laboratories, Columbus, Ohio, 1974.

81. *Task Force Report from the National Heart and Lung Institute: Genetic Factors in Atherosclerotic Disease.* DHEW Publ. No. (NIH) 76-922. Supt. of Documents, U.S. Government Printing Office, Washington, D.C., 1976.

82. Glueck, C. J., and R. C. Tsang. Pediatric familial type II hyperlipoproteinemia: Effects of diet on plasma cholesterol in the first year of life. *Am. J. Clin. Nutr. 25*:224–230, 1972.

83. Mueller, J. F. Current Recommended Dietary Allowances for Adolescents. In: McKigney, J. I., and H. N. Munro. (Eds.) *Nutrient Requirements in Adolescence.* MIT Press, Cambridge, Mass. 1976.

84. Munro, H. N. How well recommended are the Recommended Dietary Allowances? *J. Am. Dietet. Assoc. 71*:490–494, 1977.

85. Harper, A. E. Recommended Dietary Allowances: Are they what we think they are? *J. Am. Dietet. Assoc. 64*:151–156, 1974.

86. Leverton, R. M. The RDAs are not for amateurs. *J. Am. Dietet. Assoc. 66*:9–11, 1975.

87. *Recommended Dietary Allowances.* Eighth Edition. National Academy of Sciences, Washington, D.C., 1974.

88. *Dietary Standard for Canada.* Bureau of Nutritional Sciences, Department of National Health and Welfare, Ottawa, 1976.

89. *Recommended Dietary Allowances for the Caribbean.* Caribbean Food and Nutrition Institute, Kingston, Jamaica, 1976.

90. FAO/WHO Handbook on Human Nutritional Requirements, 1974. *Nutr. Rev. 33*:147-157, 1975.

91. Heald, F. P., P. S. Remmell, and J. Mayer. Caloric protein and fat intakes in children and adolescents. In: Heald, F. P. (Ed.) *Adolescent Nutrition and Growth.* Appleton-Century-Crofts, New York, 1969.

92. Nutritional Status USA. *California Agric. Expt. Station Bull. 769,* University of California, Berkeley, 1959.

93. Abraham, E., M. D. Carroll, C. M. Dresser, and C. L. Johnson. *Dietary Intake Findings, United States, 1971-1974.* DHEW Publ. No. (HRA) 77-1647. Supt. of Documents, U.S. Government Printing Office, Washington, D.C., 1977.

94. Burke, B. S., R. B. Reed, A. S. van den Berg, and H. C. Stuart. Caloric and protein intakes of children between 1 and 18 years of age. *Pediat. 24*(Suppl. Part II): 922–940, 1959.

95. Beal, V. A. Nutritional Intake. In: McCammon, R. W. (Ed.) *Human Growth and Development.* Charles C Thomas, Springfield, Ill., 1970.

96. *Ten-State Nutrition Survey, 1968–1970. V. Dietary.* DHEW Publ. No. (HSM) 72-8133. Supt. of Documents, U.S. Government Printing Office, Washington, D.C., 1972.

97. Smith, N. J. *Food for Sport.* Bull Publ. Co., Palo Alto, Calif., 1976.

98. Bergström, J., and E. Hultman. Nutrition for maximal sports performance. *JAMA 221*:999–1006, 1972.

99. Johnston, J. A. Protein requirements of adolescents. *Ann. N.Y. Acad. Sci. 69*:881–892, 1958.

100. Heald, F. P., and S. M. Hunt. Caloric dependency in obese adolescents as affected by degree of maturation. *J. Pediat. 66*:1035–1041, 1965.

101. World Health Organization. *Energy and Protein Requirements.* Tech. Report Series 522. FAO/WHO, Geneva, 1973.

102. Garn, S. M., and B. Wagner. The adolescent growth of the skeletal mass and its implications to mineral requirements. In: Heald, F. P. (Ed.) *Adolescent Nutrition and Growth.* Appleton-Century-Crofts, New York, 1969.

103. Ohlson, M. A., and G. Stearns. Calcium intake of children and adults. *Fed. Proc. 18*:1076–1085, 1959.

104. Thomas, J. A., and D. A. Call. Between-meal eating: A nutrition problem among teenagers? *Nutr. Rev. 31*:137–139, 1973.

105. Cook, J. D., and E. R. Monson. Food absorption in human subjects: III. Comparison of the effect of animal proteins on nonheme iron absorption. *Am. J. Clin. Nutr. 29*:859–867, 1976.

9

THE
ADULT
AND
THE
ELDERLY

Growth, development, maturity, and aging are phases in the continuum of life of the cells, tissues, organs, and the whole organism. From conception to maturity the major phenomenon is one of increase of mass and development of function. The peak may be maintained for some time during maturity, but in subtle ways many functions decline after reaching their maximum. Aging is a fundamental intrinsic characteristic, with gradual loss of operational efficiency, vitality, and resistance to stress. No type of cell or tissue is unaffected by age, but there is wide variation among cells and tissues in their ability to maintain normal function and to resist deterioration. The degree and rate of change vary among tissues within the individual, among individuals within a species, and among species.

The life span is genetically determined.[1] The life span of the mouse is 3 to 4 years, of the guinea pig 7 to 8 years, of the horse 45 to 50 years, and of the human perhaps 100 to 120 years. Large mammals tend to live longer than smaller animals. With most animals life span seems to be inversely related to metabolic rate; small animals have higher metabolic rates but shorter life spans. Humans, however, do not fit this pattern, since their lifetime energy expenditure is high. It has, therefore, been theorized that the size of the brain and learning capacity, as well as genetics, influence longevity, and that life span is longer for species with a slower rate of growth and attainment of maturity.[1]

Within each organism some cells and tissues have life spans unrelated to that of the whole organism. The placenta, for example, is a tissue that grows, matures, and then deteriorates and is discarded when its specialized function has been completed. The fetal red blood cell has a life span of 70 days and the mature red blood cell's span is 120 days from formation to destruction. It has been estimated that in the 70-kg man 2.3×10^{11} erythrocytes die and are replaced daily.[1] In the epidermis, cells are replaced every four to eight days as they are sloughed off; they are therefore replaced about 60 times every year. Epithelial cells of the gastrointestinal tract are constantly aging, being discarded, and replaced. These cells are, in general, unable to reproduce themselves, and the body is dependent on *de novo* synthesis of cells for maintenance of its functions.

In contrast, nerve and muscle cells, which are also incapable of cell division, have a longer life span and they must be maintained with functional efficiency for the health of the total organism. Liver and kidney cells are capable of cell division. Although mitosis is rare in liver cells, the liver retains the ability to replace damaged or lost cells to restore its mass.

Aging, then, begins in the fetal period even when anabolism and hyperplasia are the dominant characteristics of the organism. The degree, timing, and rate of loss vary with the type of cell or tissue. The body can synthesize and replace essential cells and thereby maintain functional ability throughout the period of growth and into maturity. This is followed by a gradual decline in cell efficiency and in the capacity of the organism to adapt to its environment.

As a process of change, aging involves all aspects of the body. Deterioration may begin within the cell as a result of changes in the nucleus, organelles, or cytoplasm, in the cell wall, or in the extracellular environment. Since the organism is integrated at several levels, the consequences of cell aging may range from altered structure and function of body tissues to the total interrelationships of the organism to its physical and social environment. The gradual decrement in physiological function, such as cardiac output, renal blood flow, antibody formation, or response to insulin, may reduce the ability of the body to adjust to challenge or stress. Susceptibility to disease is increased, and disease further speeds the rate of deterioration.

Aging is a progression of changes that occur to all individuals if they live long enough, although at different rates for different individuals. Disease, in contrast, is a pathological state which may occur at any age but is more likely to strike the elderly because of their decreased resistance. As a result of the greater prevalence of disease in the elderly, the study of the aging process itself is complicated by concomitant alterations in the body as a result of disease or its treatment. However, it is important to distinguish between the intrinsic effects of aging, which may not be subject to modification, and the associated effects of disease, which are presently or potentially subject to intervention.

LIFE EXPECTANCY IN THE UNITED STATES

An infant born in 1900 could anticipate an average life span of 49 years. By 1930 this had risen to 59 years, by 1950 to 68 years, and by 1970 to 71 years. In 1977 life expectancy had further increased to 73 years.[2] The lengthening

382

of the average life span was due primarily to a general reduction in mortality, especially in the infant death rate. As a result more people live to an older age than was true earlier in the century. However, there has been less increase in life expectancy at older ages. For example, an adult who reached the age of 65 years in 1900 could anticipate living an additional 12 years. An adult who is now 65 years old can expect to live an average of 16 additional years, an increase of only 4 years.

Life expectancy is greater for women than for men at every period of life. At birth the life expectancy of females is 76.9 years and of males 69.2 years, a difference of 7.7 years. The female advantage decreases with advancing age, and at the age of 70 years the female's expected remaining life is 14.4 years and the male's 10.9 years, a difference of 3.4 years.[2] Longevity is less for blacks than for whites at all ages,[3] and the sex difference is also apparent in black individuals, as shown in Table 9.1. Longevity is less for American Indians than for other population groups in the United States.

The age distribution of the United States population in this century has shifted toward the right, and the median age is now close to 30 years. This movement toward older ages has resulted from a combination of a lower birth rate, decreased mortality in early and middle life, and therefore marked increments in the number of elderly. In 1900 less than four million people were over 65 years of age, constituting slightly less than 4 percent of the population. Between 1900 and 1960 the total population doubled, but the number over 65 quadrupled. At the present time more than 20 million persons are over 65, and they constitute approximately 11 percent of the population. Even within the age category over 65, there is a shift, with an increasing number older than 75 years. It has been estimated that approximately 8000 persons in this country are over 100 years of age. The ratio of women to men above 65 years is now 100:72.

Despite the fact that larger numbers of people live to older ages, there is no evidence that the maximum age attained has changed over the centuries. It is difficult to authenticate ages, since birth certificates are a relatively new development and not universally available, and exaggeration of age is not uncommon. Reports in 1973 that large numbers of the populations of three remote mountain areas in Pakistan, Ecuador, and Russia were more than 100 years of age led to much speculation about the factors that led to such extended life spans. However, a more recent investigation[4] of the elderly in Vilcabamba, Ecuador, led to the conclusion that the oldest person in the village was really 96 years of age, rather than close to 150. Exaggeration of age seemed to begin at about 70 years, and as many as 20 to 40 years were added to the true age, compounded by the confusion of identical names of parents and children and immigration of elderly from surrounding areas. The oldest authenticated age in the world is 113 years, and the oldest in the United States nearly 113 years.[5]

Table 9.1 *Average Remaining Lifetime in Years at Specified Ages, by Color and Sex: 1900–1902, 1969–1971, and 1976 (For 1900–1902, data are for 10 States and the District of Columbia; for 1969–1971 and 1976 data are for the United States)*

Age in Years	1976	1969–1971	1900–1902[a]	1976	1969–1971	1900–1902[a]
	White, Male			White, Female		
0	69.7	67.94	48.23	77.3	75.49	51.08
1	69.8	68.33	54.61	77.2	75.66	56.39
5	66.0	64.55	54.43	73.4	71.86	56.03
10	61.1	59.69	50.59	68.5	66.97	52.15
15	56.2	54.83	46.25	63.6	62.07	47.79
20	51.6	50.22	42.19	58.7	57.24	43.77
25	47.1	45.70	38.52	53.9	52.42	40.05
30	42.4	41.07	34.88	49.1	47.60	36.42
35	37.7	36.43	31.29	44.2	42.82	32.82
40	33.1	31.87	27.74	39.5	38.12	29.17
45	28.7	27.48	24.21	34.9	33.54	25.51
50	24.4	23.34	20.76	30.4	29.11	21.89
55	20.5	19.51	17.42	26.1	24.85	18.43
60	16.9	16.07	14.35	22.0	20.79	15.23
65	13.7	13.02	11.51	18.1	16.93	12.23
70	10.9	10.38	9.03	14.4	13.37	9.59
75	8.5	8.06	6.84	11.2	10.21	7.33
80	6.6	6.18	5.10	8.5	7.59	5.50
85	5.1	4.63	3.81	6.4	5.54	4.10

The increase in the elderly population has given rise to two special areas of study. Gerontology is the study of the aging process, and geriatrics is a medical specialty dealing with the prevention and treatment of disease in the elderly. Both terms are derived from the Greek word *geron*, meaning old man. The shift in distribution of the population has led to acute awareness of the economic, social, and political implications and has stimulated attention to the problems and needs of the elderly.

THE AGING PROCESS

There is no clear definition of "old." Professional athletes may have passed their peak performance at 30 or 35 years. Pension from the military services is possible as early as 37 years of age. Retirement with pension from employment may occur at any age between 50 and 75 years. No age limit has been set for artists, craftsmen, judges, statesmen, scholars, and the self-em-

Table 9.1 Continued

Age in Years	1976	1969–1971	1900–1902[a]	1976	1969–1971	1900–1902[a]
	All Other, Male			All Other, Female		
0	64.1	60.98	32.54	72.6	69.05	35.04
1	64.9	62.13	42.46	73.3	70.01	43.54
5	61.1	58.48	45.06	69.5	66.34	46.04
10	56.3	53.67	41.90	64.6	61.49	43.02
15	51.4	48.84	38.26	59.7	56.60	39.79
20	46.8	44.37	35.11	54.9	51.85	36.89
25	42.5	40.29	32.21	50.2	47.19	33.90
30	38.2	36.20	29.25	45.5	42.61	30.70
35	34.0	32.16	26.16	40.9	38.14	27.52
40	30.0	28.29	23.12	36.4	33.87	24.37
45	26.1	24.64	20.09	32.1	29.80	21.36
50	22.5	21.24	17.34	28.0	25.97	18.67
55	19.2	18.14	14.69	24.3	22.37	15.88
60	16.3	15.35	12.62	20.7	19.02	13.60
65	13.8	12.87	10.38	17.6	15.99	11.38
70	11.3	10.68	8.33	14.3	13.30	9.62
75	9.7	8.99	6.60	12.3	11.06	7.90
80	8.6	7.57	5.12	10.9	9.01	6.48
85	7.2	6.04	4.04	9.1	7.07	5.10

[a]Figures for the All Other group cover only Negroes. However, the Negro population comprised 95 percent of the corresponding All Other population.

Source: National Center for Health Statistics. *Facts of Life and Death.* DHEW Publ. No. (PHS) 79-1222. Supt. of Documents, U.S. Government Printing Office, Washington, D.C., 1978.

ployed. The selection of the age of 65 years, which has been most common, is attributed to Otto von Bismarck, who arbitrarily chose that age in establishing Germany's social security program in the 1880s, and for a century that age level has persisted. The lack of a clearly defined physiological age of transition into a category that might be termed "elderly" is reflected in the range of age distinctions currently used for various purposes.

Individual variation, which is characteristic of life at all ages, becomes more pronounced with the advancement of age. If aging is the result of decrement in the ability of molecules, organelles, and the cells themselves to maintain normal functions, the number of factors that can influence that ability is very large and grows as time passes. The genetic component is evident from studies of family patterns of age at death, subject to secular changes in longevity already discussed. Age at death and natural causes of death are more similar for monozygotic twins than for dizygotic twins, other siblings, or unrelated individuals.[1] However, environmental factors play a large role in both the timing and the rate of aging changes. As age increases, the individuality of experiences and history also increases. Physical size, medical history, environmental stress, intake of food and drugs, and motor activity, as well as the social, cultural, and psychological experiences that are unique to each individual result in marked differences in body status and functions. Therefore the decline in ability and the appearance of signs of aging vary widely from one person to another. Some individuals lose functional capacities at an early age while others retain them throughout life. Chronological age is not synonymous with biological or physiological age. Despite the common tendency to categorize all persons past a given age as "elderly," differences between individuals in capacity, handicaps, and needs must be recognized.

THEORIES OF THE CAUSES OF AGING

Many age-related changes occur in the structure and function of cells and tissues which are deleterious, resulting in a decline in vitality, ability to resist infections, adjustment to stress, and maintenance of homeostasis. The process of change may start long before the results become apparent. The body may adapt to small changes, especially if there are alternate physiological mechanisms that can compensate for these changes. The functions that show the greatest change usually involve the coordinated activity of a number of organ systems. Because the elderly have greater susceptibility to disease, studies of humans are plagued by the complexity of distinguishing between inevitable alterations of structure and function due to the passage of time and the deleterious effects on structure and function caused by disease or its treatment, or by environmental stress of other kinds. It is also difficult to distinguish between the causes and effects of the aging process, since the original alteration may not be recognized until after it has caused disruption of function. Some effects can be identified only after a sufficient period of progression.

In age-related deterioration, cells become less efficient, affecting not only the cell itself but also tissue mass and body functions which are dependent on the activity of those cells. When homeostatic control of one tissue is compromised, the change in enzyme or hormone production or the accumulation of metabolites in that tissue may affect other parts of the body. Aging may occur in many tissues, but with different rates at different ages, and the interrelationships of metabolism may create a domino effect, obscuring the basic or first change. In addition, alterations may occur simultaneously or in sequence at several different levels of body functioning. Since the initiating changes cannot be readily recognized, the first measurable difference in function may be at a different level of organization from the basic cause.

Investigations of the aging process have been approached from a variety of medical and paramedical specialties, and a number of theories of the causes and processes of aging have been proposed.[1,6,7] These hypotheses have been based on both human and animal studies, are not clearly differentiated, and may be mutually interdependent. The following discussion will not explore in depth the bases and consequences of age-related change, but is intended only to indicate some of the current approaches to increase our understanding.

Cellular Mutation

It has long been recognized that the mutation of germ cells becomes more frequent with increasing age, often with deleterious results. It has also been hypothesized that mutations may occur in somatic cells. Suggested causes of mutation include ionizing radiation, mechanical or thermal alterations, chemical mutagens, accumulation of the pigment lipofuscin, and a variety of other factors which cause injury to cell membrane, cytoplasm, or organelles. Mutation then decreases the efficiency of the cell in performing its essential functions. Mutations may be of minor importance in cells capable of division or replacement, but may be of major importance in nondividing, nonreplacing cells, such as nerve or muscle cells. Loss or interference with cell function may then cause structural or functional changes in nervous, endocrine, vascular, and immunologic systems and thus may have widespread effects.

Cross-Linkage

Closely related to the theory of cell mutation is the hypothesis that cross-linkages may be formed within or between molecules, preventing their normal function. If these cross-linkages occur in DNA or RNA molecules, the ability of the cell to replicate proteins is altered, and the resulting mutagens may be incapable of the expected function of those proteins. Linkages may occur in protein molecules themselves, such as enzymes or hormones, thus inhibiting or altering their metabolic activity.

Collagen and elastin are essential components of connective tissue and necessary for normal body function. Collagen is a major constituent of skin, blood vessels, bone, cartilage, and tendons, and comprises more than one-fourth of total body protein. In the adult most collagen seems to be relatively inert metabolically and has a slow rate of turnover. In aging, the amount of readily soluble collagen decreases, possibly due to an increase in cross-linkages. This change in collagen may result in some of the characteristics of aging, including loss of skin elasticity, reduction in vital capacity of the lungs, and rigidity of blood vessel walls. Thus alteration in collagen may affect many parts of the body.

Free Radicals

Free radicals are very reactive unpaired electrons produced as transient intermediates in normal metabolism, as in oxidative processes in the mitochondria. If they react with organic molecules, this may lead to polymerization and peroxidation. It has been suggested that malfunction and destruction of the cell may be caused by an increase in free radicals. Intracellular membranes are especially susceptible to damage by free radicals because of their high content of polyunsaturated fatty acids. Damage to mitochondrial membranes may interfere with cell metabolism. Damage to lysosome membranes may allow the release of hydrolytic enzymes, which in turn damage cytoplasmic or nuclear components of the cell, and alteration of the cell membrane may result in damage to extracellular materials. Because vitamin E is an antioxidant and may slow the destruction by stabilizing membranes, it has been speculated that a deficiency of vitamin E may enhance the action of free radicals on unsaturated lipids.

Programmed Cell Replication

In vitro studies using cultures of human diploid cells (lung fibroblasts) led to a theory that cells are genetically programmed for a finite number of divisions, with gradual slowing and finally cessation of mitotic activity. However, the experimental problems associated with the techniques of transplantation and culture may alter results, and there is some doubt about the validity of this theory.

Neuroendocrine Alterations

Interrelationships of the central nervous system and hormonal function develop early in life, are relatively stable during young adulthood, and undergo change during the aging process. Cortical centers of the CNS, primarily through norepinephrine, dopamine, and serotonin, exert a regulatory effect on the neurosecretory centers of the hypothalamus. The hypothalamus in turn stimulates the anterior pituitary toward synthesis and secretion of tropic hormones, which then stimulate their target endocrine glands to secrete specific hormones, such as the thyroid, adrenal, and gonadal hormones.

Except for the decrease in circulating testosterone in men and estrogen in women, few changes in hormonal production have been demonstrated with increasing age. The plasma level of triiodothyronine (T_3) decreases in the elderly, but the concentration of thyroxine (T_4) remains relatively normal, and the significance of the change in T_3 is unknown.

It has been hypothesized that, with aging, changes may occur at any stage of the neurohormonal chain of events. An increase in inhibitory synapses in the cortical centers, production of abnormal hormones, a decrease in the metabolic response of tissues to hormones, or impairment of the negative and positive feedback mechanisms may interfere with normal metabolism. This could result in specific or generalized alterations in function, including a decrease in muscle tone or function, changes in secretions, cardiovascular impairment, suppression of immunologic response, atrophy of organs, or other aspects of failure of the homeostatic and adaptive ability of the body.

Immune System

The immunologic capacity of the body increases during childhood, is maximal in the young adult, and then declines steadily. Immunocompetent lymphocytes are probably derived from bone marrow stem cells. T cells, which are thymus-dependent, are involved in cell-mediated immunity, and B cells, which are thymus-independent, are responsible for the production of circulating antibodies; both proliferate in response to antigen. Animal studies have shown that with aging there is a decline in immunologic capacity, that lymphoid tissue tends to be replaced by fat and fibrous tissue, and that an imbalance between T cells and B cells may develop. It has been hypothesized that, in addition to being a factor in reduced resistance to disease, the decreased competence of the immune system may also be a pacemaker for aging changes.

It has also been suggested that errors in the immune system may result in the inability of immunocompetent cells to distinguish between exogenous antigens and the body's own constituents. The body then produces antibodies to normal body compounds, resulting in autoimmunity.

Generalized Errors

Since there is no evidence that one single failure of metabolism is responsible for the total phenomenon of aging, it is likely that a combination of these occurrences may lead to progressive changes in many body systems. There may be an accumulation of errors, such as formation of abnormal proteins, enzyme release from lysosomes, increase of lipofuscin or other metabolites, and failure of the immune system. Such a combination or chain reaction would lead to generalized failure of normal metabolism.

PHYSIOLOGICAL CHANGES WITH AGING

Individuals who live to old age are biologically elite. Whatever the combination of genetic and environmental influences may be, those who survive early death possess traits that contribute to survival. Most of the data presently available on the changes in physiological function observed during aging have been obtained from cross-sectional studies, many on institutionalized subjects. These studies perforce include only the survivors at each age, and the observed alterations in group distributions at each additional decade of chronological age may not reflect true individual changes but merely represent the characteristics of those who are still alive. For example, a decrease in the range of body weights may be due to death of the most obese. Studies of the elderly are also selective in that two groups are most available for study: those who are physically mobile and mentally capable of cooperation in a study, and those who are institutionalized or in some other group setting. As a result, any one study is unlikely to represent the spectrum of population at a given age.

A true understanding of the characteristics that contribute either to early death or to survival will be possible when data become available from systematic longitudinal studies that trace the same individuals from an early age, prior to clinically detectable signs of aging, through the entire aging process. Such studies can be expected to sort out alterations in metabolism and function that are invariant transformations of age from those that are sequelae of disease. For example, a longitudinal study in progress at the National Institute of Mental Health (NIMH)[8] selected men who were presumably healthy for longitudinal follow-up. When extensive clinical testing showed that some had evidence of disease states, they were divided into two groups: those who were "optimally healthy" with no evidence of disease that might be expected to affect aging, and those who were "healthy" without clinical symptoms but with laboratory evidence of atherosclerotic or other pathological changes. Such longitudinal studies can be expected to provide insight into factors associated with individual variations in aging characteristics and therefore may lead to measures that can be applied to retard the effects of the aging process.

Many published studies of physiological changes have not distinguished between the normal sequence due to the aging process and those changes either caused or accelerated by disease. As a result, differences in findings at successive ages are often attributed to age. In addition, in cross-sectional studies the use of different subjects in each age group casts doubt on whether the apparent changes are real. As more carefully obtained and evaluated data become available, and as techniques for measurement of early changes are developed, concepts of aging have been revised and refined. Further progress will undoubtedly result in new concepts in the future. However, some common characteristics of aging populations have been identified in a combination of cross-sectional and semi-longitudinal studies, and will be summarized here.[1,6-11] Although body functions and systems will be arbitrarily classified for ease of presentation, the changes are interrelated and interdependent.

Cardiovascular system

Both the heart rate and the resting cardiac output decrease with age. Arteriosclerosis, the decline in arterial distensibility, is an age-related occurrence which has been observed in all populations and is progressive,[11] possibly related to the change in collagen. As a result of the decreased elasticity of the blood vessels, peripheral resistance decreases. In the elderly, exercise causes a marked acceleration in the cardiac rate and a rise in blood pressure, compensations that may not be sufficient to meet the demands of the exercising muscle.

Elevation of blood pressure with age is a common finding. In the 1971–1974 Health Examination Survey of the NCHS,[12] mean systolic pressure (sexes combined) rose from 119 mm Hg at 20 years to 150 mm at 70 years, with most of the rise observed in subjects over 35 years of age. Women had lower values than men to 55 years, and higher values thereafter. Therefore the rate of increase was faster during the adult years in women. Mean blood pressure readings of blacks were higher than those of whites in both sexes. Greater variability in the distributions was found with increasing age. However, the NCHS fifth and tenth percentiles showed little change with age between 20 and 70 years in men. This may be consistent with the lack of increase in systolic pressure of the "optimally healthy" men of the NIMH study,[8] while the "healthy" men with evidence of atherosclerosis had an increase after 65 years. The elevation of blood pressure may be an adaptive mechanism to preserve functional integrity when blood flow is restricted.

No consistent changes with age in blood volume, hemoglobin concentration, hematocrit, white blood cell count, and blood urea nitrogen have been observed in several studies. In the NIMH study, minimal changes were seen in total serum protein, but a decrease in albumin was offset by an increase in alpha-2-globulin and beta globulin. In the HANES findings[13] the prevalence of low serum protein values was higher in subjects 45 to 59 years of age than in those over 60 years. Consistent with many other studies, blacks in the HANES survey had lower hemoglobin and hematocrit levels than whites.

The lack of change with increasing age in fasting blood glucose may be due to the availability of alternate control mechanisms, but there is a decrease in the body's response to challenge. The glucose tolerance curve of older adults is often delayed in its return to normal after a glucose load when compared to the curve of younger adults.

Sex differences are apparent in the changes in total serum cholesterol from early maturity to old age. In the NCHS data,[14] median levels of both sexes were between 180 and 190 mg/100 ml at 18 to 24 years. Levels rose more rapidly in men to 44 years, and then were stabilized at 230 to 235 mg/100 ml from 45 to 74 years. In contrast, the rise in levels of women was steepest after 45 years, reaching a median of approximately 250 mg/100 ml in the 65- to 75-year age group. Mean levels of both sexes were lower in 1971–1974 than in the 1960–1962 survey.

Respiratory System

Maximal breathing capacity has usually been reported in most studies to decrease with age, with losses of as much as 40 to 60 percent between 20 and 80 years. However, only a slight decrease in maximal breathing capacity was observed among "optimally healthy" men in the NIMH study,[8] but subjects with arteriosclerotic disease showed a definite decrease. This suggests that some respiratory changes may be related more closely to pathological developments than to normal aging. Other respiratory changes usually associated with advancing age include a decrease in vital capacity, increases in residual volume and resistance to air flow in peripheral airways, and a fall in the uptake of oxygen into blood. As a result, exercise imposes a stress on respiratory function.

Renal Function

It has been clearly demonstrated that renal function deteriorates with age. Parallel to a progressive reduction in the number of functioning nephrons, decreases occur in glomerular filtration rate, renal blood flow, maximal capacity to concentrate para-aminohippuric acid, ability to resorb glucose, and ability to concentrate or dilute urine.

Gastrointestinal Function

Parietal cells lose their efficiency in secreting hydrochloric acid. This could be expected to have an effect on the digestion and absorption of several nutrients, but such effects have not been clearly demonstrated. The relative achlorhydria and decrease in the intrinsic factor may, however, be related to the greater prevalence of vitamin B_{12} deficiency in the elderly. There is some evidence that digestion of protein may become less efficient, possibly as a result of lower secretion of pepsin and other proteolytic enzymes. The absorption of calcium may also decrease.

Muscles

After 35 years a decrease in strength has been demonstrated by tests of hand grip; whether this is due to alterations in hormonal or neural factors or to intrinsic change in muscle structure is unknown. There is some evidence of decrease in the number and efficiency of muscle fibers. Lower gastric motility may prolong transit time in the gastrointestinal tract and contribute to constipation, which is often a complaint of the elderly.

Nervous System

It is through the integrative functions of the CNS that the body compensates for changes and regulates itself for continued survival, and the nervous system is considered to be an important influence on aging. The evidence of a decrease in the number of brain cells is controversial, but there is a decrease in the functional capacity of neurons. The response to stimuli is slowed, possibly due to less efficient synaptic connections or to alterations in cell function as a result of lipofuscin accumulation or free radical damage.

Several senses are altered with age. The number or efficiency of olfactory and taste receptors declines, and there is loss of both visual and auditory acuity, especially after 40 years of age.

Skeletal System

Density of long bones and vertebrae decreases with a loss of calcium from bone. A decrease in stature and breadth or depth of bony structures, such as the shoulders and the chest, may be related to a modification of the protein matrix of the skeleton. Decrement of bone in the jaw and loss of teeth are interdependent.

Hormonal Secretion

A gradual decrease in testosterone and increase in gonadotropin secretion have been reported in males after 25 years of age.

Menopause in the female results in a decrease in circulating levels of estrogen and progesterone and in the number of ovarian follicles and corpora lutea. There may also be changes in secondary sex characteristics, including the amount and texture of hair and the appearance of the breasts. In the NCHS study[15] of 1960–1962, mean age at menopause was in the fiftieth year, with fewer than 2 percent experiencing menopause before 40 years and fewer than 4 percent after 55 years. Age at menopause was unrelated to height, age at menarche, and probably to parity, but women considered lean by skinfold measurements tended to have menopause at earlier ages than heavier women. The mean age in the NCHS study was comparable to ages reported from Europe, South Africa, and other United States studies, which ranged from 47 to 50 years.

Basal Metabolic Rate

Due either to loss or to decrease in functional capacity of cells, the basal metabolic rate falls with age. Shock[11] estimated that BMR decreased 20 percent between 30 and 90 years of age. The lower metabolic needs may be related to the progressive loss of lean body mass, which is accompanied by an increase in adipose tissue.

CHANGES IN HEIGHT, WEIGHT, AND BODY COMPOSITION

Since data on body measurements are not available on the same individuals from early adulthood to old age, information currently available on the changes that occur is derived from cross-sectional studies. These data do not necessarily represent the changes that can be expected in individuals. They are subject to the usual limitations of cross-sectional data, which depend on the availability and selection of different individuals in successive age groups. For the elderly such data have the additional qualification of being the measurements of survivors in each age group, and a distribution of parameters studied may reflect characteristics which are conducive to survival. For example, a decrease in weight measurements may be the result of death of the obese and survival of the lean. In addition, the secular changes in height which were discussed in Chapter 1 must be considered; younger adults may be expected to be taller than those whose childhood growth occurred during a period of lesser growth rates. Therefore, some of the decrease in height with advancing age may be the result of secular changes in heights of population groups.

The largest assembly of data on adults in the United States population has been collected in the Health Examination Surveys of NCHS at intervals between 1960 and 1974. These surveys were based on a scientifically designed sample representative of the civilian noninstitutionalized population and may be expected to have wider application than data from insurance applicants or other selected groups.

Height

The mean height of males between 18 and 74 years in the 1971–1974 survey[17] was 176 cm. However, age trends were apparent, with a decrease of slightly more than 1 cm/decade in mean height. The mean height of males decreased from 177 cm at 18 to 24 years to 171 cm in the group 65 years and older. Mean heights of black males were approximately 1 cm shorter than those of white subjects. Heights in this survey were slightly higher than those found in the 1960–1962 survey, reflecting secular change.

Mean heights of women were also slightly higher than a decade earlier. The overall mean was 162 cm for women between 18 and 74 years. The mean of 163 cm at 18 to 24 years showed little change until 44 years, after which mean heights of women dropped to 158 cm in the 65 and older age group. No consistent differences in mean heights of black and white women were observed.

The decrease in stature with age may also reflect postural changes with atrophy of intervertebral discs.[6] This is consistent with the decline in sitting height relative to total height after 45 years in males and 55 years in females observed in the NCHS data of 1960–1962.[16]

Weight

The mean weight of males was 78.2 kg for the entire span of 18 to 74 years in the 1971–1974 NCHS survey,[17] but the pattern of change in weight was different from the pattern of change in height. At 18 to 24 years the mean weight of males was 70.5 kg, followed by an increase to a peak of 80.9 kg at 35 to 44 years. Thereafter mean weights decreased to slightly under 70.5 kg in men 65 years and older. Minimal differences in weight were found between black and white men.

Women also increased in weight following young adulthood, with the mean rising from 60.0 kg at 18 to 24 years to a peak of 67.7 kg at 45 to 64 years, then declining to 66.8 kg after 65 years. Mean weights were higher for black women than for white at all ages; the maximum difference was 9 to 10 kg between 35 and 64 years, when the mean for black women was 76 kg and for white women approximately 66.5 kg.

Measurements of weight within a population group show greater variability at all ages than do measurements of height. The distribution of weights becomes wider and standard deviations greater as age progresses. Therefore, while the mean values show trends with age, sex, or race, it must be remembered that there is more skewing to the right, especially during the ages when peaks in mean weights are observed.

Ponderal Index and Skinfold Measurements

The ponderal index (height/weight$^{1/3}$) reflected the weight changes in the 1960–1962 NCHS data.[18] The mean index for males 18 to 24 years of age was 12.67. As weight measurements increased, the index fell to 12.30 for men between 45 and 64 years. As mean weights decreased, the ponderal index then rose to 12.42 for men 75 to 79 years of age. At 18 to 24 years the mean ponderal index of women was 12.66, nearly identical to that of men. However, the index dropped more steeply for women, to a level of 11.72 at 65 to 74 years, with a final rise to 11.88 for women 75 to 99 years of age.

Subcutaneous fat has been estimated to comprise approximately 50 percent of total body fat in the young adult. However, with increasing age more fat is added internally and skinfold measurements in the elderly require a different evaluation. There is an increase in subcutaneous fat, which can be measured simply by calipers, but there is a further increase in total body fat which can be measured indirectly by methods that were described in Chapter 1.

In the 1960–1962 NCHS data,[17] mean triceps skinfold measurements of males rose slightly more than 25 percent in young adults, maintained a relatively constant level between 30 and 44 years, and then declined. The mean measurement of men at 75 to 79 years approached the mean at 18 to 24 years. Women had consistently higher mean skinfolds at the triceps level and their increase during maturity was steeper, with a 40-percent increase in the mean to a peak at 55 to 64 years before declining; their mean at 75 to 79 years was slightly higher than the mean at 18 to 24 years. Changes in subscapular skinfold measurements were smaller and sex differences were less marked. There were wide individual variations in all skinfold measurements of fat.

Subcutaneous fat has been estimated to comprise a mean of 13 percent of total body weight in men at 25 years and 26 percent of weight at 55 years. In women comparable calculations suggest that subcutaneous fat comprises 26 percent of total weight at 25 years, rising to 38 percent at 55 years. The added inner fat of the older individual would be at least partially offset by the decline in subcutaneous fat.

NUTRITIONAL ASPECTS OF HEALTH

There is a tendency to assume that all elderly people suffer from a variety of degenerative diseases and are in poor heath. On the contrary, the majority of people over 65 years of age are relatively healthy and are functioning with little or no limitation to their activity. Fewer than 5 percent are in institutions or nursing homes. The majority live independently or with family or friends. Two-thirds of the population over 65 own their own homes. More than one-half have no physical limitation to activity, and less than 20 percent are unable to carry on major activities because of health problems, due primarily to heart conditions and arthritis.

The health problems of adults and especially of the elderly have different characteristics from those of children, however. With lower body reserves and less resistance, they become less able to cope with infection and other illnesses. They tend to have more than one disabling condition at a time and the multiplicity may be interreactive. The diseases that are of primary concern seldom have a single cause but are of multiple etiology, often poorly understood with the present state of medical knowledge. These diseases are most commonly heart disease, cancer, hypertension, arteriosclerosis, diabetes mellitus, and obesity. The prevalence rates of some diseases by age are shown in Table 9.2. They are chronic rather than temporary, and therapy tends to be palliative rather than curative.

No attempt will be made here to discuss in detail the etiology, diagnosis, and therapy of these diseases, but only to present an understanding of some of the nutritional aspects of development and effects on nutritional status and requirements of selected health problems of adults and elderly persons. This discussion must be tempered by the increase in life expectancy in the United States as indicated earlier in this chapter.

Table 9.2   Prevalence Rates of Heart Disease, Hypertension, and Arthritis by Age and Sex: 1960 to 1962 (Rates per 100 persons in specified group)

Diagnosis and Sex	Total	Age Group in Years							
		18-24	25-34	35-44	45-54	55-64	65-74	75-79
Definite heart disease, total[a]								
Both sexes	13.2	1.2	2.4	6.7	13.2	25.3	39.9	42.3
Men	12.6	1.4	2.9	7.4	13.8	24.2	33.2	38.8
Women	13.7	1.1	2.0	6.1	12.5	26.2	45.2	45.8
Suspect heart disease total[a]								
Both sexes	11.7	4.0	4.9	8.8	15.3	19.4	20.7	25.2
Men	13.9	6.4	6.6	11.4	18.3	18.5	25.3	27.1
Women	9.7	2.0	3.3	6.4	12.4	20.1	17.1	23.3
Definite hypertensive heart disease								
Both sexes	9.5	0.3	1.3	4.7	9.6	17.9	30.3	31.8
Men	7.7	0.4	1.4	5.2	9.7	13.6	18.9	24.6
Women	11.1	0.2	1.2	4.2	9.5	21.9	39.5	39.0
Suspect hypertensive heart disease								
Both sexes	4.3	0.7	1.1	2.6	4.4	8.4	10.4	14.1
Men	5.1	1.5	1.7	4.2	5.0	7.8	12.8	16.1
Women	3.5	—	0.6	1.1	3.8	9.0	8.5	12.1
Definite coronary heart disease								
Both sexes	2.8	—	0.3	0.7	2.5	7.1	9.5	6.8
Men	3.7	—	0.4	1.1	3.5	9.7	11.6	9.1
Women	2.0	—	0.2	0.5	1.6	4.7	7.9	4.5

Continued

397

Table 9.2 *Continued*

Diagnosis and Sex	Total	Age Group in Years						
		18–24	25–34	35–44	45–54	55–64	65–74	75–79
Suspect coronary heart disease								
Both sexes	2.2	—	0.1	0.9	3.0	4.8	5.9	5.7
Men	2.2	—	—	1.3	3.4	4.4	5.3	3.8
Women	2.2	—	0.2	0.5	2.5	5.2	6.4	7.5
Definite hypertension								
Both Sexes	15.3	1.4	3.9	10.9	18.2	26.9	38.5	38.8
Men	14.1	1.7	4.8	13.5	18.3	22.3	27.1	32.4
Women	16.4	1.2	3.1	8.5	18.2	31.2	47.6	45.1
Borderline hypertension								
Both sexes	14.6	5.7	7.4	11.5	16.5	25.9	24.5	27.5
Men	17.2	10.9	11.9	14.2	17.7	27.5	24.8	26.7
Women	12.2	1.4	3.2	9.0	15.3	24.5	24.3	28.3
Rheumatoid arthritis								
Both sexes	3.2	0.3	0.3	1.3	3.0	6.3	9.2	18.8
Men	1.7	0.2	—	0.5	1.5	4.2	3.1	14.1
Women	4.6	0.3	0.6	2.1	4.4	8.3	14.1	23.5
Osteoarthritis								
Both sexes	37.4	4.1	9.7	24.7	46.6	69.4	80.7	85.4
Men	37.4	7.2	13.6	30.2	47.0	63.2	75.8	80.9
Women	37.3	1.6	6.2	19.6	46.3	75.2	84.7	89.8

aIncludes persons with other types of heart disease not shown separately.

Source: National Center for Health Statistics. *Facts of Life and Death.* DHEW Publ. No. (PHS) 79–1222. Supt. of Documents, U.S. Government Printing Office, Washington, D.C., 1978.

OBESITY

Calculations of body composition from anthropometric measurements, estimations of total body potassium and body water compartments, and determination of basal oxygen comsumption all indicate that functional cellular mass decreases with advancing age. As a component of body weight, muscle is replaced by connective and adipose tissue.[19] As a result, energy needs for body maintenance decrease. In addition, physical activity is progressively less in most individuals. Therefore, unless caloric intake is comparably decreased, the relative excess of energy intake causes further accumulation of body fat and increase in body weight.

In the HANES survey of 1971–1974,[17] the peak in mean weight of males was found in the age group 35 to 44 years, and in females the highest mean weight occurred between 35 and 65 years. There was no consistent difference between black and white men in mean weights, but black women had consistently higher mean weights than white women throughout the span from 18 to 74 years. Mean weights and heights were higher in both sexes in the 1971–1974 survey than had been found in the sample of population surveyed in 1960–1962.

Damon et al.,[20] in a cross-sectional study of healthy adult males between 20 and 80 years of age, found that the redistribution of fat from peripheral to internal sites was reflected in decreased triceps skinfolds but increased abdominal measurements. The interpretation of changes in skinfold measurements in adults must take into consideration that with advancing age subcutaneous fat becomes progressively less reliable as an index of total body fat. In the HANES survey[18] the peak in mean triceps skinfold measurements of men was slightly earlier than the peak in weight, occurring at 30 to 40 years. The peak for women, however, was observed at 60 years. In the TSNS findings,[21] peak median triceps skinfold measurement was at 50 years in both sexes.

Racial differences in skinfold measurements were more pronounced in women than in men in both surveys. White males tended to be heavier with wider skinfold measurements, but the differences were relatively small. In contrast, black females were significantly heavier and had higher median skinfolds than white females throughout the span from 20 to 70 years. However, black women showed a wider range of measurements of triceps skinfolds.[21] At the seventy-fifth and ninetieth percentiles measurements of the two racial groups were similar; at the median black women had more fat than white women; at the fifth percentile black women had less subcutaneous fat than white women. In other words, racial differences were most apparent among the leanest women. Obesity was more common among low income women than among those in the middle income group, but the reverse was found in men, for whom fatness increased as income increased.

One may speculate about weight consciousness in upper income women and greater physical activity of low income men as possible factors in these differences.

Obesity of itself has not usually been shown to create a health hazard or to increase mortality. But obesity is frequently associated with conditions that threaten health and increase mortality, and obese individuals with disease have a higher mortality rate than normal weight individuals with that disease. For example, diabetes mellitus is three times more common among the obese, and hypertension is twice as common among obese as among individuals of normal weight.[22] The mortality from heart and circulatory diseases and from gall bladder and renal diseases is higher when obesity is also present. In the Framingham heart study,[23] excessive weight itself did not increase the risk of coronary heart disease in women unless hypertension and/or hypercholesteremia were also present, but obesity itself was a risk factor in men. A slight or moderate degree of obesity adds very little to the risk of disease, but the risk is increased greatly when overweight is marked.

The contribution of overweight to the development of disease may come from a variety of metabolic changes. Respiratory difficulties increase, limiting oxygenation of the blood and restricting oxygen supply to tissues. Excess weight increases the work load on the heart, which may be critical if arteriosclerotic or atherosclerotic changes in the blood vessels impede the flow of blood. Blood pressure may increase in the individual who gains excessive weight, and often returns to normal with a significant weight loss. The measurement of blood pressure with a standard cuff may be in error when there is a thick layer of fat on the upper arm, but the changes in blood pressure with weight seem to be significant even when this is taken into account. Obese individuals also have impaired carbohydrate tolerance, when compared to those of normal weight. With the changes in respiratory and circulatory function in combination with a heavier body, the obese individual may also be less tolerant to the stress of exercise. This commonly leads to reduction of physical activity, which compounds the tendency toward obesity.

Obesity may also have a deleterious effect on existing diseases. Added weight places greater stress on osteoporotic bones and on joints which already have their functional ability altered by osteoarthritis. Other disorders of either the circulatory or locomotor system may be exacerbated by excessive increase in body weight.

CORONARY HEART DISEASE, ATHEROSCLEROSIS, AND HYPERTENSION

The interplay of changes associated with normal aging and those resulting from pathology are evident in the complexities of arteriosclerosis, atherosclerosis, and hypertension as they relate to heart function. The heart muscle decreases in strength and possibly in size as a normal result of aging. Cardiac output decreases, but the circulatory requirements of the body are also less, due to decrease in muscle and other functioning tissue and a lower metabolic rate. Arteriosclerosis occurs as a consequence of aging, and the loss of elasticity of blood vessel walls limits the ability of the arteries to transport blood. There may be compensatory use of collateral vessels to supply blood to cardiac muscle. However, if atheromatous plaques accumulate in the intima of arteries and constrict the lumen, circulation of blood is further compromised. The work of the heart is increased to maintain blood flow to organs and tissues, and blood pressure is elevated. Elevation of blood pressure is a signal of reduced blood flow.[9]

Reduction of blood supply to tissues results in ischemia and is particularly serious to the heart, kidneys, and brain. Continuation of deficient blood flow to the heart results in an infarct as the tissue dies. Myocardial infarction is known as a heart attack, and its severity depends on the extent of the heart tissue involved. When arteriosclerosis and atherosclerosis affect the renal arteries, the inelasticity and occlusion result in ischemic kidney tissue and the loss of function may lead to kidney failure. Reduced blood flow to the brain may cause hypoxia, with initial symptoms like headache, impaired memory, and disorientation, and if severe may lead to cerebrovascular accident, or stroke.

Atherosclerosis

The relationship of the development of atheromatous plaques in coronary artery intima and the prevalence of coronary artery disease and mortality from heart disease have been studied extensively. Atheromatous plaques are localized cell alterations and deposits of materials on the interior walls of arteries. The endothelial cell layer becomes thickened and connective tissue is formed. Some plaques remain small and do not impede blood flow materially. Some may cause ulceration of the cell wall and invasion of the adventitia, followed by rupture and hemorrhage into surrounding spaces. Some increase in size, narrowing the lumen and causing occlusion of the artery or permitting blockage by thrombus formation or embolism. The plaques contain not only triglycerides, phospholipids, and cholesterol esters, but also a variety of other substances, including protein, sulfated polysaccharides, and collagen.[6] These fibrous plaques have been identified in arteries as early as the second decade of life. There are conflicting opinions about whether they are related to fatty streaks which have been observed as early as three years of age, as discussed in Chapter 8.

The origins of the atheromatous plaques are unknown. Bierman[24] has speculated that the initial damage to smooth muscle cells of the endothelial lining of the arterial walls may be due to a reaction to injury by any of several risk factors, followed by platelet aggregation, proliferation of smooth muscle cells into the intimal lining, exposure of cells and connective tissue layers to circulating lipoproteins and hormones, and alteration of cell metabolism, with the lesion eventually healing with a thickened intima. Alternate theories include proliferation of a single smooth muscle cell, failure of the feedback control system of cells as a result of aging, or deficiency of lysosomal cholesterol ester hydrolase, permitting the accumulation of cholesterol esters in the cells and thus leading to altered cell metabolism and cell death.

Atherosclerosis is a multifactorial disease. Its relation to heart attacks and mortality from heart disease has led to study of risk factors observed with heart disease, since atherosclerosis itself cannot be easily measured. Although a number of risk factors have been proposed, there is not universal agreement about their influence. Most data have been derived from epidemiological studies of population groups and do not permit clear-cut separation of single factors, or from animal experiments which are subject to questions about species differences. Many of the risk factors are interrelated and interdependent, giving rise to further differences of opinion about their relative importance. According to Kannel,[25] the identified risk factors even taken together do not entirely explain the variance within or between populations, suggesting major risk factors not yet identified.

Genetic susceptibility has been suggested by the difference in the prevalence of heart disease in various populations of the world. However, there are no distinctive genetic markers[26] and the populations differ in various environmental characteristics. Since the prevalence of heart disease is higher among men than among women in middle adult life,[3] but rises in women after menopause (Table 9.2), sex hormone secretion has been considered a factor. The increase in the prevalence of heart disease with age is clearly seen in Table 9.2. Arteriosclerosis progresses with advancing age, but it is unclear whether or not atherosclerosis is necessarily a concomitant of healthy aging. There is general agreement that cigarette smoking, hypertension, and diabetes increase the risk of both atherosclerosis and coronary heart disease. Obesity is an added risk, which may be related to the increased work load on the heart, alteration in metabolism, or other associated factors. Physical inactivity may be a risk factor. Studies have also categorized personality characteristics and patterns of reaction to stress which may distinguish individuals subject to heart attacks.

The relationship of dietary factors to atherosclerosis and heart disease has been subjected to much controversy.[25-27] Despite intensive studies in the past three decades, there is little unanimity of opinion on the influence of diet, and dietary theories have had waves of popularity, refutation, and revision. Some of the controversy arises from the lack of a definitive link between dietary factors, elevation of critical biochemical changes in blood, and ultimate atherosclerosis and heart disease. On the one hand, dietary intake of some nutrients influences plasma levels of cholesterol, triglycerides, and lipoproteins. In turn, high concentrations of plasma cholesterol have been identified as a risk factor in heart disease. "The unproven hypothesis that man's diet is related through the process of atherogenesis in his coronary arteries to the problem of ischemic heart disease is almost irresistible."[28] However, the search for a direct relationship between diet and heart disease has led to investigation of several nutrients, formulation of many hypotheses, and little agreement.

Dietary intake of cholesterol represents only 10 to 20 percent of the body's supply[27] since endogenous synthesis is greater than the amount in most American diets. In animal experimentation, increase in cholesterol intake causes elevation of plasma cholesterol, which is reversible by dietary manipulation, but species differences in cholesterol metabolism have raised doubts about the applicability of animal findings to humans. Fat intake was one of the earliest nutrients associated with heart disease, with concern at first about total fat intake and the proportion of its contribution to energy intake. Later studies suggested that saturated fatty acids increased the risk of heart disease while polyunsaturated fatty acids were protective, and the ratio of saturated to unsaturated fatty acids was shown to be important. Human studies in which dietary cholesterol has been severely limited, total fat intake decreased, with a larger proportion of fat from unsaturated fatty acids, have resulted in 5 to 20 percent lowering of plasma cholesterol, a decrease which is less than can be accomplished by the administration of some drugs.[27] In addition, some questions have been raised about the effects of inclusion in the diet of corn oil that has been hydrogenated, since that product contains 15 to 40 percent of the unnatural trans fatty acids.[27] The effects of reduced serum cholesterol on mortality are equivocal.[25,28]

The recommendations in the Dietary Goals for the United States, proposed by the Select Committee on Nutrition and Human Needs of the U.S. Senate,[29] that fat intake should be restricted to 30 percent of total calories, with equal contributions from saturated, monounsaturated, and polyunsaturated fats and that cholesterol intake should be limited to 300 mg/day elicited further controversy. Reviews of the literature have failed to reach a consensus on the relationship between fat intake and heart disease or on the effect of dietary change on coronary artery disease mortality,[26,27,30] and the Dietary Goals stirred further disagreement.[31,32]

Protein was proposed as a factor in atherogenesis when statistical analysis showed that the differences in mortality from heart disease could be correlated with levels of protein consumption as well as with levels of fat.[32] Additional studies have shown that mean plasma cholesterol levels are higher in persons who consume animal protein than in vegetarians.[26] However, diets that differ in protein sources also differ in types of lipids, in cholesterol, and in other nutrients and fiber, and other variations in life style tend to be associated with these dietary patterns.

Differences in the prevalence of heart disease have also been related to carbohydrate intake. It has been hypothesized that high intakes of refined sugars (disaccharides) are more atherogenic than high intakes of complex carbohydrates. Since refinement of foods eliminates some of the fiber, attention was also given to fiber content of diets. Fiber is composed of a variety of substances, including cellulose, hemicellulose, pectin, and lignin. Dietary fiber from different sources is not physically and chemically uniform, and different components of fiber have dissimilar biological effects.[34] Therefore, further clarification is needed of the mechanisms by which high-fiber diets may lower serum cholesterol and triglycerides in some subjects.

Many of the epidemiological studies on which hypotheses have been based were conducted on population groups that differed in so many respects it is difficult to identify and evaluate influential parameters. Not only do dietary intakes differ, but genetics, geography, physical activity, income, and other characteristics are different. Two studies of relatively homogeneous populations in the United States were carried out in Framingham[35] and Tecumseh.[36] In neither study was a significant relationship found between dietary factors and plasma levels of cholesterol or triglycerides. Dietary methodologies were limited to recent or recalled intakes and are subject to qualifications as discussed in Chapter 2. The development of critical plasma levels and especially the development of atherosclerosis occur over an extended period of time, and recent intake may not accurately reflect long-term intakes. Longitudinal studies of food consumption of individuals who do or do not develop coronary artery disease at later ages may be the only method of resolving the controversy.

Inter- and intra-individual metabolic responses to dietary components need to be clarified, and critical plasma levels more carefully defined. If the risk of coronary heart disease is elevated only when plasma cholesterol concentration exceeds 250 mg/100 ml,[30] early identification of individuals with higher levels could be expected to decrease the mortality from heart disease. Recent findings suggest that this identification can be modified further by the measurement of the density of lipoprotein carriers of cholesterol. If such a massive screening program were feasible, attention to diet and other therapeutic measures could be limited to individuals at risk. The major controversy is whether the diets of large population groups should be altered as a preventive measure. Until the metabolic and physical causes of atherosclerosis are better understood, differences of opinion on the practicality and benefits of major dietary changes of the population will continue.

Most of the emphasis in dietary studies has been placed on factors which influence the genesis and progress of the atherosclerotic process. Once the condition is manifest, there is little evidence that dietary manipulation can reverse the process, although it may lower plasma cholesterol concentration. This suggests that dietary changes after perhaps 55 years of age[25] may alter the increase in atherosclerosis but not reverse it, and that alteration of intake after that age may have minimal effects on mortality rates. Epidemiological data indicate that a high level of physical activity may not only prevent or delay atherosclerosis, but also enlarge atherosclerotic vessels so that the capacity of coronary arteries is increased.[37] However, this may be an indirect influence since ability or willingness to exercise is also related to health and personality factors, as well as to body weight.

Hypertension

Mean blood pressure levels rise with age, with the sharpest increase in both sexes after 45 years. Wide variations in blood pressure are observed, both between individuals and from time to time within one individual, dependent in part on conditions under which it is measured. Mild hypertension may remain asymptomatic and benign for years. However, severe and prolonged hypertension may be associated with chronic kidney disease, cerebral hemorrhage, or cardiac failure. There is no commonly accepted standard that divides the normotensive from the hypertensive. Upper limits of "normal" for systolic pressure vary from 140 to 170 mm Hg and for diastolic pressure from 90 to 95 mm Hg.[9,28]

If hypertension is secondary to renal, endocrine, or other disease, its treatment is based on therapy for the underlying disease. More common is essential or idiopathic hypertension, for which an organic cause cannot be identified. In addition to age, associated factors that have been investigated include obesity, excessive salt intake, genetic predisposition, hyperlipidemia, cigarette smoking, and psychological stress. Elevation of blood pressure is more commonly seen in obese individuals than in those of normal weight; some studies have reported a decrease in hypertension with weight loss. It has been speculated that an excessive salt intake over an extended period of years may lead to hypertension in genetically susceptible individuals,[37] but neither salt intake nor genetic susceptibility can be measured readily. Stress tends to cause a temporary increase in blood pressure, and it has been hypothesized that continued or repeated stress may cause persistent hypertension in some individuals. There is no unequivocal evidence, however, that either excessive salt intake or stress actually causes hypertension.

Treatment may include the use of drugs that lower blood pressure by vasodilation through action on the peripheral sympathetic nervous sytem. In some hypertensive individuals blood pressure may be lowered by significant reduction of total body salt content, which may be accomplished by restricting salt intake and by administration of diuretics to increase sodium excretion. Since drugs may have undesirable side effects, and continued use of diuretics may jeopardize potassium status, current therapy for hypertension requires continued follow-up of the patient. Recently behavioral modification methods of relaxation and biofeedback have resulted in small decreases in blood pressure; such methods are still experimental. Like other multifactorial diseases of older persons, the etiology remains elusive and a variety of therapeutic approaches have been explored to find the most effective treatment after the disease has been identified.

OSTEOPOROSIS

Following the termination of linear growth, bone density and cortical thickness continue to increase slightly into the fourth decade of life, after which there is a gradual loss in the absolute amount of bone. Although total bone mass diminishes, bones retain the same histological structure and chemical composition as osteoporosis progresses.[28] In this respect osteoporosis differs from osteomalacia, which is similar to rickets in children and is due to decreased absorption and deposition of calcium as a result of vitamin D deficiency. In osteomalacia hydroxyapatite formation is decreased, particularly in the shafts of the long and flat bones; the structural rigidity of bone is compromised, and the softening results in deformities. Treatment of osteomalacia is the provision of vitamin D, calcium, and phosphorus, since it is a deficiency disease.

Osteoporosis is a gradual process. Whether it is a normal occurrence with advancing age, due to alterations in hormone production or in body metabolism, or can be prevented has been the subject of debate. The prevalence is four times higher in females than in males.[38] Its onset is earlier in females, starting often at 35 to 45 years; in males, changes are estimated to begin after 45 years. The rate of loss tends to be greater in females. Blacks are less susceptible to osteoporosis than whites. The condition is often asymptomatic and is usually not diagnosed until one-third or more of bone mass has been lost. It often comes to medical attention after fracture of a bone, usually the femoral neck or a vertebra. Therefore the true prevalence of osteoporosis is unknown but is estimated as affecting 10 to 50 percent of the United States population over 50 years of age.[38] The compression of the vertebral column results in a decrease in height and may cause back pain and incapacitation. Thus far efforts to reverse the process once it has been diagnosed have had minimal success, but some theorize that the progression may be slowed.

The basic cause of osteoporosis seems to be a change in the ratio of new bone formation by osteoblasts and bone resorption by osteoclasts. When resorption exceeds formation, bone mass diminishes. The loss proceeds at varying rates within individuals of the same age, sex, and race, and in this respect it is typical of conditions with multifactorial etiology. Factors that have been investigated include hormones (primarily estrogen and parathyroid hormone), inactivity or immobilization, physical stress on bones, and dietary or metabolic aspects of calcium, phosphorus, protein, vitamins C and D, and fluorine.

Estrogen has been implicated in osteoporosis because of the sex difference in prevalence and the accelerated decrease in bone mass in women following menopause, or earlier in some women with ovariectomy.[28] Once osteoporosis has been diagnosed, however, there is little evidence that hormone administration either slows or reverses the process. Since parathyroid hormone stimulates resorption of calcium from bone, it has been investigated in relation to calcium and phosphate metabolism. Osteoporosis has been observed in other endocrine disorders, such as Cushing's syndrome, acromegaly, and hyperthyroidism, so endocrine involvement is probable.

Much research has centered on calcium intake, absorption, and utilization. It has been estimated that in the adult 700 mg calcium enters and leaves bone daily.[28] A small negative calcium balance over a period of years could result in gradual loss of bone calcium as it is withdrawn to maintain plasma calcium homeostasis and support essential functions of calcium, such as muscle contraction, nerve conduction, and membrane transport. Although calcium absorption has been reported to decrease with age, there is no evidence that absorption is poorer in individuals with osteoporosis than in those without osteoporosis. There is also no evidence that increased intake or calcium supplementation in the adult affects skeletal mass. The prevalence is higher in women, and it has been speculated that repeated depletion of calcium reserves as a result of pregnancies and lactation may contribute to later development of the condition,[38] but there seems to be no higher prevalence in women of higher parity.

Phosphorus has been studied, in relation both to its effect on production of parathyroid hormone and to its ratio with calcium. Experiments with several species of animals have shown that osteoporosis can be produced by a low-calcium, high-phosphorus diet.[39] However, bone density remains normal on varying levels of calcium and phosphorus so long as calcium intake is higher than phosphorus intake.[40] If an excess of phosphorus in the diet increases bone loss, recent changes in the United States diet have obvious implications. A higher phosphorus intake has accompanied increased consumption of meat, carbonated beverages, snack foods, and processed foods to which phosphates have been added. When adults or the elderly decrease milk intake, the ratio of calcium to phosphorus becomes progressively lower.

Vitamin D functions in the metabolism of calcium and phosphorus and may be inadequate in older adults if their intake of fortified milk is decreased and no other supplements are taken, or in derangement of absorption as a result of gastric surgery. However, there is no indication that vitamin D deficiency is a significant cause of osteoporosis in the United States. Vitamin C is essential to the formation of healthy bone matrix, but the majority of adults in the United States are unlikely to be deficient. Protein is also essential to collagen formation for bone matrix, and osteoporosis has been observed in children with severe protein-energy malnutrition, but the relatively high protein intake of most Americans makes this an unlikely cause of osteoporosis.

Fluorine produces a higher degree of crystallinity in bone formation, resulting in more stable bone mineral. Fluorine appears to be the only substance known to stimulate osteoblasts and to cause the change in cellular behavior in bone that could achieve the increased mass essential for correction of osteoporosis.[40] However, the level of fluorine administered must be higher than that recommended for prevention of dental caries,[9] and fluorine is effective only in combination with calcium.[40] Studies on fluorine are still experimental, and the advantages and risks of this treatment need further study.

Inactivity causes bone loss. The decreased activity of adults and especially of the elderly has been implicated as one of the causative factors in osteoporosis. With total immobility the rate of bone loss is rapid and urinary excretion of calcium increases, but these alterations seem to be reversible with resumption of activity. Bones with weight-bearing functions tend to be somewhat protected from calcium loss.[40] It has been speculated that activity may stimulate osteoblastic function.

Like many other conditions of the elderly, osteoporosis often is not recognized until well along in its progression. Since the basic metabolic mechanisms have not been identified, programs for prevention cannot be established on firm ground. The recommendation to maintain adequate calcium intake throughout adult life seems logical and has been a factor in the decision of the Food and Nutrition Board[41] to retain a higher recommended allowance for calcium than most other countries. To date therapeutic measures after diagnosis of osteoporosis have had little effect on slowing or reversing the degenerative changes.

ALCOHOLISM

The interrelationships of nutrient metabolism and the clinical or biochemical sequellae of acute or chronic alcoholism have long been recognized and many of the organic, neuromuscular, and mental alterations of alcoholism have been attributed to dietary deficiencies. Recent studies have suggested that the relationship is more complex and that the ingestion of ethanol may have a primary toxic effect on many body tissues, causing alteration in absorption and utilization of nutrients and leading to biochemical and clinical manifestations of malnutrition even when the dietary intake seems adequate.[42]

Frank deficiency diseases are now observed in less than three percent of alcoholics admitted to hospitals in the United States.[43] The decrease in deficiency diseases since World War II has been attributed to the enrichment of bread and cereal products with B-complex vitamins. Another factor in the low prevalence of deficiency diseases is that chronic alcoholics are usually intermittent, not continuous, drinkers, so that periods of low intake associated with heavy alcohol consumption may be alternated with periods of better eating. It has been estimated that mild malnutrition as evidenced by biochemical findings may not exceed 20 percent prevalence in chronic alcoholics.[43] There is wide variation among individuals in the amount and frequency of alcohol consumption, in dose-dependency, in sensitivity to the effects of alcohol, and in dietary intake.

Nutrient deficiencies most often observed, either clinically or biochemically, involve protein, vitamins of the B complex, magnesium, and zinc. Alcohol ingestion may have a direct effect on appetite, inhibiting desire for food, or may displace other sources of calories, thereby limiting intake of nutrients. In addition, alcohol has a direct toxic effect on many organs of the body which then indirectly influence nutriture. Impairment of absorption as a result of ingestion of alcohol has been demonstrated for thiamin and folacin. Fatty liver may be a result of nutrient deficiency or a direct effect of alcohol; the development of alcoholic liver disease is not prevented by an adequate diet. Similarly, the megaloblastosis often observed in alcoholism may be the direct toxic effect of ethanol on bone marrow or a symptom of folacin deficiency. Alcohol may produce acute pancreatitis and hyperglycemia. Its diuretic effect has been shown to be related to increased urinary excretion of magnesium and zinc and other electrolytes, resulting in nutritional imbalances. Therefore, alcoholism may produce nutritional deficiencies directly by its effect on body organs or indirectly by its effect on limiting food intake.

The rate of oxidation of ethanol in the body does not seem to be affected by nutritional status as much as by the amount of alcohol dehydrogenase present.[43] The rate is normally slow, and the effects of ethanol are usually greater with frequent intakes of large amounts. An excessive intake may precipitate deficiency symptoms in a body that is in a state of precarious balance due to chronic depletion. Clinical symptoms vary with the severity of the deficiency, and usually represent multiple rather than single nutrient deficiencies. Most vulnerable are the liver, pancreas, skeletal and cardiac muscle, and nerve tissue. Protein deficiency has been related to the development of fatty liver, thiamin deficiency to neuromuscular pathology, magnesium deficiency to delirium tremens, folacin deficiency to macrocytosis, and deficiency of several B vitamins, including thiamin, niacin, and pyridoxine, to mental confusion.[42] Since simultaneous deficiencies are most likely, therapy should include provision of all nutrients.

OSTEOARTHRITIS

There is no evidence of nutritional involvement in osteoarthritis, either in its etiology or its treatment. However, the disease may limit activity and the therapeutic use of aspirin may cause gastrointestinal bleeding which predisposes to anemia, so the presence of the disease may affect nutritional status. If the individual is overweight, dietary restriction may be advised in order to limit the stress on joints.

Osteoarthritis is a degenerative joint disease characterized by softening and deterioration of the cartilage around the joints. When the smooth cartilage surface disintegrates, the underlying bone ends become thickened and may develop spurs. As the disease progresses, there may be pain on movement, stiffness, and limitation of motion. Any joint in the body may be affected, whether weight-bearing or not. In a Health Examination Survey of the NCHS,[44] more than one-third of all adults in the United States were found to have some degree of osteoarthritis by X-ray and clinical diagnosis, with the rate increasing from 4 percent in the age group of 18 to 24 years to 85 percent of those 75 to 79 years of age. Men had a higher prevalence than women under the age of 45 years, but the prevalence was slightly higher in women past 65 years of age. Not only does the rate increase with age, but the severity also increases.

The cause of this disease is unknown, although genetic, hormonal, and metabolic factors have been investigated. Its progress may be enhanced by stress or by obesity. The limitation of joint movement may inhibit mobility and lead to instability, thus increasing difficulty in walking and a tendency to fall. No cure has been found but anti-inflammatory and other drugs are often recommended for relief from pain and discomfort. In many individuals the condition does not cause symptoms; in those with symptoms, there are usually periods of remission and exacerbation.

Despite the fact that, except for gout, there is no evidence that nutritional factors or specific foods either cause or cure arthritis, a number of claims have been made for certain diets, oils, food products, and vitamins. It has been estimated that millions of dollars are spent every year in the United States for worthless products, primarily by the elderly who are most afflicted.

MATURITY-ONSET DIABETES MELLITUS

Alteration in glucose metabolism is one of the physiological changes observed with increasing age. The glucose tolerance curve becomes slower in its return to normal after a glucose load, even when the level of plasma insulin is elevated, suggesting alteration in the sensitivity of cells to insulin. The diminished insulin response to glucose presents difficulties in interpretation of glucose tolerance tests in the adult, especially when stress or medications may alter the results.[45] In addition, diabetes in the elderly is often asymptomatic and mild cases may not be diagnosed. As a result, the true prevalence of diabetes in the older population is not known. However, diabetes mellitus is among the ten leading causes of death in the United States population over 25 years of age. The mortality rate increases from 2.7/100,000 population in the 25 to 44 year age group, to 18.3 at 45 to 64 years, and to 108.1 after 65 years.[3]

Adult-onset diabetes is often gradual in its development and tends to have a milder course with fewer pathological sequelae than the childhood-onset disease.[9,46] The classical symptoms of thirst, frequent urination, weight loss, weakness, glycosuria, and elevation of fasting blood glucose may not be present. The adult may have abnormal glucose tolerance despite elevation of plasma insulin, with alteration in sensitivity of cells to insulin. The degree of carbohydrate intolerance may be minor and may remain unchanged for several years. Ketosis is not common.

Epidemiological studies of world distribution indicate that diabetes is more common in countries with a high standard of living and a high prevalence of obesity. In the individual, obesity often accompanies diabetes. Restriction of caloric intake to accomplish weight loss is usually associated with better control of blood glucose as well as lower serum lipid levels. Adult-onset diabetes in its mild form may often be managed with dietary management and weight loss alone. Oral drug treatment may be indicated, and severe cases may require insulin injections.

Complications associated with diabetes include neuropathy, renal disorders, ocular retinopathy, and peripheral vascular disease.[9] In addition to the hazards of obesity, the adult diabetic has a greater risk of atherosclerosis and coronary heart disease, and the mortality rate of diabetics after a heart attack is higher than for nondiabetics. Control of the diabetic state is important in limiting the effect of these complications.

CANCER

Mortality from heart disease in the United States has been declining, but deaths from cancer continue to increase (Figure 9.1).[47] Relationships between diet and cancer are more complex than for other multifactorial diseases and even more poorly understood. The relationship seems to exist at several levels. Aside from food additives and contaminants, dietary components or nutrient balances may be involved in the etiology of some cancers. The nutritional requirements of malignant cells during growth of the tumor

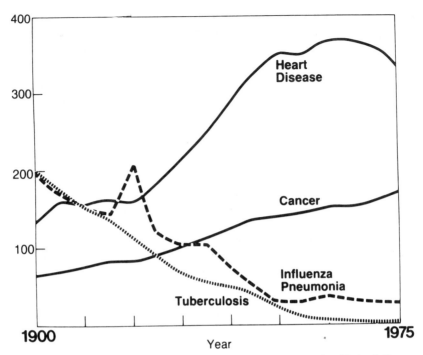

Figure 9.1   Death rates per 100,000 population in the United States from selected causes, 1900–1970. (Reprinted from Gori, G.B. Diet and cancer. J. Am. Dietet. Assoc. 71:375–379, 1977.)

may compete with the requirements of normal body tissues, thus creating imbalances or deficiencies. The presence of a carcinoma may alter digestion, absorption, and metabolism by obstruction, alteration of hormonal or enzyme synthesis, or a variety of other mechanisms. The nutritional status of a patient affects response to radiation, surgery, or chemotherapy, and in turn the therapeutic measures alter nutritional status. Some types of dietary manipulation or administration of antimetabolites play a role in treatment of certain kinds of cancer. Therefore dietary intake and nutritional status are closely interwoven with the occurrence and treatment of cancer, in ways not clearly understood with present knowledge.

Most current information about factors that initiate, inhibit, or enhance carcinogenicity is derived from epidemiological data or animal experimentation. Epidemiological studies in humans rely heavily on statistical methods to draw conclusions from a mass of often uncontrolled and uncontrollable variables; animal studies concern relatively strictly controlled populations with a minimum number of variables but present considerable difficulties when extrapolated across species to humans.[48] Cancer incidence is related both to factors intrinsic in the individual and to factors that origi-

412   THE ADULT AND THE ELDERLY

nate in the environment. Causes of cancer have not been identified, and may differ with the site within the body, so interpretation of findings to date must be tentative and subject to difference from one specialist to another.

The geographic distribution of prevalence of various types of cancer has led to many hypotheses, although the accuracy of data on incidence and mortality in many countries is limited.[49] Colon cancer is second only to lung cancer in cancer mortality rates in the United States and England, but is rare in Japan and many developing countries.[50] The prevalence increases among migrants from a country of low prevalence to one of high prevalence, and becomes similar to the rate in the host country. On the other hand, gastric cancer is less common in the United States, but is four or more times higher in Japan, Chile, Austria, Finland, and Iceland. Cancer of the liver is seen more often in China, Hawaii, and Rumania, and is the most common malignancy in sub-Saharal Africa, but the prevalence is relatively low in the continental United States. Even within the country, prevalence of some cancers varies with income and ethnic groups, and in the United States, Seventh Day Adventists and Mormons have lower mortality from cancer than the general population.

Attempts to relate the differences in prevalence of various types of cancer to customary food intakes have given rise to many theories. The data provide hypotheses on association of dietary characteristics with specific sites of cancer, but do not permit conclusions about causation. For example, the greater frequency of colonic cancer among populations in developed countries has led to speculation that since a diet high in fat and low in fiber decreases transit time, alters bacterial flora, and increases the concentration of neutral and acidic fecal steroids, such a diet enhances the induction of cancer by providing longer time for development and activity of carcinogens in the colon. However, the Western diet is also higher in energy, protein (especially of animal origin), sugar, and other refined carbohydrates, which may also affect carcinogenicity.[51] As yet there is no confirmation of relative importance of the different factors. The protective role claimed for fiber has been questioned.[52]

A different mechanism has been proposed for the higher prevalence of breast cancer in the United States than in Japan, with supporting evidence from animal studies.[53] Epidemiological studies of women suggest that breast cancer is hormone-dependent. Risk factors include nulliparity, late pregnancy, late menopause, and family history. Animal studies have shown a relationship between high intakes of fat, both saturated and unsaturated, and the timing and number of breast tumors. Fat stimulates production and release of prolactin. It has, therefore, been hypothesized that a high-fat diet increases the ratio of prolactin to estrogen, enhancing the effect of carcinogens on breast tissue.

Several specific nutrients have been investigated in animal experiments to determine their effect either in protection against or predisposing toward the genesis of tumors. Diet has been shown to alter the site and number of tumors, presumably by effects on synthesis and release of such body compounds as hormones, enzymes, and bile acids, on the conversion of precarcinogens to active forms, or on the susceptibility of body tissues to potentially carcinogenic substances. Experimental data have indicated that a deficiency of some nutrients or an excess of others may enhance carcinogenesis. Further research in this area is needed before conclusions can be drawn.

The effects of cancer on nutritional status may be far-reaching in some patients with profound derangement of body metabolism. Cachexia has been observed in one-third to two-thirds of patients with various types of cancer.[54] It is characterized by anorexia, extensive weight loss, and alterations in body composition and function. The lack of appetite and early satiation remain unexplained, despite investigation of many theories; it may be related to effects of peptides and other small molecules produced by the tumor on hypothalamic and other regulatory mechanisms.[54,55] Basal metabolic rate and energy expenditure increase, even beyond the energy needs of the tumor itself. Nitrogen is lost from body tissues, primarily from skeletal muscle as muscle mass decreases; it has been hypothesized that the nitrogen taken from the host tissue by the tumor is not released. Plasma albumin decreases as breakdown exceeds synthesis. Weight loss is accentuated as fat is mobilized from adipose tissue to meet increased energy requirements. Both intra- and extracellular body water increase, with derangement of electrolyte metabolism characterized mainly by hyponatremia and increased urinary excretion of sodium and potassium. Anemia of multifactorial origin is common, with decrease in production of hemoglobin and red blood cells and more rapid destruction of red blood cells. The activity of many enzymes is altered, particularly liver enzymes, and hormonal changes have been reported, possibly secondary to malnutrition. Hyperalimentation is often used to limit the effects of cachexia, but may be of only temporary benefit. Reversal of cachexia may be achieved only when the total malignant growth is removed or when complete remission has been accomplished by radiation or chemotherapy.[54]

Nutritional support is essential to minimize the effects of cancer on the body, to aid in the response to therapy, and to accelerate the healing process. Increasingly it is being recognized that improvement in the nutritional status of the patient lowers the mortality rate during surgery and increases the tolerance of the patient to radiation or chemotherapy. Since both radiotherapy and chemotherapy may cause anorexia, nausea, vomiting, diarrhea, loss of taste, food aversion, and weight loss, the nutriture of the patient is further compromised. Marked progress has been made in recent years in oral, tube, and total parenteral nutrition for the cancer patient.

DIET-DRUG INTERACTION

The prevalence of chronic diseases increases with age. Chronic diseases are likely to necessitate long-term or permanent treatment with drugs. Therefore the effects of drug therapy on nutritional status are a greater problem in adulthood than in childhood. The effect of many drugs is dependent on alteration of body metabolism or interruption of nutrient supply to microorganisms in the body. As a result, the absorption and utilization of nutrients may also be affected and, in turn, the ingestion of food alters the efficacy of some drugs taken by mouth. No attempt will be made here to present in detail the many complexities of diet-drug interactions, but some aspects of therapeutic medications will be summarized as they relate to nutrient requirements and interfere with normal nutrient metabolism when taken for extended periods of time.[42,56,57]

When drugs are taken with meals, the presence of food in the gastrointestinal tract enhances the effects of some drugs but decreases the efficacy of others. Usually the rate of absorption of drugs is slower when they are taken with food. For some, such as aspirin, the rate of absorption may be slower but the total net absorption is not altered. In this case, the drug is less effective since a rapid analgesic effect is desired. A slower rate of absorption is less important for drugs that are given in multiple doses to achieve a constant blood level, so long as total absorption is not decreased. However, if total absorption is decreased when a drug such as tetracycline is taken with food, the optimal effect of therapy may not be attained.

The longer transit time resulting from food consumption also affects the absorption of drugs in specific ways for each drug. Slower passage of some drugs results in higher absorption. However, drugs such as levodopa, which are metabolized or degraded by acid, are less effective when taken with acid beverages or retained for longer periods of time in the stomach. The composition of the diet may also affect the action of drugs. For example, a high fat intake stimulates bile secretion and therefore may increase the absorption of fat-soluble drugs such as the antifungal agent griseofulvin, resulting in a higher blood concentration of the drug. High intakes of vitamin K may affect the absorption of oral anticoagulants and alter prothrombin time. The chemical characteristics and the mechanisms of achieving the desired therapeutic effects of the drug must be evaluated for each medication to determine the advisability of simultaneous consumption of food.

Drugs also affect the absorption of nutrients. Those that cause nausea or vomiting interfere with digestion and decrease the availability of nutrients to the body. Antimicrobials may damage the intestinal mucosa, and antimitotic agents for cancer therapy inhibit regeneration of gastrointestinal epithelial cells, so the effect of either medication on cells and their enzyme production may result in decreased absorption of a variety of nutrients. Aspirin, commonly taken as an analgesic, may irritate the gastrointestinal wall and cause bleeding. Some drugs, such as the diuretic chlorothiazide, interfere with transport mechanism, particularly in the availability of sodium, which is necessary for the intestinal transport of many nutrients. Mineral oil may directly absorb carotene and, to a lesser extent, vitamin A, making them unavailable to the body. Hypocholesterolemic agents, such as cholestyramine and clofibrate, function by interfering with absorption of sterols, but may also interfere with the absorption of other nutrients. For example, cholestyramine, a nonabsorbable ion-exchange resin which binds bile salts, may impair the absorption of fats and fat-soluble vitamins. Drugs that interfere with the production or release of pancreatic enzymes can alter the digestion of macronutrients.

The transport and metabolic functions of nutrients within the body may be altered by a variety of medications. The efficacy of some drugs in therapy is dependent on their functions as antivitamins by combining with or inhibiting enzyme systems that are required by a vitamin for conversion to its active form or by competition for binding sites on proteins or cells. Those drugs that act by stimulation of the activity of microsomal enzymes can also stimulate catabolism of normal body constituents, including some vitamins; for example, folate or vitamin D deficiency may be caused by some anticonvulsants. Excretion of nutrients may be increased by some drugs, as shown by the higher loss of pyridoxine during treatment with the antituberculosis agent isoniazid. The interrelationships of vitamins, especially those of the B-complex, in metabolic functions for which several vitamins are required as coenzymes in various steps of conversions, may result in distortion of function at several levels when the antagonist of a single vitamin is administered.

Roe[42] has stated that alterations in the absorption and/or utilization of folate and vitamins B_6 and B_{12} account for the largest proportion of drug-induced nutritional deficiencies. She concluded that the risk is greater with drugs that cause massive malabsorption, function as vitamin antagonists, or affect nutrients with multiple metabolic functions. Greater effect on nutrient depletion can be seen when the drugs are taken for an extended period of time or if the patient's prior nutritional status was marginal.

PSYCHOSOCIAL-BIOLOGICAL INTERACTIONS

With increasing age, individuality becomes more pronounced. Each life history is unique to the individual, and the impact of specific environmental events and influences results in increasing variability between people at each succeeding chronological age. There is greater variability among adolescents than among preschool children, even greater variability among adults, and differences are most marked toward the end of the life span. The accumulated years of experiences, of challenges to health, of dietary patterns, and of all the other factors that impinge on development of physiological and psychological characteristics are specific to each person, as are that individual's reactions and adaptations to the stresses of life. If biological age could be measured, it would be a better frame of reference than chronological age for evaluating the health and needs of the adult and elderly. Some individuals begin to show signs of aging at a relatively young chronological age, while others maintain vitality throughout most of a century. Comfort[58] has described the activities of many well-known people in the fields of arts, sciences, and politics who remained creative and productive even into their eighties and nineties. They demonstrate retention of a combination of physical ability and interest in a changing world, which is the goal of extending life. The purpose of increasing longevity is not merely to add years to one's existence, but to add meaningful and enjoyable years.

The cumulative effects of genetics, disease, medical care, psychological stress, physical activity, diet, economics, and social factors throughout a lifetime result in the quality of life of the adult and of the elderly. Many of the contagious and infectious diseases have been controlled by medical advancements. Nutritional deficiency diseases in this country are now rare. Greater emphasis has been placed in recent years on the advantages to health of continued physical exertion. Attention has been directed toward the study of degenerative diseases with the hope of finding means to delay their appearance. Since these are multifactorial conditions that are involved with many aspects of life style, an understanding of the etiology of these diseases can come only from analysis of widely diverse practices and environmental influences. Even the study of dietary intake of adults requires evaluation of social, cultural, economic, and psychological factors that alter the availability and selection of food, as well as the physical characteristics that alter the consumption, digestion, and utilization of food.

Mobility is obviously a major factor influencing not only the ability to obtain food for oneself, but also the metabolism of nutrients and the maintenance of homeostasis within the body. In a 1974 survey of adults in the United States, more than 90 percent of adults under 45 years of age reported no limitation of activity, but after the age of 65 years slightly more than half of the population surveyed reported being free of conditions that limited activity.[3] As age progressed, more individuals found it necessary to restrict major activities related to work outside or inside the home. Limitation of activity was particularly severe for 29 percent of males and 9 percent of females past 65 years. The major causes were heart conditions and arthritis. Loss of gross motor ability narrows the environment of the individual, placing increasing dependence on others not only for transportation outside the home but also for accomplishing dressing, eating, and other activities in the daily routine. It also imposes psychological damage, particularly to the individual who has characteristically been active, outgoing, and independent and now must adjust to an altered life style.

Muscle loss and disease processes in bones or joints may not create major problems in activity to most individuals, but many experience a decrease in fine motor control. The ability to manipulate objects may diminish. This may lead to more frequent accidents, particularly when objects are dropped. More common is an accumulation of smaller nuisances, such as spilling foods. The embarrassment of these accidents may lead to withdrawal from social situations where they could occur.

Mental testing of adults has shown that there is no decline in intelligence with age, but that the speed of reaction is slowed.[58] However, some individuals experience mental confusion or loss of memory. When these aberrations are minor they are only a source of annoyance to the individual or family. However, if they are severe, they create real hazards and require watchfulness by another person to prevent tragic results, diminishing the independence of the individual.

Physical stress as a result of surgery, injury, fracture, burns, or other trauma causes direct loss of nutrients from the body, either through the site of the injury or through loss of muscle tissue and increased urinary excretion of metabolites.[59] Immobility after physical stress further jeopardizes electrolyte metabolism and homeostatic control. If surgery or disease involves the gastrointestinal tract, the site and extent of removal or damage determine the effect on nutrient absorption. In both chronic and acute stress nutrient absorption by the individual may need to be monitored carefully.

Psychological stress may come from a variety of sources. Decreasing physical ability may be stressful to some persons. The emotional stress of loss of companionship by the individual who outlives his or her contemporaries is increasingly recognized as a major contributing factor to change in health and nutritional status. Loneliness may lead to indifferent attitudes toward health and medical care, and the lack of motivation to prepare meals may lead to either indifference to eating or to compulsive eating to assuage loneliness.

Comfort[58] used the term "sociogenic aging" for the state produced by the role society imposes on people when they reach a certain arbitrary chronological age. They must retire, are rendered unemployed and useless, and are sometimes impoverished. In a society that denies age by resorting to face lifts, wigs, and other means of disguising age, and that indoctrinates the young to value youth rather than age and work rather than leisure, the results may be destructive to the older adult. While there have been changes in legislation that alter the age of compulsory retirement, attitudes are more difficult to change. With increasing numbers of the population living a longer life and becoming organized socially and politically, further opportunities for the elderly to remain active and to make major contributions to society can be expected. In 1972, Pelcovits[60] quoted a description of the elderly as follows:

> *The older American presents difficulties in outreach simply not found in other populations. He ordinarily pays his bills, lives within his means, obeys the laws, and is seldom found in the courts. He does not ordinarily march in the streets protesting his low pension, inadequate housing, or poor transportation. He gradually drops away from his social clubs and churches and stays within his own small circle of acquaintances and activities, calling no particular attention to his needs until he becomes hospitalized. In short, he is almost deliberately inconspicuous.*

That description of the older American has, in the intervening years, become less valid. Organizations of retired persons, federal programs providing meals and social activities for the elderly, and local councils on aging have opened opportunities which had previously been largely ignored. Although sociogenic aging is still caused by the attitudes of society, those attitudes are currently being reshaped.

During early and middle adulthood, income level is related closely to the type of employment, and the individual's or family's relative financial position is usually stabilized. However, retirement from employment may alter income status suddenly and require major adjustments. Economic problems of the elderly have been ameliorated somewhat by programs such as Social Security, Medicare, and other forms of income supplementation. In the present era, more people retire with pensions than was true with previous generations, but there are still many elderly persons with inadequate incomes or with fixed incomes which become inadequate during periods of price inflation. With advancing age medical care becomes increasingly necessary and expensive. Essential costs of housing, heat, and so on, take precedence in budgeting available money, with the result that expenditures for food sometimes are the only category that can be reduced. Protective foods, such as animal protein sources, fruits, and vegetables are more expensive than foods that are high in carbohydrate, so persons with low incomes are more likely to have higher intakes of carbohydrates and may not meet their needs for proteins and some minerals and vitamins. A limitation of income may also necessitate moving to housing that may not have adequate facilities for preparation and storage of food, thereby placing further constraints on the availability of an adequate diet.

Individual dietary patterns develop during childhood and tend to become well established by maturity. Although a number of factors may alter dietary patterns, there is a strong tendency to retain the familiar. Food is not only a source of nutrients, but represents the sum of the individual's culture and traditions. Food is a means of communication and a symbol of economic and social status. It has increasing meaning to the individual as the years pass since it is a link to childhood and family. Eating provides relief from stress, a feeling of gratification, and a sense of security, especially if the foods are familiar and well liked. The social and psychological connotations of food selection make alterations of the diet difficult when imposed for either medical or financial reasons.

Cultural characteristics of the elderly population in the United States may also be seen in the history of this country in the last century. Many of these people are foreign-born. It has been estimated that approximately 20 percent of those born between 1890 and 1900 and 10 percent of those born between 1900 and 1910 came to the United States in the wave of immigration during that period. Educational levels of the population have changed. Those born prior to 1900 averaged eight years of schooling, and the number of years of formal education has gradually risen since that time. Prior to 1920 half of the population in the United States lived on farms. Those who are now over 50 years of age lived through the depression years of the 1930s. As a result, the life experiences of individuals who now comprise the population over 65 years of age were different from those in younger age groups, with corresponding differences in health, work, relationships, social patterns, and attitudes.

In reviewing the vulnerability of the elderly to risk of nutritional deficiency, Exton-Smith[61] suggested that particular attention should be given to those who have been recently bereaved, those who are socially isolated, especially with impairment of senses, those with mental disorders, very old people, and those who have not consulted a physician for some time.

NUTRIENT REQUIREMENTS AND RECOMMENDED DIETARY ALLOWANCES

Few definitive data are available in the literature on the metabolic needs of individuals past early adulthood. Most studies of requirements and circulating blood levels of nutrients have been done on young adults, primarily males. Interest in aging adults is relatively recent and has been concentrated mainly on anthropometric and biochemical studies of males or on dietary intake studies of females. The lack of longitudinal data on individuals as they progress from early adulthood to the later years has led to assumptions about requirements based on findings from cross-sectional surveys of subjects in successive age groups. As a result, a great deal of judgment has entered into the establishment of levels of recommended intakes.

Metabolic and dietary studies of the elderly are especially difficult to interpret. The increasing prevalence of degenerative diseases with age is superimposed on alterations in nutrient requirements due to the slowing of metabolic functions. The effects of medications for chronic diseases also influence the need for nutrients. Even studies of presumably healthy adults must be subjected to question, as was shown by the NIMH study[8]; initial screening identified "healthy" men who were later divided into two groups when further clinical and biochemical examinations showed that some had evidence of degenerative diseases not identified in the first screening process. When low concentrations of circulating nutrients are found, the interpretation must consider not only the possibility of malnutrition, but also the impairment of homeostatic mechanisms due to either age or disease and the results of stress due to pathological processes.[62] Evaluation of nutritional status becomes more complex with age, and the establishment of nutrient requirements and recommended allowances progressively more difficult.

It is generally assumed from available data that energy requirements decrease with age but that there is little or no change in the need for protein and micronutrients between early and late maturity. The decrease in lean body mass, metabolic rate, and physical activity can be expected to lower nutrient requirements, but in practical application to dietary intake this may be offset by less efficient digestion and absorption as a result of decreased production of enzymes, bile acids, and other compounds essential to utilization of the nutrients in foods.

The tendency in published reports of research to place into a single category all individuals over a given age, such as 50, 60, or 65 years, has also made it difficult to identify progressive changes in intake, requirement, or metabolic functions. For example, until recently little attempt has been made to distinguish between the 60-year-old and the 80-year-old. This lack of definitive age data is also reflected in the varying age categories in current tables of dietary allowances. In all tables a differentiation is made for women before and after the menopause because of their decrease in iron need, with the age categories divided at 50 or 55 years. After the age of 18 to 20 years, three age categories are classified for the RDA of the United States, although the 1979 RDA recommends a decrease in energy intake after 75 years, and the text of the Canadian standard provides a lower figure for energy after 66 years. Four age categories are listed in the United Kingdom table,[64] with the oldest at 75-plus years, and five categories in the Caribbean standards,[65] with the oldest at 70-plus years.

In addition to the change in iron allowance for women, all of the tables provide for decreasing caloric and thiamin intakes at successive ages. In all except the British standards allowances for riboflavin and niacin also decrease with age. Only the British standard recommends a decrease in protein intake. Other nutrients that are lowered in some but not all tables of recommendations are iodine, zinc, and vitamin E. None recommends a decrease with age in intakes of calcium, phosphorus, magnesium, vitamin A, ascorbic acid, pyridoxine, folate, or vitamin B_{12}. The inadequacy of data on the elderly does not permit clear delineation of changing requirements with age, and the recommendations reflect the best judgment of the committees involved and can be expected to change as new studies are reported.

None of the standards of recommended allowances include therapeutic needs arising from infections, metabolic disorders, chronic diseases, or other conditions that require attention for the individual. Nor are they formulated to cover alterations in absorption or utilization of nutrients resulting from continued use of pharmaceutical preparations, including oral contraceptives, antibiotics, anticoagulants, and other drugs. These special problems must be evaluated when considering the nutrient needs of the individual.

ENERGY

The rates of synthesis of body compounds and of cell turnover decrease with age during adulthood. Increasing body fat and decrease in lean mass lower the energy needs for maintenance. Therefore, both total requirement and requirement per unit of body size become progressively less. The major factor of difference in individual requirement of energy is physical activity. McGandy et al.[66] concluded that average energy need is relatively constant for men in light occupations between 20 and 45 years of age, but 200 kcal/day less between 45 and 75 years, and 500 kcal/day less after 75 years. There is, however, wide variation in physical activity, due only partly to limitations of the skeletomuscular system of the elderly. Few data are available on the range of energy expenditure of older adults. Energy needs are lower for the adult whose life style is sedentary, both in occupation and in leisure activities, than for the individual performing manual labor or strenuous athletics. While the general tendency in adulthood is for decreasing physical activity, some adults maintain a high level of activity and a high energy requirement.

The RDA for males decreases from 2900 kcal (12.2 MJ) at 19 to 22 years to 2700 kcal (11.3 MJ) between 23 and 50 years, a decrease of 10 percent. A decrease of 11 percent to 2400 kcal (10.1 MJ) between 51 and 75 years of age and a further decrease of 14.5 percent to 2050 kcal (8.6 MJ) are provided in the 1979 RDA. For females the RDA decreases from 2100 kcal (8.8 MJ) at 19 to 22 years to 2000 kcal (8.4 MJ) at 23 to 50 years, a decrease of less than 5 percent, to 1800 kcal (7.6 MJ) at 51 to 75 years, a decrease of 10 percent, and then to 1600 kcal (6.7 MJ) after 75 years of age, a further decrease of 11 percent. Several studies in the literature have indicated that a reduction of 5 percent per decade in caloric needs occurs between 55 and 75 years, and a reduction of 7 percent after 75 years.[9] The Canadian Dietary Standard[63] suggests a decrease of 15 percent for males and of 17 percent for females after 65 years of age. The United Kingdom recommendations[64] provide for a further decrease of 12 percent for men and 7 percent for women after 75 years of age. Therefore it is clear that a reduction in energy requirement is expected, but there is little consensus on the rate of reduction.

Historically, the changes in successive editions of the RDA for energy have not followed a consistent trend for men, with only minor increases or decreases in the allowances and changes in the age categories. The RDA levels for women, however, have been lowered. Until 1948 the RDA for "adult" women was 2500 or 2400 kcal. Since the 1963 edition the RDA for young adult women has been 2000 to 2100 kcal, and the expanded age categories allow for a lower level of 1600 kcal in the oldest age group.

Except for one edition, 70 kg has been used as the body weight of the reference man in the RDA calculations. The reference woman had a weight of 56 kg through 1948, 55 kg in 1953, 58 kg between 1963 and 1974, and 55 kg in 1979. The allowance of energy per kg body weight has been lowered over the years. The 1979 RDA levels provide for 41.5 kcal/kg for males 19 to 22 years of age, decreasing to 29.3 kcal/kg after 75 years. For women of corresponding ages, the allowance decreases from 38.2 to 29.1 kcal/kg. In contrast, the standards used in evaluation of the HANES data[67] were somewhat lower for both sexes at all ages, decreasing from 40 kcal to 34 kcal/kg for males and from 35 kcal to 29 kcal/kg for females between 20 and 60-plus years of age.

Dietary studies of voluntary intake of older adults are relatively scarce, particularly for men, and are difficult to interpret as indications of energy needs. Most studies have been limited to records or recalls of 24-hour intake, usually on a single day, requiring qualification about whether such intakes are typical for the individual. In addition, memory becomes less efficient with advancing age, and errors are likely to be those of omission. However, dietary records and observed intakes tend to corroborate each other, with the overwhelming evidence that both men and women tend to consume fewer calories than recommended. If the reported intakes are accurate, it suggests that the RDA levels are higher than necessary and that energy consumption at the recommended level would increase the prevalence of obesity.

The longest age span of intakes was provided by HANES,[67] in which median intakes of women decreased steadily from nearly 1600 kcal at 20 to 24 years to less than 1250 kcal after 65 years of age. Mean intakes in other studies of women over 60 years of age have usually ranged between 1300 and 1600 kcal/day. Fewer studies of the intakes of males have been reported. The HANES medians for males decreased from 2700 kcal/day at 20 to 24 years to approximately 1700 kcal at 65-plus years.

The discrepancy between voluntary and recommended intakes has practical implications in feeding programs for the elderly. Most programs plan food to meet a given percentage of the RDA levels; if voluntary consumption of energy is lower than planned, the intake of other nutrients may be proportionately low unless special attention is given to provide foods of high nutrient density.

The significance of the level of caloric intake to longevity has been extensively studied in several species of animals. Restriction of energy intake prolongs life and lowers the incidence of debilitating and life-shortening diseases. However, the level of caloric restriction most conducive to longer life changes with age.[68] The application of these studies to the human presents obvious difficulties in methodology but the findings are consistent with higher prevalence of degenerative diseases among obese humans.

CARBOHYDRATES

No recommended allowance has been established for carbohydrate. In the average United States diet carbohydrate contributes 45 to 50 percent of total energy, nearly equally divided between complex carbohydrates and sugars. The U.S. Dietary Goals[29] recommend an increase of total carbohydrate to 58 percent of calories to replace some of the fat in the diet. They also recommend that nearly three-fourths of the carbohydrate should be complex, thus reducing the intake of sugars.

LIPIDS

No recommended allowances have been established for fat in the diet. The needs of the body for fat as a source of essential fatty acids and a carrier for fat-soluble vitamins can be met by a diet containing 15 to 25 g of the proper fats. The essentail fatty acids, linoleic and arachidonic, are probably adequate when they contribute 1 to 2 percent of total energy.[41] There is no evidence that lipid requirement is altered with age, although tolerance may be reduced in some individuals or specific disease states may require limitation of dietary fat.

The relationship between coronary heart disease and intake of various fats has been investigated extensively, as discussed earlier. The role of essential fatty acids in cholesterol metabolism and transport has not yet been defined clearly. Diets high in polyunsaturated fatty acids have been shown to reduce serum cholesterol in experimental animals and in humans, although the ultimate fate of the cholesterol removed from circulation has not yet been identified.[41] In the average United States diet, fat provides 40 to 45 percent of total energy. Saturated fats supply 16 percent, monounsaturated fats 19 percent, and polyunsaturated fats 7 percent of total calories. The U.S. Dietary Goals[29] recommend a decrease of total fat to 30 percent of calories, equally divided into saturated, monounsaturated, and polyunsaturated fats. Canada's Food Guide[69] recommends restriction of fat intake to no more than 35 percent of calories, including a source of polyunsaturated fatty acid (linoleic acid).

PROTEIN

Although some early balance studies suggested an increased requirement of nitrogen with advancing age, recent investigations indicate that there is little change in requirements of protein from early adulthood to old age.[70] Young[71] hypothesized that the optimal pattern of essential amino acids may change with age, but data are lacking to confirm or reject this hypothesis. The physical and physiological changes in body composition and function make this hypothesis logical. Body mass decreases, with the primary change in muscle mass. The rate of protein turnover declines; total body protein synthesis per unit of body weight is 30 to 40 percent lower in the elderly as compared to the young adult.[71] The proportion of protein synthesis in muscle becomes smaller while the proportion of synthesis in visceral tissues becomes larger with advancing age. Therefore there may be alteration in the amounts of various essential amino acids required for maintenance of the aging body.

There are opposing considerations in determining protein needs and intakes of the older adult.[70] With the decrease in energy requirement, a diet of higher nutrient density is recommended to supply the unchanged needs for protein and micronutrients. High protein foods are also more concentrated sources of minerals and vitamins, and therefore assume greater importance when caloric intake is restricted. On the other hand, renal function tends to deteriorate with age and the work of the kidney is increased on a high protein diet. In the absence of kidney disease, a diet in which 10 to 15 percent of energy is derived from protein seems well tolerated and protects against depletion of trace minerals.

Both psychological and physical stress have been shown to result in negative nitrogen balance. With advancing age environmental and physiological stress may increase. Infection, fever, and surgical trauma may increase urinary nitrogen loss and raise the body's requirement for protein.[41] The RDA values do not include provision for the added protein to meet the needs created by stress, so individual evaluation is essential in working with the elderly.

Throughout adulthood, from 19 to 51-plus years, the RDA is based on a calculation of 0.8 g protein/kg body weight for both sexes. The Canadian Dietary Standard[63] provides 0.80 g/kg for men but 0.73 g/kg for women, and the Caribbean Allowances[65] are similar to the Canadian. The allowances are based largely on factorial calculations and balance studies on young adults, with extrapolation to estimated allowances for older age categories. For the reference 70 kg man, the RDA and Canadian Dietary Standard recommend 56 g protein; for the 65 kg male in the Caribbean Allowances, 53 g protein is recommended. For the 55 kg reference woman with a protein level of 0.8 g/kg, the RDA recommendation is 44 g. For both the Canadian reference woman of 56 kg and the Caribbean woman of 55 kg, the allowance is 41 g, based on the lower allowance per kg. All of the recommendations have been adjusted for the quality of protein commonly consumed in each area.

Dietary intakes in both the United States and Canada tend to exceed the recommended allowances. Surveys in both countries have shown that some women have intakes below the recommended levels, but mean intakes tend to be well above the standards. Although caloric intakes may be used, with some qualifications, to indicate energy needs of the population, protein intakes tend to reflect availability of animal and vegetable proteins and socio-economic factors, and are less indicative of physiological need. The recommended protein intakes represent 8.3 to 11.0 percent of calories, showing an increase with age and slightly higher levels for women than for men. In contrast, mean dietary protein consumption in both the United States and Canada has ranged between 12 and 15 percent in a number of dietary surveys.[72,73]

Minerals

The only mineral for which recommendations have been lowered for the older adult is iron, for women only. For other minerals the recommended intakes are the same for young and older adults (Appendix 1). However, there are specific conditions that must be considered in relation to needs for some minerals.

Calcium

Both the United States and Canadian recommendations for males throughout the adult years are 800 mg/day. For females the RDA is 800 mg and the Canadian Dietary Standard is 700 mg. The recommendations of the Caribbean Food and Nutrition Institute and the United Kingdom are 500 mg for both sexes, and the FAO/WHO recommendation is 400 to 500 mg.

In retaining the higher allowance for calcium, the committee of the Food and Nutrition Board[41] stated that it was based on daily obligatory losses of 320 mg calcium per day; assuming 40 percent absorption of dietary calcium, 800 mg is required to maintain equilibrium. While recognizing that some standards recommend lower intakes, the committee considered that the studies that showed that lower levels could maintain equilibrium were primarily in tropical or semitropical countries with abundant sunlight and possibly unrecognized dietary sources of calcium, and decided that it was unwise to recommend such low calcium intakes for the United States. The Canadian committee[63] placed total daily obligatory calcium losses at 4.3 mg/kg and also used 40 percent as average absorption, reaching a recommendation of 11 mg/kg for maintenance.

Other factors influenced the United States committee to retain the 800 mg recommendation. The United States diet is relatively high in protein and phosphorus, suggesting the need for a high calcium intake. Although a high calcium intake may not increase bone density once osteoporosis has developed, there is evidence that when calcium intake is high retention improves and symptoms may be alleviated. Calcium intake in early adulthood may affect bone loss at a later age. If absorption of calcium becomes less efficient with age, a higher intake may be safer for the elderly person. Therefore, despite the fact that some individuals can remain in balance on intakes below the RDA, the committee considered it prudent to retain the recommendation of 800 mg.

Iron

The recommendation for the adult male is 10 mg/day in the United States, Canadian, and United Kingdom tables, 6 mg in the Caribbean table, and 5 to 9 mg in the FAO/WHO[74] table. As discussed in Chapter 8, the recommendations for women between menarche and menopause vary widely from one standard to another. The United States and Caribbean values are 18 and 19 mg respectively, and the Canadian and United Kingdom standards are 14 and 12 mg respectively. FAO/WHO provides a range of 14 to 28 mg. After menopause the United States and United Kingdom recommendations are 10 mg. the Canadian Standard is 9 mg. and the Caribbean standard is 6 mg/day.

Individuals with regular use of medications, such as aspirin, or physical conditions, such as diverticular disease, who suffer blood loss, should be evaluated for iron nutriture. The recommended allowances are established for healthy persons and do not provide for therapeutic levels of intake. However, in dealing with the elderly, the increased prevalence of conditions which involve chronic or intermittent blood loss must be considered.

The prevalence of anemia has been reported to increase among some elderly, but whether this is due to increased need for iron, vitamin B_{12}, or folacin, or a combination of these nutrients is not clear. There is some evidence that iron-deficiency anemia may be less common after 65 to 70 years and that deficiencies of either of the two B vitamins may be more common after that age.[69]

Iodine
A decrease in the recommendation for iodine is provided in the Canadian Standard but not in the United States allowances. The RDA level is 150 μg for both sexes during adulthood. The Canadian Standard drops from 150 ug to 140 μg for males and from 110 μg to 100 μg for females after 35 years of age.

Potassium
The estimated "safe and adequate" dietary intake of potassium for adults is between 1875 and 5625 mg (Appendix 1). Excessive urinary losses due to diuretic therapy, renal disease, diarrhea, and other health problems of the elderly may jeopardize potassium nutriture. In such cases particular attention to dietary sources or to supplementation is indicated.

VITAMINS

The only vitamins for which a decrease in allowances with advancing age is suggested are those based on energy allowances, specifically thiamin, riboflavin, and niacin. The decrease in riboflavin allowance may be equivocal, since its requirement may be related equally well to protein needs. However, there are few studies from which requirements can be defined clearly. There is no evidence to suggest that needs of other vitamins change with increasing age, although there are conditions that may alter the need of specific vitamins.

Fat-soluble Vitamins

The recommendations for vitamin A are identical in both the United States and Canadian standards. For the adult male at all ages 5000 I.U. (1000 R.E.) is recommended, and for the adult female 4000 I.U. (800 R.E.).

For the first time an allowance for vitamin D was specified for adults in the 1979 RDA. An intake of 5 μg (200 I.U.) is recommended for all adults after 23 years of age. The Canadian Standard allows for 100 I.U. (2.5 μg cholecalciferol) for adults, with an increase to 200 I.U. (5.0 μg cholecalciferol) for the elderly, sick, or housebound if they are shielded from the sun. Harper[69] has stated that, in view of the evidence of lowered efficiency of calcium absorption and the continuous loss of calcium from the skeleton, it would seem appropriate to recommend a vitamin D allowance for the older adult.

The RDA for vitamin E is 10 mg for adult males and 8 mg for adult females at all ages. The Canadian Standard is slightly lower.

Water-soluble Vitamins

The decrease in allowances for thiamin, riboflavin, and niacin is progressive with age in males, with the lowest recommendation for the 51-plus age group. The thiamin allowance for males decreases from 1.4 to 1.2 mg, the riboflavin allowance decreases from 1.6 to 1.4 mg, and the niacin allowance decreases from 18 to 16 mg. The allowances for females are 1.0 mg thiamin, 1.2 mg riboflavin, and 13 mg niacin equivalents, and do not change with age.

There are some indications that the need for pyridoxine may be increased with advancing age, possibly as a result of less efficient absorption. With inadequate basis for altering the allowance, the United States recommendation of 2.2 mg for males and 2.0 mg for females is maintained throughout the adult years. The Canadian Standard provides for 2.0 mg for adult males and 1.5 mg for adult females. As discussed in Chapter 8, there may be increased need for pyridoxine for women taking oral contraceptives containing estrogens.

Folacin allowances for both sexes have been set at 400 μg in the RDA and 200 μg in the Canadian Standard, with no changes from early to late adulthood. For some adults folacin intake may need special attention. Megaloblastic anemia may result from a combination of folacin and ascorbic acid deficiencies, and has been observed especially in alcoholics and in individuals taking drugs that interfere with folacin metabolism.

Both the RDA and the Canadian Standard recommend 3.0 μg of vitamin B_{12} for both sexes during the adult years. There is no evidence that a dietary deficiency of B_{12} may occur when the diet contains animal foods, but B_{12}

nutriture may be jeopardized if all animal foods are excluded from the diet. Special consideration may be needed if surgery or atrophy has affected the gastric mucosa, which normally secretes the intrinsic factor, a glycoprotein that binds B_{12} for transport to mucosal cells. In the absence of the intrinsic factor B_{12} absorption may be compromised, resulting in pernicious anemia. The prevalence of pernicious anemia is higher in the elderly than in young adults. Supplementation of the diet with folacin for treatment of megaloblastic anemia should not be undertaken without further diagnostic tests, since folacin alone does not prevent or cure the neurological damage of pernicious anemia.

There is no evidence of a change with age in the requirements for ascorbic acid, although stress or drug therapy may affect its metabolism in some individuals who will require individual evaluation. The 1979 RDA for adults is 60 mg for both sexes at all ages, reflecting an increase over the 1974 value of 45 mg. The Canadian Standard is 30 mg.

MEETING NUTRIENT NEEDS

For the young adult advice about dietary intake to meet nutrient needs is relatively simple. The recommended allowances are based on more extensive research than for younger or older persons, and can readily be adapted for physical activity or other special needs. As age advances and chronic diseases become more prevalent, individualization in dietary counseling is necessary. The accumulated life experiences of the elderly have created greater variability in nutrient needs and in the complexity of factors that may interfere with meeting nutrient requirements. As a result, greater attention must be given to the needs of the elderly with regard to the economic, social, physical, and physiological circumstances of the individual. Each of these factors must be taken into account if nutrition counseling of the older adult is to be effective. The recommended diet should be adapted to physiological demands within the economic and social constraints of the individual.

Adjustment to a lower income with retirement from paid employment commonly limits allowable expenditures for food. The Social Security Act of 1935 and the amendment to the act which established Medicare and Medicaid programs in 1965 have provided some measure of economic security to older adults. The addition in 1972 of Title VII to the 1965 Older Americans Act made available meal service and recreational activities for the elderly in areas where local programs were established. These programs, in addition to other programs of income maintenance, allow at least a basic income to many elderly persons. Although pension plans of private industry and public institutions have become more common in recent years, they do not extend to all, and are often inadequate during periods of price inflation. As a result, some elderly people have severe economic restrictions which limit their ability to purchase foods to meet all nutrient requirements. Animal products, fruits, and vegetables are high in nutrients but also high in cost. Limited income may dictate housing without adequate facilities for storage and preparation of foods. Therefore nutrition counseling for those on limited budgets should be directed toward obtaining low-cost foods with the highest nutrient value, assistance in shopping, and simplicity of meal preparation.

Sociocultural differences among individuals are more pronounced with age. Food patterns have become long-standing habits; food likes and dislikes are well established and resistant to change except with alteration in food tolerance. The association of specific foods and meal patterns with cultural background and earlier experiences provides security and familiarity which become increasingly important to the elderly person, so the meaning of foods to the individual must be a factor in dietary advice.

Recent change in status may cause an abrupt or gradual alteration of food intake and should alert the professional counselor to probe for its effects. For example, death of family members or close friends, retirement from work, or physical incapacity may result in social withdrawal. Some studies have shown that elderly persons who eat alone tend to have lower nutrient intakes,[75] while other studies show no effect,[76] suggesting individual reactions which differ in their influence on eating. Most of the population who are now over 65 years of age were not exposed to nutrition education in their youth and may have little knowledge of the relationship between food and health. They are, however, prime targets for food faddists and salesmen who promise extended life and relief from chronic diseases, and they may spend a disproportionate amount of their income on special foods or nutritional supplements.

Physical and physiological status may impose a variety of limitations on food consumption and nutrient needs. Loss of neuromuscular control and coordination or inhibition of mobility make shopping for food and manipulation of utensils difficult. Appetite and interest in food may be depressed by decrease in the senses of taste, smell, and vision. Lack of teeth or the use of dentures, along with diminution in saliva secretion, make chewing more difficult. Food intolerance, whether physiologically or psychologically based, increases with age. Anxiety, depression, or alcoholism may alter intake, digestion, or absorption. Disease states may have multiple effects, including dietary prohibitions or restrictions, medications, and the influences of surgery or other therapeutic procedures.

It is obvious, then, that diverse influences on food selection, consumption, and metabolic capability increase with age and must be considered in dietary counseling to meet the nutrient needs of the individual. The following discussion is based on general recommendations for the adult but must be adapted for the individual.

Since most nutrient requirements remain constant throughout the adult years, the nucleus of the diet to provide those nutrients is unchanged from early maturity to old age. Extra provision needs to be made for increased iron intake of the woman until menopause. Energy allowances are less for women, for sedentary persons, and for the elderly, all of whom should select foods of high nutrient density as the major core of the diet. Greater leeway is possible for young adults, men, and very active individuals whose energy needs are higher.

Dairy products deserve emphasis in the diet of adults, but are frequently neglected because of a common belief that calcium is not needed after linear growth is complete. Calcium is needed by the adult, not only for its functions in blood clotting, muscle contraction, transmission of nerve impulses, cell permeability, and as a catalyst in many metabolic reactions, but also for replacement of bone calcium. A daily obligatory loss of 320 mg/day, with average absorption of 40 percent of dietary calcium,[41] cannot be met by a diet excluding dairy products, since such a diet rarely provides more than 300 mg of calcium per day. A chronic negative calcium balance is likely to result in loss of bone mineral and may be a factor in the development of osteoporosis. In addition, milk is an excellent source of protein and other nutrients. At least 16 ounces of milk or its equivalent in other dairy products should be included in the daily diet. The milk may be whole, low-fat, skim, evaporated, dried, or buttermilk, and replacements may include cheese, ice cream, or yogurt. Despite the evidence from lactose load tests that non-Caucasian individuals may have some degree of lactose intolerance, most individuals can comfortably take moderate amounts of milk without symptoms. In the HANES survey of 1971–1974,[77] levels of milk consumption of black and white adults were similar. However, the recommended intake of two or more servings daily was recorded for only 26 percent of young adults and 15 percent of older subjects. The high nutrient density of milk, particularly low-fat milk, makes it especially valuable in the diet when caloric intake must be limited.

Two or more servings daily of meat, fish, poultry, eggs, legumes, or nuts are recommended for the adult. Each serving of meat should be two to three ounces or more, with comparable protein content of the substitutes. Not only do these foods supply protein of good or excellent amino acid content, but they are major sources of trace elements and vitamins of the B complex. The visible fat of meat may be removed for those on energy or fat restrictions. Egg intake is restricted for those on low-cholesterol diets, but for healthy individuals there is not conclusive evidence that eggs provide a greater risk of atherosclerosis or coronary heart disease. Persons on vegetarian diets vary widely in the degree of exclusion of animal products; vegans need special guidance to provide the essential amino acid balance and vitamin B_{12}.

Four or more servings daily of fruits and vegetables should be encouraged. One serving daily of a fruit high in vitamin C and at least three to four servings weekly of vegetables high in carotene are recommended, since surveys have often shown that vitamins A and C tend to be low in the diets of adults. Not only do fruits and vegetables supply minerals and vitamins, but most are high in fiber, which helps to maintain normal bowel function.

Three or more servings of whole grain or enriched bread or cereal are recommended, primarily for their contribution of trace elements and vitamins of the B complex. Whole grain products have higher nutrient content than the refined products; the enrichment of bread and cereal may be limited to iron and three B vitamins although more nutrients and some fiber are lost in the refinement process.

Butter and margarine supply vitamin A. They also enhance the flavor of foods and help to stimulate appetite and enjoyment of foods. Personal tastes and dietary restrictions may limit total intake, but two to three teaspoons or more per day may be recommended.

Fiber has recently been recognized again as an essential component of the diet to maintain normal gastrointestinal function. Many other health claims have been made for fiber, and its ultimate role in disease processes remains to be elucidated. There is, however, good evidence that moderate amounts of fiber improve bowel function, and this becomes of greater importance to older adults with decreased function of smooth muscles.

Water is also important in gastrointestinal function at all ages, but especially to the elderly who may have decreased secretion of saliva and gastrointestinal fluids. Total fluid intake of six to eight glasses a day should be encouraged.

Other foods, or larger amounts of the foods already listed, should be provided to meet energy needs. It is important that enjoyment of foods should be a major emphasis in nutrition counseling, which requires recognition of those foods and flavors which have particular significance to the individual. If appetite is poor, it can often be stimulated by serving favorite foods. Too often the nutritional value of the diet is stressed to the exclusion of enjoyment. Even the adaptation of special diets as a therapeutic measure should be aimed at making minimum essential changes in the habitual diet of the individual. Dietary advice is more likely to be followed when the patient is allowed to cling to the familiar; adjustment to illness and its problems may be difficult without adding the trauma of major changes in diet.

The older adult may be more comfortable with several small feedings during the day rather than three larger meals. Care should be taken, however, that the same balance of foods is maintained. Unfortunately, the temptation is great to make the smaller feedings easy to prepare and they often tend to be readily available snacks high in carbohydrate. Guidance in selection of cheese, fruit, juices, raw vegetables, peanut butter sandwiches, or other high-nutrient foods that do not require cooking is often helpful to the older adult.

The use of vitamin and/or mineral supplements depends on the nutritional status and physical or physiological constraints of the individual. Supplements are indicated when they are essential for meeting nutrient requirements, particularly when food intake is low or when malabsorption or increased destruction or excretion of nutrients places greater demand on their supply. However, most healthy persons may obtain all necessary nutrients from a well-chosen diet. The money spent for supplements that provide a limited number of nutrients might better be spent for foods that contain a broader spectrum of nutrients. As knowledge about trace elements increases, it becomes ever more obvious that the greatest protection lies in consuming a wide variety of foods subjected to minimal processing.

Nutrition is important to health and vitality at all stages of the life span. Within the limits of genetic inheritance and environment, good nutritional status is the best insurance policy for optimal growth and for attaining adulthood with maximum physical capability. With medical advances in diagnosis and treatment of diseases, a longer life has become possible for more people. It is now important to ensure that the added years are characterized by the greatest possible degree of health and vigor. Therefore, maintaining good nutritional status is a basic component of a long and enjoyable life.

REFERENCES

1. Lamb, M. J. *Biology of Ageing.* John Wiley and Sons, New York, 1977.
2. Gains in longevity continue. *Statistical Bull. 59:*7–9, 1978. Metropolitan Life Insurance Co., New York.
3. National Center for Health Statistics. *Facts of Life and Death.* DHEW Publ. No. (PHS) 79-1222. Supt. of Documents, U.S. Government Printing Office, Washington, D.C., 1978.
4. Staff report. Paradise lost. *Nutr. Today 13:*6–9, 1978.
5. McWhirter, N., and R. McWhirter. *Guinness Book of World Records.* Bantam Books, New York, 1973.
6. Timiras, P. S. *Developmental Physiology and Aging.* Macmillan, New York, 1972.
7. Timiras, P. S. Biological perspectives on aging. *Amer. Scientist 66:*605–613, 1978.

8. Birren, J. E., R. N. Butler, S. W. Greenhouse, L. Sokoloff, and M. R. Yarrow. *Human Aging: A Biological and Behavioral Study.* National Institute of Mental Health Publ. No. (HSM) 71-9051. Supt. of Documents, U.S. Government Printing Office, Washington, D.C., 1971.

9. Kart, C. S., E. S. Metress, and J. F. Metress. *Aging and Health: Biologic and Social Perspectives.* Addison-Wesley, Menlo Park, Calif., 1978.

10. Masoro, E. Physiologic changes with aging. In: Winick, M. (Ed.). *Nutrition and Aging.* John Wiley and Sons, New York, 1976.

11. Shock, N. W. Physiologic aspects of aging. *J. Am. Dietet. Assoc.* *56*:491–496, 1970.

12. Roberts, J., and K. Maurer. *Blood Pressure Levels of Persons 6–74 Years, United States, 1971–1974.* DHEW Publ. No. (HRA) 78-1648. Supt. of Documents, U.S. Government Printing Office, Washington, D.C., 1977.

13. Abraham, S., F. W. Lowenstein, and C. L. Johnson. *Preliminary Findings of the First Health and Nutrition Examination Survey, United States, 1971–1972: Dietary Intake and Biochemical Findings.* DHEW Publ. No. (HRA) 74-1219-1. Supt. of Documents, U.S. Government Printing Office, Washington, D.C., 1974.

14. Abraham, S., C. L. Johnson, and M. D. Carroll. *Total Serum Cholesterol Levels of Adults 18–74 Years, United States, 1971–1974.* DHEW Publ. No. (PHS) 78-1652. Supt. of Documents, U.S. Government Printing Office, Washington, D.C., 1978.

15. McMahon, B., and J. Worcester. *Age at Menopause, United States, 1960–1962.* DHEW Publ. No. (HSM) 73-1268. Supt. of Documents, U.S. Government Printing Office, Washington, D.C., 1966.

16. Stroudt, H. W., A. Damon, R. McFarland, and J. Roberts. *Weight, Height and Selected Body Dimensions of Adults, United States, 1960–1962.* Public Health Service Publ. No. 1000, Series 11, No. 8. Supt. of Documents, U.S. Government Printing Office, Washington, D.C., 1965.

17. *Height and Weight of Adults 18–74 Years of Age in the United States.* Advance Data from Vital and Health Statistics of the National Center for Health Statistics. *3*:1–8, 1976.

18. Stroudt, H. W., A. Damon, R. A. McFarland, and J. Roberts. *Skinfolds, Body Girths, Biacromial Diameter, and Selected Anthropometric Indices of Adults, United States, 1960–1962.* DHEW Publ. No. (HRA) 74-1281. Supt. of Documents, U.S. Government Printing Office, Washington, D.C., 1973.

19. Novak, L. P. Aging, total body potassium, fat-free mass, and cell mass in males and females between ages 18 and 85 years. *J. Gerontol.* *27*:438–443, 1972.

20. Damon, A., C. C. Seltzer, H. W. Stroudt, and B. Bell. Age and physique in healthy white veterans at Boston. *J. Gerontol. 27*:202–208, 1972.

21. Garn. S. M., and D. C. Clark. Trends in fatness and the origins of obesity. *Pediat. 57*:443–456, 1976.

22. *Obesity and Health.* Public Health Service, U.S. Dept. of Health, Education, and Welfare, Arlington, Va., 1966.

23. Kannel, W. B., E. J. LeBauer, T. R. Dawber, and P. M. McNamara. The relation of body weight to development of coronary heart disease: The Framingham study. *Circulation 35*:734–744, 1967.

24. Bierman, E. L. Atherosclerosis and aging. *Fed. Proc. 37*:2832–2836, 1978.

25. Kannel, W. B. State of coronary heart disease risk factors. *J. Nutr. Educ. 10*:10–14, 1978.

26. Glueck, C. J., and W. E. Connor. Diet-coronary heart disease relationships reconnoitered. *Am. J. Clin. Nutr. 31*:727–737, 1978.

27. Mann, G. V. Diet-heart: End of an era. *N. E. J. Med. 297*:644–650, 1977.

28. Davidson, S., R. Passmore, and J. F. Brock. *Human Nutrition and Dietetics,* Fifth Edition. Williams and Wilkins, Baltimore, Md., 1973.

29. Select Committee on Nutrition and Human Needs, U.S. Senate. *Dietary Goals for the United States, Second Edition.* Supt. of Documents, U.S. Government Printing Office, Washington, D.C., Dec., 1977.

30. Reiser, R. Oversimplification of diet : coronary heart disease relationships and exaggerated diet recommendations. *Am. J. Clin. Nutr. 31*:865–875, 1978.

31. Harper, A. E. Dietary Goals: A skeptical view. *Am. J. Clin. Nutr. 31*:310–321, 1978.

32. Hegsted, D. M. Dietary Goals: A progressive view. *Am. J. Clin. Nutr. 31*:1504–1509, 1978.

33. Yerushalmy, J., and H. E. Hilleboe. Fat in the diet and mortality from heart disease. A methodologic note. *N.Y. State J. Med. 57*:2343–2354, 1957.

34. The Nutritional Significance of Fiber. Life Sciences Research Office, *Fed. Am. Soc. Exp. Biol.,* Bethesda, Md., 1977.

35. Kannel, W. B., and T. Gordon. *Framingham Study, Epidemiological Investigation of Cardiovascular Disease: Diet and Regulation of Serum Cholesterol.* Class no. HE 20.3002: F84/Sect. 24. Supt. of Documents, U.S. Government Printing Office, Washington, D.C., 1970.

36. Nichols, A. B., C. Ravenscroft, D. E. Lamphiar, and L. D. Ostrander, Jr. Daily nutritional intake and serum lipid levels. The Tecumseh Study. *Am. J. Clin. Nutr. 29*:1384–1392, 1976.

37. Dahl, L. K. Salt and hypertension. *Am. J. Clin. Nutr.* 25:231–244, 1972.
38. Avioli, L. V. The osteoporosis problem. In: Winick, M. (Ed.) *Nutritional Disorders of American Women.* John Wiley and Sons, New York, 1977.
39. Lutwak, L. Periodontal disease. In: Winick, M. (Ed.) *Nutrition and Aging.* John Wiley and Sons, New York, 1976.
40. Jowsey, J. Prevention and treatment of osteoporosis. In: Winick, M. (Ed.) *Nutrition and Aging.* John Wiley and Sons, New York, 1976.
41. *Recommended Dietary Allowances, Eighth edition.* National Academy of Sciences, Washington, D.C., 1974.
42. Roe, D. A. *Drug-induced Nutritional Deficiencies.* Avi Publishing Company, Westport, Conn., 1978.
43. Olson, R. E. Nutrition and Alcoholism. In: Goodhart, R. S., and M. E. Shils (Eds.). *Modern Nutrition in Health and Disease, Fifth edition.* Lea and Febiger, Philadelphia, 1975.
44. Roberts, J., and T. A. Burch. *Osteoarthritis Prevalence in Adults by Age, Sex, Race, and Geographic Area, United States, 1960–1962.* Public Health Service Publ. No. 1000—Series 11— No. 15. Supt. of Documents, U.S. Government Printing Office, Washington, D.C., 1966.
45. Moss, J. M. Pitfalls to avoid in diagnosing diabetes in the elderly. *Geriatrics 31*:52–55, 1976.
46. Friedman, G. J. Diet in the treatment of diabetes mellitus. In: Goodhart, R. S., and M. E. Shils (Eds.). *Modern Nutrition in Health and Disease, Fifth edition.* Lea and Febiger, Philadelphia, 1975.
47. Gori, G. B. Diet and cancer. *J. Am. Dietet. Assoc. 71*:375–379, 1977.
48 Clayson, D. B. Nutrition and experimental carcinogenesis. In: Winick, M. (Ed.). *Nutrition and Cancer.* John Wiley and Sons, New York, 1977.
49. Walker, A. R. P. Colon cancer and diet, with special reference to intakes of fat and fiber. *Am. J. Clin. Nutr. 29*:1417–1426, 1976.
50. Shils, M. E. Nutrition and neoplasia. In: Goodhart, R. S., and M. E. Shils (Eds.). *Modern Nutrition in Health and Disease, Fifth edition.* Lea and Febiger, Philadelphia, 1975.
51. Oace, S. M. Diet and cancer. *J. Nutr. Educ. 10*:106–108, 1978.
52. Wynder, E. L., and B. S. Reddy. Diet and cancer of the colon. In: Winick, M. (Ed.). *Nutrition and Cancer.* John Wiley and Sons, New York, 1977.
53. Carroll, K. K. Dietary factors and hormone-dependent cancers. In: Winick, M. (Ed.). *Nutrition and Cancer.* John Wiley and Sons, New York, 1977.

54. Theologides, A. Cancer cachexia. In: Winick, M. (Ed.). *Nutrition and Cancer.* John Wiley and Sons, New York, 1977.

55. Munro, H. N. Tumor-host competition for nutrients in the cancer patient. *J. Am. Diet. Assoc. 71*:380–384, 1977.

56. Hathcock, J. N. *Nutrition and Drug Interrelations.* Academic Press, New York, 1977.

57. Visconti, J. A. *Drug-food Interaction.* Ross Laboratories, Columbus, Ohio, 1977.

58. Comfort, A. *A Good Age.* Crown Publ., New York, 1976.

59. Balsley, M., M. F. Brink, and E. W. Speckman. Nutrition in disease and stress. *Geriatrics 26* (3):87–93, 1971.

60. Pelcovits, J. Nutrition to meet the human needs of older Americans. *J. Am. Dietet. Assoc. 60*:297–300, 1972.

61. Exton-Smith, A. N. Nutritional needs of the elderly. In: Hollingsworth, D., and M. Russell (Eds.). *Nutrition Problems in a Changing World.* Halsted Press, New York, 1973.

62. Exton-Smith, A. N. Physiological aspects of aging: Relationship to nutrition. *Am. J. Clin. Nutr. 25*:853–859, 1972.

63. *Dietary Standard for Canada.* Supply and Services Canada, Ottawa, 1976.

64. *Recommended Intakes of Nutrients for the United Kingdom.* Report on Public Health and Medical Subjects No. 120: 18–19, 1969.

65. *Recommended Dietary Allowances for the Caribbean.* Caribbean Food and Nutrition Institute, Kingston, Jamaica, 1976.

66. McGandy, R. B., C. H. Barrows, Jr., A. Spanias, A. Meredith, J. L. Stone, and A. H. Norris. Nutrient intakes and energy expenditure in men of different ages. *J. Gerontol. 21*:581–587, 1966.

67. Abraham, S., M. D. Carroll, C. M. Dresser, and C. L. Johnson. *Dietary Intake Findings, United States, 1971–1974.* DHEW Publ. No. (HRA) 77-1647. Supt. of Documents, U.S. Government Printing Office, Washington, D.C., 1977.

68. Ross, M. H. Dietary behavior and longevity. *Nutr. Rev. 35*:257–265, 1977.

69. *Recommendations for Prevention Programs in Relation to Nutrition and Cardiovascular Disease.* Bureau of Nutritional Sciences, Dept. of National Health and Welfare, Ottawa, Canada, June, 1977.

70. Harper, A. E. Recommended dietary allowances for the elderly. *Geriatrics 33*(5):13–15, 1978.

71. Young, V. R. Protein metabolism and needs in elderly people. In: Rockstein, M., and M. L. Sussman (Eds.). *Nutrition, Longevity, and Aging.* Academic Press, New York, 1976.

72. O'Hanlon, P., and M. B. Kohrs. Dietary status of older Americans. *Am. J. Clin. Nutr. 31*:1257–1269, 1978.
73. Nutrition Canada. *Food Consumption Patterns Report.* Bureau of Nutritional Sciences, Dept. of National Health and Welfare, Ottawa, Canada, 1977.
74. FAO/WHO Handbook on Human Nutritional Requirements, 1974. *Nutr. Rev. 33*:147–157, 1975.
75. Grotowski, M. L., and L. Sims. Nutritional knowledge, attitudes, and dietary practices of the elderly. *J. Am. Dietet. Assoc. 72*:499–506, 1978.
76. Todhunter, E. N. Life style and nutrient intake in the elderly. In: Winick, M. (Ed.) *Nutrition and Aging.* John Wiley and Sons, New York, 1976.
77. *Selected Findings: Food Consumption Profiles of White and Black Persons 1–74 Years of Age in the United States, 1971–1974.* Advance Data from Vital and Health Statistics of the National Center for Health Statistics, No. 21, June 26, 1978. U.S. Dept. of Health, Education and Welfare, Washington, D.C.

Appendix 1

RECOMMENDED DIETARY ALLOWANCES, REVISED, 1979

Source: Food and Nutrition Board, National Academy of Sciences—National Research Council, Washington, D.C.

Table 1   Food and Nutrition Board, National Academy of Sciences—National
Designed for the Maintenance of Good Nutrition of Practically All Healthy

	Age (years)	Weight (kg)	Weight (lb)	Height (cm)	Height (in.)	Protein (g)	Fat-Soluble Vitamins Vitamin A (μg R.E.)[b]	Fat-Soluble Vitamins Vitamin D (μg)[c]	Fat-Soluble Vitamins Vitamin E (mg α T.E.)[d]	Water-Soluble Vitamins Vitamin C (mg)	Water-Soluble Vitamins Thiamin (mg)
Infants	0.0–0.5	6	13	60	24	kg × 2.2	420	10	3	35	0.3
	0.5–1.0	9	20	71	28	kg × 2.0	400	10	4	35	0.5
Children	1–3	13	29	90	35	23	400	10	5	45	0.7
	4–6	20	44	112	44	30	500	10	6	45	0.9
	7–10	28	62	132	52	34	700	10	7	45	1.2
Males	11–14	45	99	157	62	45	1000	10	8	50	1.4
	15–18	66	145	176	69	56	1000	10	10	60	1.4
	19–22	70	154	177	70	56	1000	7.5	10	60	1.5
	23–50	70	154	178	70	56	1000	5	10	60	1.4
	51 +	70	154	178	70	56	1000	5	10	60	1.2
Females	11–14	46	101	157	62	46	800	10	8	50	1.1
	15–18	55	120	163	64	46	800	10	8	60	1.1
	19–22	55	120	163	64	44	800	7.5	8	60	1.1
	23–50	55	120	163	64	44	800	5	8	60	1.0
	51 +	55	120	163	64	44	800	5	8	60	1.0
Pregnant						+30	+ 200	+ 5	+ 2	+20	+0.4
Lactating						+20	+ 400	+ 5	+ 3	+40	+0.5

[a]The allowances are intended to provide for individual variations among most normal persons as they live in the United States under usual environmental stresses. Diets should be based on a variety of common foods in order to provide other nutrients for which human requirements have been less well defined.

[b]Retinol equivalents. 1 retinol equivalent = 1 μg retinol or 6 μg β carotene.

[c]As cholecalciferol. 10 μg cholecalciferol = 400 I.U. vitamin D.

[d]α tocopherol equivalents. 1 mg d α - tocopherol = 1 α T.E.

[e]1 NE (niacin equivalent) is equal to 1 mg of niacin or 60 mg of dietary tryptophan.

[f]The folacin allowances refer to dietary sources as determined by *Lactobacillus casei* assay after treat-

Table 2   Estimated Safe and Adequate Daily Dietary Intakes of Additional

	Age (years)	Vitamins Vitamin K (μg)	Vitamins Biotin (μg)	Vitamins Pantothenic Acid (mg)	Trace Elements[b] Copper (mg)	Trace Elements[b] Manganese (mg)
Infants	0–0.5	12	35	2	0.5–0.7	0.5–0.7
	0.5–1	10–20	50	3	0.7–1.0	0.7–1.0
Children	1–3	15–30	65	3	1.0–1.5	1.0–1.5
and	4–6	20–40	85	3–4	1.5–2.0	1.5–2.0
adolescents	7–10	30–60	120	4–5	2.0–2.5	2.0–3.0
	11 +	50–100	100–200	4–7	2.0–3.0	2.5–5.0
Adults		70–140	100–200	4–7	2.0–3.0	2.5–5.0

[a]Because there is less information on which to base allowances, these figures are not given in the main table of the RDA and are provided here in the form of ranges of recommended intakes.

[b]Since the toxic levels for many trace elements may be only several times usual intakes, the upper levels for the trace elements given in this table should not be habitually exceeded.

442

Research Council Recommended Daily Dietary Allowances,[a] Revised 1979. People in the U.S.A.

Water-Soluble Vitamins					Minerals					
Riboflavin (mg)	Niacin (mg N.E.)[c]	Vitamin B$_6$ (mg)	Folacin[f] (μg)	Vitamin B$_{12}$ (μg)	Calcium (mg)	Phosphorus (mg)	Magnesium (mg)	Iron (mg)	Zinc (mg)	Iodine (μg)
0.4	6	0.3	30	0.5[g]	360	240	50	10	3	40
0.6	8	0.6	45	1.5	540	360	70	15	5	50
0.8	9	0.9	100	2.0	800	800	150	15	10	70
1.0	11	1.3	200	2.5	800	800	200	10	10	90
1.4	16	1.6	300	3.0	800	800	250	10	10	120
1.6	18	1.8	400	3.0	1200	1200	350	18	15	150
1.7	18	2.0	400	3.0	1200	1200	400	18	15	150
1.7	19	2.2	400	3.0	800	800	350	10	15	150
1.6	18	2.2	400	3.0	800	800	350	10	15	150
1.4	16	2.2	400	3.0	800	800	350	10	15	150
1.3	15	1.8	400	3.0	1200	1200	300	18	15	150
1.3	14	2.0	400	3.0	1200	1200	300	18	15	150
1.3	14	2.0	400	3.0	800	800	300	18	15	150
1.2	13	2.0	400	3.0	800	800	300	18	15	150
1.2	13	2.0	400	3.0	800	800	300	10	15	150
+0.3	+2	+0.6	+400	+1.0	+400	+400	+150	h	+5	+25
+0.5	+5	+0.5	+100	+1.0	+400	+400	+150	h	+10	+50

ment with enzymes ("conjugases") to take polyglutamyl forms of the vitamin available to the test organism.

[g]The RDA for vitamin B$_{12}$ in infants is based on average concentration of the vitamin in human milk. The allowances after weaning are based on energy intake (as recommended by the American Academy of Pediatrics) and consideration of other factors such as intestinal absorption.

[h]The increased requirement during pregnancy cannot be met by the iron content of habitual American diets nor by the existing iron stores of many women; therefore the use of 30–60 mg of supplemental iron is recommended. Iron needs during lactation are not substantially different from those of nonpregnant women, but continued supplementation of the mother for 2–3 months after parturition is advisable in order to replenish stores depleted by pregnancy.

Selected Vitamins and Minerals[a]

Trace Elements[b]				Electrolytes		
Fluoride (mg)	Chromium (mg)	Selenium (mg)	Molybdenum (mg)	Sodium (mg)	Potassium (mg)	Chloride (mg)
0.1–0.5	0.01–0.04	0.01–0.04	0.03–0.06	115–350	350–925	275–700
0.2–1.0	0.02–0.06	0.02–0.06	0.04–0.08	250–750	425–1275	400–1200
0.5–1.5	0.02–0.08	0.02–0.08	0.05–0.1	325–975	550–1650	500–1500
1.0–2.5	0.03–0.12	0.03–0.12	0.06–0.15	450–1350	775–2325	700–2100
1.5–2.5	0.05–0.2	0.05–0.2	0.1 –0.3	600–1800	1000–3000	925–2775
1.5–2.5	0.05–0.2	0.05–0.2	0.15–0.5	900–2700	1525–4575	1400–4200
1.5–4.0	0.05–0.2	0.05–0.2	0.15–0.5	1100–3300	1875–5625	1700–5100

Source: Recommended Dietary Allowances, Revised 1979. Food and Nutrition Board National Academy of Sciences—National Research Council, Washington, D.C.

Table 3   Mean Heights and Weights and Recommended Energy Intake

Category	Age (years)	Weight (kg)	Weight (lb)	Height (cm)	Height (in.)	Energy Needs (with Range) (kcal)	Energy Needs (with Range) (MJ)
Infants	0.0–0.5	6	13	60	24	kg × 115 (95–145)	kg × .48
	0.5–1.0	9	20	71	28	kg × 105 (80–135)	kg × .44
Children	1–3	13	29	90	35	1300 (900–1800)	5.5
	4–6	20	44	112	44	1700 (1300–2300)	7.1
	7–10	28	62	132	52	2400 (1650–3300)	10.1
Males	11–14	45	99	157	62	2700 (2000–3700)	11.3
	15–18	66	145	176	69	2800 (2100–3900)	11.8
	19–22	70	154	177	70	2900 (2500–3300)	12.2
	23–50	70	154	178	70	2700 (2300–3100)	11.3
	51–75	70	154	178	70	2400 (2000–2800)	10.1
	76+	70	154	178	70	2050 (1650–2450)	8.6
Females	11–14	46	101	157	62	2200 (1500–3000)	9.2
	15–18	55	120	163	64	2100 (1200–3000)	8.8
	19–22	55	120	163	64	2100 (1700–2500)	8.8
	23–50	55	120	163	64	2000 (1600–2400)	8.4
	51–75	55	120	163	64	1800 (1400–2200)	7.6
	76+	55	120	163	64	1600 (1200–2000)	6.7
Pregnancy						+300	
Lactation						+500	

The data in this table have been assembled from the observed median heights and weights of children shown in Table 1, together with desirable weights for adults given above for the mean heights of men (70 inches) and women (64 inches) between the ages of 18 and 34 years as surveyed in the U.S. population (HEW/NCHS data).

The energy allowances for the young adults are for men and women doing light work. The allowances for the two older age groups represent mean energy needs over these age spans, allowing for a 2% decrease in basal (resting) metabolic rate per decade and a reduction in activity of 200 kcal/day for men and women between 51 and 75 years, 500 kcal for men over 75 years and 400 kcal for women over 75. The customary range of daily energy output is shown for adults in parentheses, and is based on a variation in energy needs of ± 400 kcal at any one age, emphasizing the wide range of energy intakes appropriate for any group of people.

Energy allowances for children through age 18 are based on median energy intakes of children these ages followed in longitudinal growth studies. The values in parentheses are 10th and 90th percentiles of energy intake, to indicate the range of energy consumption among children of these ages.

Source: Recommended Dietary Allowances, Revised 1979. Food and Nutrition Board National Academy of Sciences—National Research Council, Washington, D.C.

Appendix 2

GROWTH PERCENTILES, NATIONAL CENTER FOR HEALTH STATISTICS*

Source: Tables 1 to 5 from P. V. V. Hamill, T. A. Drizd, C. L. Johnson, R. B. Reed, and A. F. Roche. *NCHS Growth Curves for Children Birth–18 years*. DHEW Publication No. (PHS) 78-1650. Supt. of Documents, U. S. Government Printing Office, Washington, D.C., 1977.

445

Table 1   Smoothed Percentiles of Recumbent Length (in Centimeters), by Sex and Age: Statistics from National Center for Health Statistics and Data from Fels Research Institute, birth–36 months

Sex and Age	Smoothed[a] Percentile						
	5th	**10th**	**25th**	**50th**	**75th**	**90th**	**95th**
Male	Recumbent Length in Centimeters						
Birth	46.4	47.5	49.0	50.5	51.8	53.5	54.4
1 month	50.4	51.3	53.0	54.6	56.2	57.7	58.6
3 months	56.7	57.7	59.4	61.1	63.0	64.5	65.4
6 months	63.4	64.4	66.1	67.8	69.7	71.3	72.3
9 months	68.0	69.1	70.6	72.3	74.0	75.9	77.1
12 months	71.7	72.8	74.3	76.1	77.7	79.8	81.2
18 months	77.5	78.7	80.5	82.4	84.3	86.6	88.1
24 months	82.3	83.5	85.6	87.6	89.9	92.2	93.8
30 months	87.0	88.2	90.1	92.3	94.6	97.0	98.7
36 months	91.2	92.4	94.2	96.5	98.9	101.4	103.1
Female							
Birth	45.4	46.5	48.2	49.9	51.0	52.0	52.9
1 month	49.2	50.2	51.9	53.5	54.9	56.1	56.9
3 months	55.4	56.2	57.8	59.5	61.2	62.7	63.4
6 months	61.8	62.6	64.2	65.9	67.8	69.4	70.2
9 months	66.1	67.0	68.7	70.4	72.4	74.0	75.0
12 months	69.8	70.8	72.4	74.3	76.3	78.0	79.1
18 months	76.0	77.2	78.8	80.9	83.0	85.0	86.1
24 months	81.3	82.5	84.2	86.5	88.7	90.8	92.0
30 months	86.0	87.0	88.9	91.3	93.7	95.6	96.9
36 months	90.0	91.0	93.1	95.6	98.1	100.0	101.5

[a]Smoothed by cubic-spline approximation.

446

Table 2   Smoothed Percentiles of Weight (in Kilograms), by Sex and Age: Statistics from National Center for Health Statistics and Data from Fels Research Institute, birth–36 months

Sex and Age	Smoothed[a] Percentile						
	5th	10th	25th	50th	75th	90th	95th
Male	Weight in Kilograms						
Birth	2.54	2.78	3.00	3.27	3.64	3.82	4.15
1 month	3.16	3.43	3.82	4.29	4.75	5.14	5.38
3 months	4.43	4.78	5.32	5.98	6.56	7.14	7.37
6 months	6.20	6.61	7.20	7.85	8.49	9.10	9.46
9 months	7.52	7.95	8.56	9.18	9.88	10.49	10.93
12 months	8.43	8.84	9.49	10.15	10.91	11.54	11.99
18 months	9.59	9.92	10.67	11.47	12.31	13.05	13.44
24 months	10.54	10.85	11.65	12.59	13.44	14.29	14.70
30 months	11.44	11.80	12.63	13.67	14.51	15.47	15.97
36 months	12.26	12.69	13.58	14.69	15.59	16.66	17.28
Female							
Birth	2.36	2.58	2.93	3.23	3.52	3.64	3.81
1 month	2.97	3.22	3.59	3.98	4.36	4.65	4.92
3 months	4.18	4.47	4.88	5.40	5.90	6.39	6.74
6 months	5.79	6.12	6.60	7.21	7.83	8.38	8.73
9 months	7.00	7.34	7.89	8.56	9.24	9.83	10.17
12 months	7.84	8.19	8.81	9.53	10.23	10.87	11.24
18 months	8.92	9.30	10.04	10.82	11.55	12.30	12.76
24 months	9.87	10.26	11.10	11.90	12.74	13.57	14.08
30 months	10.78	11.21	12.11	12.93	13.93	14.81	15.35
36 months	11.60	12.07	12.99	13.93	15.03	15.97	16.54

[a]Smoothed by cubic-spline approximation.

*Table 3   Smoothed Percentiles of Head Circumference (in Centimeters),
by Sex and Age: Statistics from National Center for Health Statistics and
Data from Fels Research Institute, birth–36 months*

Sex and Age	Smoothed[a] Percentile						
	5th	**10th**	**25th**	**50th**	**75th**	**90th**	**95th**
Male	Head circumference in Centimeters						
Birth	32.6	33.0	33.9	34.8	35.6	36.6	37.2
1 month	34.9	35.4	36.2	37.2	38.1	39.0	39.6
3 months	38.4	38.9	39.7	40.6	41.7	42.5	43.1
6 months	41.5	42.0	42.8	43.8	44.7	45.6	46.2
9 months	43.5	44.0	44.8	45.8	46.6	47.5	48.1
12 months	44.8	45.3	46.1	47.0	47.9	48.8	49.3
18 months	46.3	46.7	47.4	48.4	49.3	50.1	50.6
24 months	47.3	47.7	48.3	49.2	50.2	51.0	51.4
30 months	48.0	48.4	49.1	49.9	51.0	51.7	52.2
36 months	48.6	49.0	49.7	50.5	51.5	52.3	52.8
Female							
Birth	32.1	32.9	33.5	34.3	34.8	35.5	35.9
1 month	34.2	34.8	35.6	36.4	37.1	37.8	38.3
3 months	37.3	37.8	38.7	39.5	40.4	41.2	41.7
6 months	40.3	40.9	41.6	42.4	43.3	44.1	44.6
9 months	42.3	42.8	43.5	44.3	45.1	46.0	46.4
12 months	43.5	44.1	44.8	45.6	46.4	47.2	47.6
18 months	45.0	45.6	46.3	47.1	47.9	48.6	49.1
24 months	46.1	46.5	47.3	48.1	48.8	49.6	50.1
30 months	47.0	47.3	48.0	48.8	49.4	50.3	50.8
36 months	47.6	47.9	48.5	49.3	50.0	50.8	51.4

[a]Smoothed by cubic-spline approximation.

Table 4   Smoothed Percentiles of Stature (in Centimeters), by Sex and Age: Data and Statistics from National Center for Health Statistics, 2 to 18 years

Sex and Age	Smoothed[a] Percentile						
	5th	10th	25th	50th	75th	90th	95th
Male	Stature in Centimeters						
2.0 years[b]	82.5	83.5	85.3	86.8	89.2	92.0	94.4
2.5 years	85.4	86.5	88.5	90.4	92.9	95.6	97.8
3.0 years	89.0	90.3	92.6	94.9	97.5	100.1	102.0
3.5 years	92.5	93.9	96.4	99.1	101.7	104.3	106.1
4.0 years	95.8	97.3	100.0	102.9	105.7	108.2	109.9
4.5 years	98.9	100.6	103.4	106.6	109.4	111.9	113.5
5.0 years	102.0	103.7	106.5	109.9	112.8	115.4	117.0
5.5 years	104.9	106.7	109.6	113.1	116.1	118.7	120.3
6.0 years	107.7	109.6	112.5	116.1	119.2	121.9	123.5
6.5 years	110.4	112.3	115.3	119.0	122.2	124.9	126.6
7.0 years	113.0	115.0	118.0	121.7	125.0	127.9	129.7
7.5 years	115.6	117.6	120.6	124.4	127.8	130.8	132.7
8.0 years	118.1	120.2	123.2	127.0	130.5	133.6	135.7
8.5 years	120.5	122.7	125.7	129.6	133.2	136.5	138.8
9.0 years	122.9	125.2	128.2	132.2	136.0	139.4	141.8
9.5 years	125.3	127.6	130.8	134.8	138.8	142.4	144.9
10.0 years	127.7	130.1	133.4	137.5	141.6	145.5	148.1
10.5 years	130.1	132.6	136.0	140.3	144.6	148.7	151.5
11.0 years	132.6	135.1	138.7	143.3	147.8	152.1	154.9
11.5 years	135.0	137.7	141.5	146.4	151.1	155.6	158.5
12.0 years	137.6	140.3	144.4	149.7	154.6	159.4	162.3
12.5 years	140.2	143.0	147.4	153.0	158.2	163.2	166.1
13.0 years	142.9	145.8	150.5	156.5	161.8	167.0	169.8
13.5 years	145.7	148.7	153.6	159.9	165.3	170.5	173.4
14.0 years	148.8	151.8	156.9	163.1	168.5	173.8	176.7
14.5 years	152.0	155.0	160.1	166.2	171.5	176.6	179.5
15.0 years	155.2	158.2	163.3	169.0	174.1	178.9	181.9
15.5 years	158.3	161.2	166.2	171.5	176.3	180.8	183.9
16.0 years	161.1	163.9	168.7	173.5	178.1	182.4	185.4
16.5 years	163.4	166.1	170.6	175.2	179.5	183.6	186.6
17.0 years	164.9	167.7	171.9	176.2	180.5	184.4	187.3
17.5 years	165.6	168.5	172.4	176.7	181.0	185.0	187.6
18.0 years	165.7	168.7	172.3	176.8	181.2	185.3	187.6

449

Table 4   Continued

Sex and Age	5th	10th	25th	50th	75th	90th	95th
			Smoothed[a] Percentile				
Female			Stature in Centimeters				
2.0 years[b]	81.6	82.1	84.0	86.8	89.3	92.0	93.6
2.5 years	84.6	85.3	87.3	90.0	92.5	95.0	96.6
3.0 years	88.3	89.3	91.4	94.1	96.6	99.0	100.6
3.5 years	91.7	93.0	95.2	97.9	100.5	102.8	104.5
4.0 years	95.0	96.4	98.8	101.6	104.3	106.6	108.3
4.5 years	98.1	99.7	102.2	105.0	107.9	110.2	112.0
5.0 years	101.1	102.7	105.4	108.4	111.4	113.8	115.6
5.5 years	103.9	105.6	108.4	111.6	114.8	117.4	119.2
6.0 years	106.6	108.4	111.3	114.6	118.1	120.8	122.7
6.5 years	109.2	111.0	114.1	117.6	121.3	124.2	126.1
7.0 years	111.8	113.6	116.8	120.6	124.4	127.6	129.5
7.5 years	114.4	116.2	119.5	123.5	127.5	130.9	132.9
8.0 years	116.9	118.7	122.2	126.4	130.6	134.2	136.2
8.5 years	119.5	121.3	124.9	129.3	133.6	137.4	139.6
9.0 years	122.1	123.9	127.7	132.2	136.7	140.7	142.9
9.5 years	124.8	126.6	130.6	135.2	139.8	143.9	146.2
10.0 years	127.5	129.5	133.6	138.3	142.9	147.2	149.5
10.5 years	130.4	132.5	136.7	141.5	146.1	150.4	152.8
11.0 years	133.5	135.6	140.0	144.8	149.3	153.7	156.2
11.5 years	136.6	139.0	143.5	148.2	152.6	156.9	159.5
12.0 years	139.8	142.3	147.0	151.5	155.8	160.0	162.7
12.5 years	142.7	145.4	150.1	154.6	158.8	162.9	165.6
13.0 years	145.2	148.0	152.8	157.1	161.3	165.3	168.1
13.5 years	147.2	150.0	154.7	159.0	163.2	167.3	170.0
14.0 years	148.7	151.5	155.9	160.4	164.6	168.7	171.3
14.5 years	149.7	152.5	156.8	161.2	165.6	169.8	172.2
15.0 years	150.5	153.2	157.2	161.8	166.3	170.5	172.8
15.5 years	151.1	153.6	157.5	162.1	166.7	170.9	173.1
16.0 years	151.6	154.1	157.8	162.4	166.9	171.1	173.3
16.5 years	152.2	154.6	158.2	162.7	167.1	171.2	173.4
17.0 years	152.7	155.1	158.7	163.1	167.3	171.2	173.5
17.5 years	153.2	155.6	159.1	163.4	167.5	171.1	173.5
18.0 years	153.6	156.0	159.6	163.7	167.6	171.0	173.6

[a]Smoothed by cubic-spline approximation.
[b]Because of a logistic problem the percentiles of stature for children under 2.5 years are not highly reliable. The age interval represented is 2.00–2.25 years.

450

Table 5   Smoothed Percentiles of Weight (in Kilograms), by Sex and Age: Data and Statistics from National Center for Health Statistics, 1.5 to 18 years

Sex and Age	_Smoothed[a] Percentile						
	5th	10th	25th	50th	75th	90th	95th
Male	Weight in Kilograms						
1.5 years	9.72	10.18	10.51	11.09	12.02	12.95	14.42
2.0 years	10.49	10.96	11.55	12.34	13.36	14.38	15.50
2.5 years	11.27	11.77	12.55	13.52	14.61	15.71	16.61
3.0 years	12.05	12.58	13.52	14.62	15.78	16.95	17.77
3.5 years	12.84	13.41	14.46	15.68	16.90	18.15	18.98
4.0 years	13.64	14.24	15.39	16.69	17.99	19.32	20.27
4.5 years	14.45	15.10	16.30	17.69	19.06	20.50	21.63
5.0 years	15.27	15.96	17.22	18.67	20.14	21.70	23.09
5.5 years	16.09	16.83	18.14	19.67	21.25	22.96	24.66
6.0 years	16.93	17.72	19.07	20.69	22.40	24.31	26.34
6.5 years	17.78	18.62	20.02	21.74	23.62	25.76	28.16
7.0 years	18.64	19.53	21.00	22.85	24.94	27.36	30.12
7.5 years	19.52	20.45	22.02	24.03	26.36	29.11	32.73
8.0 years	20.40	21.39	23.09	25.30	27.91	31.06	34.51
8.5 years	21.31	22.34	24.21	26.66	29.61	33.22	36.96
9.0 years	22.25	23.33	25.40	28.13	31.46	35.57	39.58
9.5 years	23.25	24.38	26.68	29.73	33.46	38.11	42.35
10.0 years	24.33	25.52	28.07	31.44	35.61	40.80	45.27
10.5 years	25.51	26.78	29.59	33.30	37.92	43.63	48.31
11.0 years	26.80	28.17	31.25	35.50	40.38	46.57	51.47
11.5 years	28.24	29.72	33.08	37.46	43.00	49.61	54.73
12.0 years	29.85	31.46	35.09	39.78	45.77	52.73	58.09
12.5 years	31.64	33.41	37.31	42.27	48.70	55.91	61.52
13.0 years	33.64	35.60	39.74	44.95	51.79	59.12	65.02
13.5 years	35.85	38.03	42.40	47.81	55.02	62.35	68.51
14.0 years	38.22	40.64	45.21	50.77	58.31	65.57	72.13
14.5 years	40.66	43.34	48.08	53.76	61.58	68.76	75.66
15.0 years	43.11	46.06	50.92	56.71	64.72	71.91	79.12
15.5 years	45.50	48.69	53.64	59.51	67.64	74.98	82.45
16.0 years	47.74	51.16	56.16	62.10	70.26	77.97	85.62
16.5 years	49.76	53.39	58.58	64.39	72.46	80.84	88.59
17.0 years	51.50	55.28	60.22	66.31	74.17	83.58	91.31
17.5 years	52.89	56.78	61.61	67.78	75.32	86.14	93.73
18.0 years	53.97	57.89	62.61	68.88	76.04	88.41	95.76

451

Table 5   Continued

Sex and Age	Smoothed[a] Percentile						
	5th	**10th**	**25th**	**50th**	**75th**	**90th**	**95th**
Female			Weight in Kilograms				
1.5 years	9.02	9.16	9.61	10.38	10.94	11.75	12.36
2.0 years	9.95	10.32	10.96	11.80	12.73	13.58	14.15
2.5 years	10.80	11.35	12.11	13.03	14.23	15.16	15.76
3.0 years	11.61	12.26	13.11	14.10	15.50	16.54	17.22
3.5 years	12.37	13.08	14.00	15.07	16.59	17.77	18.59
4.0 years	13.11	13.84	14.80	15.96	17.56	18.93	19.91
4.5 years	13.83	14.56	15.55	16.81	18.48	20.06	21.24
5.0 years	14.55	15.26	16.29	17.66	19.39	21.23	22.62
5.5 years	15.29	15.97	17.05	18.56	20.36	22.48	24.11
6.0 years	16.05	16.72	17.86	19.52	21.44	23.89	25.75
6.5 years	16.85	17.51	18.76	20.61	22.68	25.50	27.59
7.0 years	17.71	18.39	19.78	21.84	24.16	27.39	29.68
7.5 years	18.62	19.37	20.95	23.26	25.90	29.57	32.07
8.0 years	19.62	20.45	22.26	24.84	27.88	32.04	34.71
8.5 years	20.68	21.64	23.70	26.58	30.08	34.73	37.58
9.0 years	21.82	22.92	25.27	28.46	32.44	37.60	40.64
9.5 years	23.05	24.29	26.94	30.45	34.94	40.61	43.85
10.0 years	24.36	25.76	28.71	32.55	37.53	43.70	47.17
10.5 years	25.75	27.32	30.57	34.72	40.17	46.84	50.57
11.0 years	27.24	28.97	32.49	36.95	42.84	49.96	54.00
11.5 years	28.83	30.71	34.48	39.23	45.48	53.03	57.42
12.0 years	30.52	32.53	36.52	41.53	48.07	55.99	60.81
12.5 years	32.30	34.42	38.59	43.84	50.56	58.81	64.12
13.0 years	34.14	36.35	40.65	46.10	52.91	61.45	67.30
13.5 years	35.98	38.26	42.65	48.26	55.11	63.87	70.30
14.0 years	37.76	40.11	44.54	50.28	57.09	66.04	73.08
14.5 years	39.45	41.83	46.28	52.10	58.84	67.95	75.59
15.0 years	40.99	43.38	47.82	53.68	60.32	69.54	77.78
15.5 years	42.32	44.72	49.10	54.96	61.48	70.79	79.59
16.0 years	43.41	45.78	50.09	55.89	62.29	71.68	80.99
16.5 years	44.20	46.54	50.75	56.44	62.75	72.18	81.93
17.0 years	44.74	47.04	51.14	56.69	62.91	72.38	82.46
17.5 years	45.08	47.33	51.33	56.71	62.89	72.37	82.62
18.0 years	45.26	47.47	51.39	56.62	62.78	72.25	82.47

[a]Smoothed by cubic-spline approximation.

452

Appendix 3

TABLE
OF
CURRENT
GUIDELINES
FOR
CRITERIA
OF
NUTRITIONAL
STATUS
FOR
LABORATORY
EVALUATION

Source: Christakis, G. (Ed.) Nutritional Assessment in Health Programs. *Am. J. Public Health 63*: Supplement, November, 1973.

Nutrient and Units	Age of Subject (years)	Criteria of Status		
		Deficient	Marginal	Acceptable
[a]Hemoglobin (gm/100ml)	6–23 mos.	Up to 9.0	9.0–9.9	10.0+
	2–5	Up to 10.0	10.0–10.9	11.0+
	6–12	Up to 10.0	10.0–11.4	11.5+
	13–16M	Up to 12.0	12.0–12.9	13.0+
	13–16F	Up to 10.0	10.0–11.4	11.5+
	16+M	Up to 12.0	12.0–13.9	14.0+
	16+F	Up to 10.0	10.0–11.9	12.0+
	Pregnant (after 6+ mos.)	Up to 9.5	9.5–10.9	11.0+
[a]Hematocrit (Packed cell volume in percent)	Up to 2	Up to 28	28–30	31+
	2–5	Up to 30	30–33	34+
	6–12	Up to 30	30–35	36+
	13–16M	Up to 37	37–39	40+
	13–16F	Up to 31	31–35	36+
	16+M	Up to 37	37–43	44+
	16+F	Up to 31	31–37	38+
	Pregnant	Up to 30	30–32	33+
[a]Serum albumin (gm/100ml)	Up to 1	—	Up to 2.5	2.5+
	1–5	—	Up to 3.0	3.0+
	6–16	—	Up to 3.5	3.5+
	16+	Up to 2.8	2.8–3.4	3.5+
	Pregnant	Up to 3.0	3.0–3.4	3.5+

		Deficient		Acceptable
[a]Serum protein (gm/100ml)	Up to 1	—	Up to 5.0	5.0+
	1–5	—	Up to 5.5	5.5+
	6–16	—	Up to 6.0	6.0+
	16+	Up to 6.0	6.0–6.4	6.5+
	Pregnant	Up to 5.5	5.5–5.9	6.0+
[a]Serum ascorbic acid (mg/100ml)	All ages	Up to 0.1	0.1–0.19	0.2+
[a]Plasma vitamin A (mcg/100ml)	All ages	Up to 10	10–19	20+
[a]Plasma carotene (mcg/100ml)	All ages	Up to 20	20–39	40+
	Pregnant	—	40–79	80+
[a]Serum iron (mcg/100 ml)	Up to 2	Up to 30	—	30+
	2–5	Up to 40	—	40+
	6–12	Up to 50	—	50+
	12+M	Up to 60	—	60+
	12+F	Up to 40	—	40+
[a]Transferrin saturation (percent)	Up to 2	Up to 15.0	—	15.0+
	2–12	Up to 20.0	—	20.0+
	12+M	Up to 20.0	—	20.0+
	12+F	Up to 15.0	—	15.0+
[b]Serum folacin (ng/ml)	All ages	Up to 2.0	2.1–5.9	6.0+
[b]Serum vitamin B$_{12}$ (pg/ml)	All ages	Up to 100	—	100+

Continued

455

Nutrient and Units	Age of Subject (years)	Criteria of Status		
		Deficient	Marginal	Acceptable
[a]Thiamin in urine (mcg/g creatinine)	1–3	Up to 120	120–175	175+
	4–5	Up to 85	85–120	120+
	6–9	Up to 70	70–180	180+
	10–15	Up to 55	55–150	150+
	16+	Up to 27	27– 65	65+
	Pregnant	Up to 21	21– 49	50+
[a]Riboflavin in urine (mcg/g creatinine)	1–3	Up to 150	150–499	500+
	4–5	Up to 100	100–299	300+
	6–9	Up to 85	85–269	270+
	10–16	Up to 70	70–199	200+
	16+	Up to 27	27– 79	80+
	Pregnant	Up to 30	30– 89	90+
[b]RBC transketolase-TPP-effect (ratio)	All ages	25+	15– 25	Up to 15
[b]RBC glutathione reductase-FAD-effect (ratio)	All ages	1.2+	—	Up to 1.2
[b]Tryptophan load (mg xanthurenic acid excreted)	Adults (Dose: 100mg/kg body weight)	25 + (6 hrs.) 75 + (24 hrs.)	— —	Up to 25 Up to 75

		Deficient	Acceptable	High
[b]Urinary pyridoxine (mcg/g creatinine)	1–3	Up to 90	—	90+
	4–6	Up to 80	—	80+
	7–9	Up to 60	—	60+
	10–12	Up to 40	—	40+
	13–15	Up to 30	—	30+
	16+	Up to 20	—	20+
[a]Urinary N'methyl nicotinamide (mg/g creatinine)	All ages	Up to 0.2	0.2–5.59	0.6+
	Pregnant	Up to 0.8	0.8–2.49	2.5+
[b]Urinary pantothenic acid (mcg)	All ages	Up to 200	—	200+
[b]Plasma vitamin E (mg/100ml)	All ages	Up to 0.2	0.2–0.6	0.6+
[b]Transaminase index (ratio)				
[c]EGOT	Adult	2.0 +	—	Up to 2.0
[d]EGPT	Adult	1.25 +	—	Up to 1.25

[a]Adapted from the Ten State Nutrition Survey
[b]Criteria may vary with different methodology
[c]Erythrocyte Glutamic Oxalacetic Transaminase
[d]Erythrocyte Glutamic Pyruvic Transaminase

457

Index

Acne vulgaris, 355
Adipose tissue, in adolescence, 326, 327
  in aging, 46, 395
  fetal deposition of, 126–131
  growth of, 45–46
  in infancy, 211–212, 214
  measurement of, 74, 101–105
  in middle childhood, 299–300
  in preschool period, 266–267
  see also Obesity
Adolescence, 321–329
  definition of, 321–322
  development in,
    in female, 178, 334–342
    in male, 342, 344
  hormones in, 330–334
  physiological maturation in, 343–348
  pregnancy in, 140, 155–156, 358–361
  timing of, 17
Adrenal cortical steroids, 332
Aging, causes of, 386–389
  decline of function in, 17
  height in, 21, 394
  individuality of, 3
  physiological changes in, 389–395

  process of, 381–382, 385–395
  psychosocial-biological interactions, 416–420
  skinfold measurements in, 46, 395, 399
  weight in, 21, 394–395
Alcohol consumption, 147–148, 408–409
American Academy of Pediatrics, statement on infant formulas, 250–251
  statement on iron in infancy, 236–238
Amniotic fluid, 124
Androgens, 333
Anemia,
  iron-deficiency, in adolescence, 353–354
  causes and clinical significance of, 90–100
  in infancy, 235–238
  in pregnancy, 133–134
  in preschool period, 268–270, 284–285
  racial differences in, 95–96
  see also Iron

megaloblastic,
in aging, 429
in pregnancy, 161–162
pernicious, 429–430
see also Folacin; Vitamin B$_{12}$
Anorexia nervosa, 352–353
Anthropometric measurements, body
composition in relation to, 51
head circumference, 73
selection of, 36–37, 71–76
see also Height and Length; Obesity;
Weight
Appetite, in adolescence, 371
in cancer, 414
in preschool period, 270–275
Arteriosclerosis, 402
Ascorbic acid, in adolescence, 370
in adulthood, 430
biochemical tests for, 77–78, Appendix 3
in breast milk, 189, 193, 238
deficiency of, 69
effect of oral contraceptives on, 356
in infancy, 238
in osteoporosis, 406–407
in pregnancy, 152
in preschool period, 285–287
Recommended Dietary Allowances,
Appendix 1
Atherosclerosis, 361–362, 401–404, 411

Basal metabolic rate, in adolescence,
345
in aging, 393
in pregnancy, 136–137
Biochemical measurements, 76–80, Appendix 3
Blood volume, 133–135, 346
Body composition, direct measurement
of, 46–47
indirect measurement of, 47–52
Bonding, maternal-infant, 212,
222–224, 240
Breast feeding, 171–210, 240–242
amenorrhea in, 186
contraindications to, 179

in developing countries, 2, 171, 199
duration of, 174
factors in decision of, 174–177
factors in successful, 1–2, 184–186
frequency of, 183–184
hormonal control of, 179–181
let-down reflex in, 181
nutrient requirements for, 198–205
prevalence in United States, 172–173
Breast milk, 185–201
contraceptives, effects on, 186
non-nutritive components in,
186–187
nutrient content of, 188–198, 201,
238
species specificity of, 171
volume of, 185–186, 199
Breasts, development of, 177–179,
334–336
British Perinatal Mortality Survey, 140

Calcium, in breast milk, 192–198
dietary standards for, 86
fetal deposition of, 130–131
in infant formulas, 243
in osteoporosis, 406–408, 432
recommended allowances of, in
adolescence, 368–369
in adulthood, 427
in infancy, 234–235
in lactation, 201, 203–204
in middle childhood, 312
in pregnancy, 156–157
in preschool period, 282–284
Recommended Dietary
Allowances, Appendix 1
serum levels of, 78, 135
urinary excretion of, 432
Calcium, phosphorus ratio, 235, 369,
407
Calories, *see* Energy
Canadian Dietary Standard, basis of,
86–89
in adolescence, 364–369
in adulthood, 421–423, 426–429
iron absorption rate in, 100, 237